CANCER RESEARCH PERSPECTIVES

CANCER RESEARCH PERSPECTIVES

LARISSA S. PEREIRA
EDITOR

Nova Biomedical Books
New York

For permission to use material from this book please contact us:
Telephone 631-231-7269; Fax 631-231-8175
Web Site: http://www.novapublishers.com

LIBRARY OF CONGRESS CATALOGING-IN-PUBLICATION DATA

Cancer research perspectives / Larissa S. Pereira, editor.
p.; cm.
Includes bibliographical references and index.
ISBN-13: 978-1-60021-980-1 (hardcover)
ISBN-10: 1-60021-980-2 (hardcover)
1. Cancer. I Pereira, Larissa S.
[DNLM: 1. Neoplasms. 2. research--trends. QZ 206 C2158 2008]
RC261.C2747 2008
616.99'4--dc22

2007034862

Published by Nova Science Publishers, Inc. ; New York

CONTENTS

PREFACE

Cancer is a group of different diseases (more than 100) characterized by uncontrolled growth and spread of abnormal cells. Cancer can arise in many sites and behave differently depending on its organ of origin. If a cancer spreads (metastasizes), the new tumor bears the same name as the original (primary) tumor. Significant progress has been made in recent years in the battle against cancer and in understanding its underlying biological mechanisms. This research progress has resulted in many experimental treatments and cures which establish hope for wide-spread cures.This book presents new research of importance to the field.

Chapter I - Epithelial cancer, or squamous cell carcinoma, constitutes a major proportion of all diagnosed cancers. Squamous cell carcinoma of the oral cavity and pharynx account for approximately 3% of all cancers in the United States with more than 50,000 new cases diagnosed yearly. Worldwide, head and neck cancer is the sixth most common malignancy. Oral squamous cell carcinoma (OSCC) mainly affects the older population, with a steep increase in incidence in the people aged 60 years and older. Although OSCC is generally easily accessible to early diagnosis and therapy, they are associated with a relatively high rate of mortality due to recurrence and metastasis. The overall five-year survival rate for oral and pharyngeal cancers is among the lowest of all cancers and has not significantly changed during the last two decades. Most advances in oral carcinoma treatment have been confined to surgical excision and reconstruction procedures. Previously, the therapeutic modality offered to patients was based on traditional clinical stage-predicting indices and on histologic grading. Nowadays, the advanced research in molecular biology has been exploited for a better understanding of oral carcinogenesis. Several potential markers of molecular changes in oral premalignant and malignant lesions have been studied and interest in the genetic changes associated with these lesions is increasing. Oral carcinogenesis has long been known as a multistep process involving many genetic alterations; hence, these alterations can be used in predicting the prognosis of patients and the progression of the tumor. Examples of molecular markers or alterations during oral carcinogenesis investigated include activated oncogenes, inactivated tumor suppressor genes, loss of heretozygosity (LOH) on some particular chromosomes, altered signal transducers, and DNA contents. Research on new agents, including agents that modulate signal transduction, cell-cycle progression, programmed cell death, matrix invasion, and angiogenesis are in development for oral cancer treatment. Since oral cancer is easily accessible, research on gene therapy for oral cancer and premalignant lesions are also available in many settings of clinical trials. In summary, this chapter will be focused on the review of research on molecular mechanisms of as well as molecular markers for early carcinogenesis, tumor invasion, metastasis, and prognosis of OSCC. Advanced research on the treatments of OSCC using new agents and gene therapy will also be covered.

Chapter II - From the first use of canaries in coal mines a century ago, companion animals have been useful sentinels for risk associated with environmental exposures they share with humans. There has been a great deal of inconsistency in results from studies of passive smoking and cancer in humans, due largely to misclassification of exposure levels and confounding by other factors. Evaluations of how passive smoking relates to cancers in companion animals may potentially clarify these relationships in humans.

Similarities in cancer incidence and biology make dogs and cats appropriate models for the etiology of a variety of human cancers, including breast, testes, bladder, lung, nasal/sinus, bone and lymphatic cancers. Because dogs and cats have shorter life spans, the effects of passive smoking on cancer development can be assessed more quickly than in most human studies. In humans, associations between passive smoking and cancer may be confounded by factors such as alcohol intake and occupational exposures, but because these are not relevant to pets the likelihood of confounding is greatly reduced.

Pets living in smoking households undoubtedly receive a substantial exposure dose, which may be more consistent and easily measured than in humans. Recent data suggest that dogs and cats absorb and metabolize nicotine after household exposure, and demonstrate urinary cotinine levels that increase linearly with exposure. In addition to inhalation and trans-dermal exposure, oral grooming leads to oral ingestion of particulates; therefore pets may serve as models for both adults and young children, who may be exposed through these multiple routes.

In dogs, household passive smoking exposure has been associated with increased risks of lung and nasal/sinus cancers. In one study dogs living with smokers had a 60% greater risk of lung cancer than unexposed dogs. Passive smoking also appears related to cancer incidence in cats. In a recent study, cats exposed to household passive smoking had a significant 2-fold increase in risk of malignant lymphoma. Passive smoking may also increase risk of oral cancer, perhaps by altering expression of p53.

In summary, epidemiologic studies of companion animals can make a unique and valuable contribution to knowledge of the relationship between passive smoking and cancer in humans. Though this field is still in its adolescence, provocative results from early investigations suggest that cancer risk increased with both the duration and quantity of exposure. Additional studies of the health effects of passive smoking in animal populations are clearly warranted.

Chapter III - The recent identification of endothelial progenitor cells (EPCs) in the peripheral blood of adult individuals has highlighted the possibility that vasculogenesis can take place in the postnatal life. It has been reported that circulating EPCs can be recruited and incorporated into sites of active neovascularization but they can also play a role in replacing lost endothelial cells on the vessel wall mediating a mechanism of maintenance of the normal vascular homeostasis. An accurate and unique phenotypical and functional characterization of circulating EPC subsets is still matter of debate; infact, neither a precise and unique panel of cell surface markers nor universally accepted protocols are available up to now for their in vitro growth.

Methods for the identification and characterization of circulating endothelial cells able to participate to postnatal vasculogenesis and endothelial repair will be part of the authors review, that will be focused mainly on physiological and pathological conditions characterized by a spontaneous increase of the number of circulating EPCs. The possible role of a number of soluble factors able to induce the mobilization of EPCs from the bone marrow into the peripheral blood will be also discussed.

Chapter IV - Environmental tobacco smoke (ETS) is a widespread contaminant of indoor air where smoking is not prohibited. It is a significant source of exposure to a large number of substances known to be hazardous to human health. Over the last several decades there has been a growing interest in examining the health consequences of ETS. The International Agency for Research on Cancer (IARC) has evaluated the evidence of a carcinogenic risk from exposure to ETS, and has classified it as an established human carcinogen. Except for lung cancer, the evidence of a causal association between ETS exposure and other cancers is inconclusive. In this review chapter, the authors reviewed recent publications on exposure to ETS and cancers to add more evidence of the risk of passive smoking in lung cancer, which has been established as a causal association, and in other types of cancer in adults and in children.

Chapter V - Advances in molecular genetics have provided a wealth of information relevant to the understanding of the mechanisms underlying both primary immunodeficiency diseases and lymphomas. This information provides the research community with insights into the different lymphocyte developmental stages. In this chapter the authors discuss expression profiling in lymphomas and primary immunodeficiencies affecting the B-cell lineage. In particular mantle cell lymphomas, chronic lymphocytic leukemias/small lymphocytic lymphomas and X-linked agammaglobulinemia (Btk deficiency) are discussed.

There is considerable hope that the microarray technology will lead to a better understanding of different disease processes. The results of a multitude of gene expression studies in malignant lymphomas clearly suggest that the vast majority of B-cell lymphomas emanate from antigen experienced cells or memory B-cells and not from naïve B-cells. These findings, together with preferential use of certain V heavy chain gene conformations, points to a role for antigen at some stages in lymphoma development. This seems to be of particular relevance as to the discussion of cell-of-origin for low-grade lymphomas such as B-cell chronic lymphocytic leukemia, mantle cell lymphoma and marginal zone lymphoma.

The gene expression studies conducted in primary immunodeficiencies have foremost been helpful to better understand the basic biology of the disease. Microarray analysis has also been used as an exploratory tool to study gene expression in immunodeficiency diseases of unknown cause. For X-linked agammaglobulinemia, the technique has provided better understanding of the genes influenced by Btk.

Chapter VI - Fas (APO-1/CD95) is a member of tumor necrosis factor (TNF)/nerve growth factor (NGF) receptor superfamily. Cross-linking of cell membrane Fas (mFas) by Fas ligand (FasL) transduces a death signal that results in a unique cell death, apoptosis, in which cells show chromatin condensation and nuclear fragmentation. One of the important biological roles of this system is the maintenance of immune homeostasis. Activated lymphocytes which express mFas are eliminated after appropriate immune reaction to avoid prolonged and surplus reaction. Interestingly, *lpr* and *gld* mice that show spontaneous dysfunctional mutations of Fas and (FasL), respectively, show autoimmune diseases with increased numbers of activated lymphocytes. The balance between death and survival is delicately controlled not only by the mFas expression but also by its isoform soluble Fas (sFas) and cytoplasmic apoptosis promotive and repressive molecules. Adult T-cell leukemia lymphoma (ATLL) is a unique neoplasm of activated mature T-cells caused by human T-cell leukemia virus type-1 (HTLV-1). Because of its activated T-cell nature, ATLL cells express abundant mFas. Nevertheless, ATLL cells vigorously proliferate escaping from the attack of FasL, which suggests that ATLL cells acquire strong apoptosis-resistant systems during their development. Here, the authors review the molecules involved in apoptosis resistance in ATLL and discuss their role in oncogenesis and their clinical significance.

Chapter VII - Pyrimidine analogue 5-fluorouracil (5-FU) is a standard chemotherapeutic agent in treating colorectal cancer (CRC). Occasionally fluorodeoxyuridine (FUdR) has been used; however, the third analogue fluoro uridine (FUR) has never been used in the clinic. In this study the authors compared the anti-tumorigenic activity of the above agents *in vitro* and *in vivo*. The cultured cells were protected from the cytotoxic effects of the FUdR by deoxy thymidine and FUR by uridine. Cytotoxicity of these agents as analyzed *in vitro* by cell culture demonstrated FUR to be the most potent anti-tumor agent. *In vivo* they tested the effect of 5-FU and FUR on tumor bearing mice. Intra-peritoneal administration of 5-FU or FUR proved that FUR is fifteen times more effective than 5-FU. Severe inhibitory effect of FUR on TS expression and its RNA mediated cell kill may explain its superiority over the other two fluoropyrimidines tested *in vivo*.

Chapter VIII - Gene expression profiling initially showed that it could be used to distinguish between the major variants of acute leukaemia. Several studies have now been published that have illustrated the potential of micro array analysis in the diagnosis of haematological malignancy. For acute myeloid leukaemia (AML), in particular, expression profiling has also provided novel insights into disease pathogenesis and shown it could lead to refinements in risk-stratification, prognostic markers, and eventually a more rational and personalised approach to therapy. These gene expression studies will be compared and contrasted in terms of results; with a view to speculating whether arrays can complement current laboratory methodologies for leukaemia diagnosis.

Chapter IX - Cystatins comprise a large superfamily of related proteins with diverse biological activities. They were initially characterised as inhibitors of lysosomal cysteine proteases, however, in recent years some alternative functions for cystatins have been proposed. In tumours their role was considered as protective since they are capable to impair excessive activity of cysteine proteases, associated with tumour growth, invasion, angiogenesis and metastasis. Knockout or transgenic animal models and clinical investigations of cystatins in body fluids provided the opposite, i.e. cystatins can also promote malignant disease. Their dual relation to progression of cancer, various physiological roles and differences between type I and type II cystatins with regard to possible applications in diagnosis and therapy in cancer are discussed in this review.

In: Cancer Research Perspectives
Editor: Larissa S. Pereira, pp. 1-7

ISBN 978-1-60021-980-1

Short Communication

COMBINATION OF ASPIRIN AND Ω-3 POLYUNSATURATED FATTY ACID FOR CANCER CHEMOPREVENTION

Xiaoxin Chen[*,ϒ]

Cancer Research Program, Julius L. Chambers Biomedical/Biotechnology Research Institute, North Carolina Central University, Durham, NC 27707, USA.

ABSTRACT

It has been well established that cyclooxygenase 2 (Cox2) plays a very important role in carcinogenesis, and its inhibition by specific and non-specific inhibitors produces chemopreventive effects. However, much concern has been raised on the use of Cox2 specific inhibitors for cancer chemoprevention due to their cardiovascular side effects. Here a combination of aspirin and ω-3 polyunsaturated fatty acid (PUFA) is proposed for cancer chemoprevention. Mechanistically it is based on a unique feature of aspirin, acetylation of Cox2. Once acetylated, Cox2 is essentially a lipoxygenase which converts arachidonic acid and PUFA into anti-inflammatory metabolites, lipoxins and resolvins, respectively. In the precancerous lesions where Cox2 is frequently up-regulated, the combination of aspirin and PUFA may exert synergistic inhibitory effects on inflammation-associated cancer. This combination approach may balance long-term efficacy, safety and expense of cancer chemoprevention.

* Correspondence concerning this article should be addressed to: Dr. Xiaoxin (Luke) Chen, MD, PhD, Cancer Research Program, Julius L. Chambers Biomedical/Biotechnology Research Institute, North Carolina Central University, 700 George Street, Durham, NC 27707. Tel: 919-530-6425; Fax: 919-530-7998; Email: lchen@nccu.edu.

ϒ Supported by NIH grants CA101235 and DK63650.

Keywords: Aspirin; ω-3 Polyunsaturated fatty acid; chemoprevention.

ABBREVIATIONS

AA,	arachidonic acid;
Cox2,	cyclooxygenase 2;
DHA,	docosahexaenoic acid;
EPA,	docosapentaenoic acid;
HETE,	hydroxyeicosatetraenoic acid;
LX,	lipoxin;
PUFA,	ω-3 polyunsaturated fatty acid.

Cyclooxygenase 2 (Cox2) is known to play a very important role in carcinogenesis, and its inhibition by specific and non-specific inhibitors produces chemopreventive effects. However, withdrawal of Rofecoxib (Vioxx; Merck) may cause a setback in cancer chemoprevention research [1]. On December 17, 2004, the National Cancer Institute suspended the use of Celecoxib (Celebrex; Pfizer) in a clinical trial for colon cancer prevention due to increased cardiovascular events (www.fda.gov/bbs/topics/news/2004/new01144.html). Similar side effects have been found, or serious concerns raised, on other Cox2 inhibitors, such as Valdecoxib (Bextra; Pfizer), Lumiracoxib (Bextra; Norvatis), Parecoxib (a prodrug of Lumiracoxib), Etoricoxib (Arcoxia; Merck) [2,3]. It is believed that the cardiovascular side effects of these Cox2 inhibitors result from decrease of prostacyclin synthesis in the endothelial cells and increase of thromboxane A2 synthesis in the activated platelets [4]. Since the high-risk population needing cancer prevention and patients with arthritis are known to have an increased risk of cardiovascular diseases, cardiovascular safety of long-term treatment becomes a critical factor in targeting Cox2 for cancer chemoprevention.

Here a combination of aspirin and ω-3 polyunsaturated fatty acid (PUFA) is proposed for cancer chemoprevention. Aspirin has a unique feature to acetylate the Ser^{516} residue of the Cox2 protein [5]. Once acetylated, Cox2 is essentially a lipoxygenase, which converts arachidonic acid (AA) into 15*R*-hydroxyeicosatetraenoic acid (15*R*-HETE), and 11*R*-hydroxyeicosatetraenoic acid (11*R*-HETE) to a lesser extent. 15*R*-HETE can be further metabolized into 15*R*-epi-lipoxin A4 (LXA4) and 15*R*-epi-lipoxin B4 (LXB4) by 5-lipoxygenase (5-Lox). In contrast, when the Ser^{530} residue of the Cox1 protein is acetylated by aspirin, Cox1 is inactivated [6]. LXA4 and LXB4 may also be synthesized from leukotriene A4 through the 5-Lox pathway, or 15*S*-HETE through the 15-Lox pathway. Acting on its membrane receptor, LXA4 and its analogs are anti-inflammatory *in vitro* and *in vivo* [7]. Oral, topical, or intravenous administration of LXA4, LXB4, or their analogs produces potent anti-inflammatory effects at various organ sites [8]. In an aspirin-induced gastric ulcer model, intraperitoneal administration of LXA4 reduced the severity of gastric damage, whereas a receptor antagonist exerted the opposite effects, both in a dose-dependent manner [9]. A recent study showed that a 15*R*-epi-LXA4 analog suppressed hapten-induced colitis [10]. Transgenic overexpression of LXA4 receptor attenuated inflammation [11].

Besides AA, PUFAs are also substrates of native and acetylated Cox2. Native Cox2 converts docosahexaenoic acid (DHA) and docosapentaenoic acid (EPA) into anti-inflammatory metabolites, 3-series of prostanoids and 5-series of leukotrienes [12]. Acetylated Cox2 converts DHA and EPA into resolvins D1, D2, D3, D4, and E1. These resolvins are pro-resolution or anti-inflammatory *in vitro* and *in vivo* [13].

Aspirin or PUFA alone has been tested for cancer chemoprevention in animal models and humans. In rat colon cancer models induced by carcinogens, aspirin significantly inhibited carcinogenesis [14,15]. In thc $Apc^{Min/+}$ mouse model, some reports showed dramatic effects, whereas some others marginal or no effects, on intestinal tumorigenesis, probably due to different treatment regimes, sample sizes, genetic backgrounds, and husbandry regimes [16-20]. Three randomized human clinical trials showed that low dose of aspirin prevented the occurrence of colon polyps, although it is still unclear why aspirin did not produce dose-dependent response [21-23]. PUFA has also been used for colon cancer chemoprevention [24]. In carcinogen-induced rat models, high doses of fish oil, DHA or EPA in the diet had significant preventive effects. Similar effects were also observed in the $Apc^{Min/+}$ mouse model as listed in a Colon Cancer Prevention database (www.inra.fr/reseau-nacre/sci-memb/corpet/indexan.html). Dietary supplementation of PUFA to human subjects increased the tissue level of PUFA, reduced the level of AA, and inhibited cell proliferation, in colorectal mucosa [25,26].

Combination of aspirin and PUFA has been examined for synergy in cardiovascular system, but not yet for cancer chemoprevention. In one small-scale study on normal human subjects, combination of aspirin (37.5mg) and fish oil (13.8g) had synergistic effects on AA metabolism by decreasing serum levels of thromboxane A2 and leukotriene B4 [27]. However, in a study on the moderately hypercholesterolemic cynomolgus macaques, combination of aspirin (40mg) and fish oil (1.57g PUFA) for 4 years failed to inhibit atherosclerosis in vein bypass grafts [28]. Overall, mixed results are presented in the literature regarding the combination effect of aspirin and PUFA on the cardiovascular system [29].

Based on the existing evidence, a combination of aspirin and PUFA is proposed for cancer chemoprevention. It is hypothesized that, in the precancerous lesions where Cox2 is frequently up-regulated, supplementation of aspirin and PUFA (e.g., fish oil) will produce more anti-inflammatory metabolites (i.e., lipoxins, resolvins), and may exert synergistic inhibitory effects on inflammation-associated cancer. This combination, especially a low dose of aspirin (e.g., 81mg per day) and a high dose of PUFA, may provide several additional advantages over the individual agents: *1)* generation of anti-inflammatory metabolites (i.e., lipoxins and resolvins) from AA and PUFA by acetylated Cox2; *2)* cardiovascular benefits; *3)* protection from the gastrointestinal side effects of aspirin by PUFA [30]; *4)* cost-effectiveness of aspirin and PUFA for long-term cancer chemoprevention [31,32]. An 81-mg daily dose of aspirin is known to be safe to the gastrointestinal tract and causes substantial inhibition of prostaglandins in human colorectal mucosa [33,34]. A recent clinical trial demonstrated that 81-mg aspirin initiated the synthesis of 15*R*-epi-lipoxins as well as the inhibition of thromboxane B2 in blood [35].

Modification of chemical structure and delivery mode of aspirin may further enhance its efficacy. It seems advisable to preserve the acetyl group [36]. Besides fish oil, other dietary sources of PUFA (e.g., flaxseed, canola) may also be considered for combination with aspirin. An ideal situation could be one softgel of "aspirinoil", which contains a low dose of enteric-coated aspirin (e.g., 81 mg) and a high dose of PUFA, once every day.

Several potential concerns on this combination approach need further research, especially how strong the synergy between aspirin and PUFA could be and whether the above-mentioned biochemistry takes place *in vivo* in epithelial cells. Aspirin is quickly absorbed into systemic circulation through the stomach and the upper small intestine, with about 70% in the original form and 30% salicylate. Hydrolysis may take place during absorption by esterases within the gut wall, plasma and liver. Once absorbed, aspirin is rapidly hydrolyzed to salicylate with a half-life of only 15-20 min [37]. Enteric-coated aspirin, which achieves peak plasma concentration of aspirin and salicylate in 240-360 min and 8-14 hr respectively, may be a better choice for cancer prevention. This preparation is also known to be safer to the gastrointestinal tract than conventional aspirin [38].

The combination of aspirin and PUFA may be contraindicated for patients with an excessive risk of bleeding and other aspirin-associated side effects. A recent epidemiological study associated the increase of pancreatic cancer risk with aspirin use [39], although another three independent epidemiological studies suggested no or marginal protective effects of aspirin on pancreatic cancer [40-42]. Shunting among the AA metabolizing pathways may result from aspirin's effect on the Cox pathway, and contribute to its side effects, for example, aspirin-induced asthma and allergic rhinitis [43]. Caution should be taken for these patients.

In summary, a combination of a low dose of enteric-coated aspirin (e.g., 81mg per day) and a high dose of PUFA may balance long-term efficacy, safety and expense of cancer chemoprevention.

References

[1] Vanchier C (2004) Vioxx withdrawal alarms cancer prevention researchers. *J Natl Cancer Inst 96:* 1734-1735.

[2] FitzGerald GA (2003) Cox-2 and beyond: approaches to prostaglandin inhibition in human disease. *Nat Rev Drug Disc 2:* 879-890.

[3] FitzGerald GA (2004) Coxibs and cardiovascular disease. *N Engl J Med 351:* 1709-1711.

[4] Vane JR (2002) Back to an aspirin a day? *Science 296:* 474-475.

[5] Lecomte M, Laneuville O, Ji C, DeWitt DL, Smith WL (1994) Acetylation of human prostaglandin endoperoxide synthase-2 (cyclooxygenase-2) by aspirin. *J Biol Chem 269:* 13207-13215.

[6] Rowlinson SW, Crews BC, Goodwin DC, *et al.* (2000) Spatial requirements for 15-(*R*)-hydroxy-5Z,8Z,11Z,13E-eicosatetraenoic acid synthesis within the cyclooxygenase active site of murine Cox2. *J Biol Chem 275:* 6586-6591.

[7] Kieran NE, Maderna P, Godson C (2004) Lipoxins: Potential anti-inflammatory, proresolution, and antifibrotic mediators in renal disease. *Kidney Intl 65:* 1145-1154.

[8] Bannenberg G, Moussignac R-L, Gronert K, *et al.* (2004) Lipoxins and novel 15-epi-lipoxin analogs display potent anti-inflammatory actions after oral adeministration. *Br J Pharmacol 143:* 43-52.

[9] Fiorucci S, de Lima OMJ, mencarelli A, *et al.* (2002) Cyclooxygenase-2-derived lipoxin A4 increases gastric resistance to aspirin-induced damage. *Gastroenterology 123:* 1598-1606.

[10] Fiorucci S, Wallace JL, Mencarelli A, *et al.* (2004) A beta-oxidation-resistant lipoxin A4 analog treats hapten-induced colitis by attenuating inflammation and immune dysfunction. *Proc Natl Acad Sci USA 101:* 15736-15741.

[11] Devchand PR, Arita M, Hong S, *et al.* (2003) Human ALX receptor regulates neutrophil recruitment in transgenic mice: roles in inflammation and host defense. *FASEB J 17:* 652-659.

[12] Larsson SC, Kumlin M, Ingelman-Sundberg M, Wolk A (2004) Dietary long-chain n-3 fatty acids for the prevention of cancer: a review of potential mechanisms. *Am J Clin Nutr 79:* 935-945.

[13] Serhan CN, Hong S, Gronert K, *et al.* (2002) Resolvins: a family of bioactive products of omega-3 fatty acid transformation circuits initiated by aspirin treatment that counter proinflammation signals. *J Exp Med 196:* 1025-1037.

[14] Craven PA, DeRubertis FR (1992) Effects of aspirin on 1,2-dimethylhydrazine-induced colonic carcinogenesis. *Carcinogenesis 13:* 541-546.

[15] Reddy BS, Rao CV, Rivenson A, Kelloff G (1993) Inhibitory effect of aspirin on azoxymethane-induced colon carcinogenesis in F344 rats. *Carcinogenesis 14:* 1493-1497.

[16] Chiu CH, McEntee MF, Whelan J (2000) Discordant effect of aspirin and indomethacin on intestinal tumor burden in $Apc^{Min/+}$ mice. *Prostag Leuk Esse Fatty Acids 62:* 269-275.

[17] Sansom OJ, Stark LA, Dunlop MG, Clarke AR (2001) Suppression of intestinal and mammory neoplasia by lifetime administration of aspirin in $Apc^{Min/+}$ and $Apc^{Min/+}$, $Msh^{-/-}$ mice. *Cancer Res 61:* 7060-7064.

[18] Barnes CJ, Lee M (1998) Chemoprevention of spontaneous intestinal adenomas in the adenomatous polyposis coli Min mouse model with aspirin. *Gastroenterology 114:* 873-877.

[19] Mahmoud NN, Dannenberg AJ, Mestre J, *et al.* (1998) Aspirin prevents tumors in a murine model of familial adenomatous polyposis. *Surgery 124:* 225-231.

[20] Reuter BK, Zhang X-J, Miller MJS (2002) Therapeutic utility of aspirin in the $Apc^{Min/+}$ murine model of colon carcinogenesis. *BMC Cancer 2:* 19-26.

[21] Baron JA, Cole BF, Sandler RS, *et al.* (2003) A randomized trial of aspirin to prevent colorectal adenomas. *N Engl J Med 348:* 891-899.

[22] Benamouzig R, Deyra J, Martin A, *et al.* (2003) Daily soluble aspirin and prevention of colorectal adenoma recurrence: one-year results of the APACC trial. *Gastroenterology 125:* 328-336.

[23] Sandler RS, Halabi S, Baron JA, *et al.* (2003) A randomized trial of aspirin to prevent colorectal adenomas in patients with previous colorectal cancer. *N Eng J Med 348:* 883-890.

[24] Reddy BS (2004) Omega-3 fatty acids in colorectal cancer prevention. *Intl J Cancer 112:* 1-7.
[25] Anti M, Armelao F, Marra G, *et al.* (1994) Effects of different doses of fish oil on rectal cell proliferation in patients with sporadic colonic adenomas. *Gastroenterology 107:* 1709-1718.
[26] Huang Y-C, Jessup JM, Forse A, *et al.* (1996) n-3 fatty acids decrease colonic epithelial cell proliferation in high-risk bowel mucosa. *Lipids 31:* S313-317.
[27] Engstrom K, Wallin R, Saldeen T (2001) Effect of low-dose aspirin in combination with stable fish oil on whole blood production of eicosanoids. *Prostag Leuk Esse Fatty Acids 64:* 291-297.
[28] Boerboom LE, Olinger GN, Almassi GH, Skrinska VA (1997) Both dietary fish-oil supplementation and aspirin fail to inhibit atherosclerosis in long-term vein bypass grafts in moderately hypercholesterolemic nonhuman primates. *Circulation 96:* 968-974.
[29] Svaneborg N, Kristensen SD, Hansen LM, *et al.* (2002) The acute and short-time effect of supplementation with the combination of n-3 fatty acids and acetylsalicylic acid on platelet function and plasma lipids. *Thromb Res 105:* 311-316.
[30] Al-Harbi MM, Islam MW, Al-Shabanah OA, Al-gharably NM (1995) Effect of acute administration of fish oil (Omega-3 marine triglyceride) on gastric ulceration and secretion induced by various ulcerogenic and necrotizing agents in rats. *Food Chem Toxic 33:* 553-558.
[31] Hur C, Simon LS, Gazelle GS (2004) The cost-effectiveness of aspirin versus cyclooxygenase selective inhibitors for colorectal carcinoma chemoprevention in healthy individuals. *Cancer 101:* 189-197.
[32] Franzosi MG, Brunetti M, Marchioli R, *et al.* (2001) Cost-effectiveness analysis of n-3 polyunsaturated fatty acids (PUFA) after myocardial infarction: results from Gruppo Italiano per lo Studio della Sopravvivenza nell'Infarto (GISSI)-Prevenzione Trial. *Pharmacoeconomics 19:* 411-420.
[33] Laine L, Maller ES, Yu C, Quan H, Simon T (2004) Ulcer formation with low-dose enteric-coated aspirin and the effect of Cox-2 selective inhibition: a double-blind trial. *Gastroenterology 127:* 395-402.
[34] Ruffin MT, Krishnan K, Rock CL, *et al.* (1997) Suppression of human colorectal mucosal prostaglandins: determining the lowest effective aspirin dose. *J Natl Cancer Inst 89:* 1152-1160.
[35] Chiang N, Bermudez EA, Ridker PM, Hurwitz S, Serhan CN (2004) Aspirin triggers antiinflammatory 15-epi-lipoxin A4 and inhibits thromboxane in a randomized human trial. *Proc Natl Acad Sci USA 101:* 15178-15183.
[36] Kalgutkar AS, Crews BC, Rowlinson SW, *et al.* (1998) Aspirin-like molecules that covalently inactive cyclooxygenase-2. *Science 280:* 1268-1270.
[37] Clissold SP (1986) Aspirin and related derivatives of salicylic acid. *Drugs 32:* 8-26.
[38] Banoob DW, McCloskey WW, Webster W (2002) Risk of gastric injury with enteric- versus nonenteric-coated aspirin. *Ann Pharmacother 36:* 163-166.
[39] Schernhammer ES, Kang JH, Chan AT, *et al.* (2004) A prospective study of aspirin use and the risk of pancreatic cancer in women. *J Natl Cancer Inst 96:* 22-28.

[40] Jacobs EJ, Connell CJ, Rodriguez C*, et al.* (2004) Aspirin use and pancreatic cancer mortality in a large United States cohort. *J Natl Cancer Inst 96:* 524-528.

[41] Anderson KE, Johnson TW, Lazovich D, Folsom AR (2002) Association between nonsteroidal anti-inflammatory drug use and the incidence of pancreatic cancer. *J Natl Cancer Inst 94:* 1168-1171.

[42] Menezes RJ, Huber KR, Mahoney MC, Moysich KB (2002) Regular use of aspirin and pancreatic cancer risk. *BMC Pub Health 2:* 18-23.

[43] Szczeklik A, Sanak M, Nizankowska-Mogilnicka E, Kielbasa B (2003) Aspirin intolerance and the cyclooxygenase-leukotriene pathways. *Curr Opin Pulm Med 10:* 51-56.

Research and Review Studies

In: Cancer Research Perspectives
Editor: Larissa S. Pereira, pp. 11-71

ISBN 978-1-60021-980-1

Chapter I

ORAL SQUAMOUS CELL CARCINOMA: MOLECULAR CARCINOGENESIS, MARKERS AND NOVEL TREATMENT

Anak Iamaroon[1,*] and Siribang-on Piboonniyom Khovidhunkit[2]

[1]Department of Odontology and Oral Pathology, Faculty of Dentistry, Chiang Mai University, Chiang Mai, Thailand;

[2]Department of Hospital Dentistry, Mahidol University, Bangkok, Thailand.

ABSTRACT

Epithelial cancer, or squamous cell carcinoma, constitutes a major proportion of all diagnosed cancers. Squamous cell carcinoma of the oral cavity and pharynx account for approximately 3% of all cancers in the United States with more than 50,000 new cases diagnosed yearly. Worldwide, head and neck cancer is the sixth most common malignancy. Oral squamous cell carcinoma (OSCC) mainly affects the older population, with a steep increase in incidence in the people aged 60 years and older. Although OSCC is generally easily accessible to early diagnosis and therapy, they are associated with a relatively high rate of mortality due to recurrence and metastasis. The overall five-year survival rate for oral and pharyngeal cancers is among the lowest of all cancers and has not significantly changed during the last two decades. Most advances in oral carcinoma treatment have been confined to surgical excision and reconstruction procedures. Previously, the therapeutic modality offered to patients was based on traditional clinical stage-predicting indices and on histologic grading. Nowadays, the advanced research in molecular biology has been exploited for a better understanding of oral carcinogenesis. Several potential markers of molecular changes in oral premalignant and malignant lesions have been studied and interest in the genetic changes associated with these

* Correspondence concerning this article should be addressed to: Professor Dr. Anak Iamaroon, Department of Odontology and Oral Pathology, Faculty of Dentistry, Chiang Mai University, Chiang Mai, Thailand 50200. Phone: +6653944451; Email: iamaroon@yahoo.com.

lesions is increasing. Oral carcinogenesis has long been known as a multistep process involving many genetic alterations; hence, these alterations can be used in predicting the prognosis of patients and the progression of the tumor. Examples of molecular markers or alterations during oral carcinogenesis investigated include activated oncogenes, inactivated tumor suppressor genes, loss of heretozygosity (LOH) on some particular chromosomes, altered signal transducers, and DNA contents. Research on new agents, including agents that modulate signal transduction, cell-cycle progression, programmed cell death, matrix invasion, and angiogenesis are in development for oral cancer treatment. Since oral cancer is easily accessible, research on gene therapy for oral cancer and premalignant lesions are also available in many settings of clinical trials. In summary, this chapter will be focused on the review of research on molecular mechanisms of as well as molecular markers for early carcinogenesis, tumor invasion, metastasis, and prognosis of OSCC. Advanced research on the treatments of OSCC using new agents and gene therapy will also be covered.

INTRODUCTION

Most malignant tumors of the oral cavity are squamous cell carcinoma. Carcinomas of the oral cavity are among the 10 most common cancers in the world, accounting for 3-5% of all malignancies (Parkin et al., 1993). In the past few decades, a significant increase in the incidence of oral cancer and its attributable mortality has been observed with a striking upward trend in younger population (Iamaroon et al., 2004). The World Health Organization predicts a continuing worldwide increase in the incidence of oral cancer, extending this trend into the next several decades. It is now generally accepted that oral carcinogenesis is a multistep process of accumulated genetic damage leading to cell dysregulation with disruption in cell signaling, DNA-repair and cell cycle which are fundamental to homeostasis (Williams, 2000).

Six important steps believed to be necessary for cancer development are proposed by Hanahan and Weinberg (Hanahan and Weinberg, 2000). They are as followed.

1) Acquisition of autonomous proliferative signaling
2) Inhibition of growth inhibitory signals
3) Evasion of programmed cell death
4) Immortalization
5) Acquisition of a nutrient blood supply (angiogenesis)
6) Acquisition of the ability to invade tissue

In this chapter, the molecular changes that occur during carcinogenesis of oral squamous cell carcinoma (OSCC) will be discussed. Molecular changes that have been detected include 1) the activation of cellular proto-oncogenes such as epidermal growth factor (EGF), epidermal growth factor receptor (EGFR), cyclin D1, and c-myc 2) inactivation of tumor suppressor genes, for example, genes in the pRB, the p53 and TGF-beta pathways 3) activation of telomerase which can induce immortalization of oral epithelial cells 4) induction of angiogenesis and 5) up-regulation of various proteinases leading to invasion and metastasis of tumor cells (Scully et al., 2000; Jefferies and Foulkes, 2001).

Since oral cavity is a part of the head and neck region and several studies of the head and neck cancer have also included oral cancer, the head and neck cancer will be also referred in this chapter book in addition to oral cancer.

ACTIVATION OF CELLULAR PROTO-ONCOGENES

Groups of Scientists have conducted experiments to investigate the potential role of proto-oncogenes in oral carcinogenesis, most notably the *EGFR* and the *c-myc*. Overexpression of EGFR and c-Myc has been detected in some oral carcinoma (Stanton et al., 1994; Baral et al., 1998), while high levels of expression of EGFR have been found to be associated with reduced disease-free and survival rate after treatment of head and neck squamous cell carcinoma (HNSCC) (Rubin Grandis et al., 1998). Overexpression of the *PRAD1* gene, which encodes cyclin D1, was also implicated in 30-50% of HNSCC (Callender et al., 1994). The D-type cyclins play an important role in cell cycle regulation by regulating the activity of the retinoblastoma tumor suppressor and overexpression of this protein leads to aberrant cell cycle progression. The role of this molecule will be discussed in the following section.

Epidermal Growth Factor Receptor (EGFR)

EGFR is a member of the ErbB/Her family of receptor tyrosine kinases which includes EGFR/ErbB1, ErbB2 (Her2/neu), ErbB3 (Her3) and ErbB4 (Her4). EGFR possesses an extracellular N-terminal ligand-binding domain, a transmembrane region and a C-terminal intracellular domain, which includes the kinase domain and multiple phosphorylation sites.

The *ErbB2* gene encodes a transmembrane protein of 185 kDa and has extensive sequence homology to EGFR (Schechter et al., 1985; Bargmann et al., 1986). Like EGFR, it has intrinsic tyrosine kinase activity and can interact with many different cellular proteins, such as Shc, PLC-γ, and GTP-ase activating protein, thereby mediating the signal transduction pathway (Xie et al., 1995; Chen et al., 1996). It can also form heterodimers with other members of the EGFR family. The *ErbB3* gene is the third member of the EGFR family. Its gene product is a transmembrane glycoprotein with a close structural similarity to EGFR and ErbB2 (Plowman et al., 1990; Kraus et al., 1993). ErbB3 does not have an intrinsic tyrosine kinase activity. It has been shown that ErbB3 can be transphosphorylated by EGFR, resulting in phosphatidylinositol 3-kinase (PI3K) recruitment (Fedi et al., 1994). The EGFR/ErbB3 chimeric receptor did not couple to PLC-γ or GTP-ase activating protein, thereby distinguishing the ErbB3 signaling pathway from that of other members of the EGFR family (Fedi, 1994). *ErbB4*, the fourth member of the family, encodes a 180 kDa transmembrane tyrosine kinase (Culouscou et al., 1993). Its extracellular domain is similar to that of ErbB3 whereas its cytoplasmic domain is homologous to EGFR and ErbB2.

Until now, 12 ligands of the ErbB family have been identified. Binding of ligands to EGFR induces homodimerization or heretodimerization of EGFR and other ErbBs, resulting in autophosphorylation of the receptor (Kalyankrishna and Grandis, 2006). Activated ErbBs stimulate many intracellular signaling pathways. Two main pathways activated by the receptors are the mitogen-activated protein kinase (MAPK) and the PI3K/AKT pathways (Yarden, 2001). Other important ErbB signaling effectors are the signal transducer and activator of transcription proteins (STATs) (Garcia et al., 2001), SRC tyrosine kinase (Ishizawar and Parsons, 2004), and mammalian target of rapamycin (mTOR) (Bjornsti and Houghton, 2004).

EGFR is overexpressed in most epithelial cancers including head and neck cancer (Hynes and Lane, 2005; Laimer et al., 2007). EGFR is also rendered constitutively active as a result of mutations in a subset of tumors. Deletion of exon 2 to 7 in the extracellular domain yields a constitutively active EGFRvIII which is prevalent in glioblastomas (Lorimer, 2002). EGFRvIII and the kinase domain mutants activate survival pathways such as AKT which can lead to oncogenesis. EGFR plays an important role not only in tumor cells, but also in the tumor stroma. It is implicated in tumor angiogenesis, which facilitates tumor progression. EGFR is also overexpressed in endothelial cells and the role of EGFR in endothelial cell proliferation is recognized to be of increased significance under conditions of limited vascular endothelial growth factor (VEGF) expression (Sini et al., 2005).

EGFR is crucially important in the pathogenesis of HNSCC. Overexpression of EGFR and its ligand, transforming growth factor alpha (TGF-α), are prevalent in HNSCC. EGFR and TGF-α mRNA are found to be elevated up to 92% and 87% in the tumors, respectively (Grandis and Tweardy, 1993). A dramatic upregulation of EGFR is revealed during the change from dysplasia to squamous cell carcinoma (Shin et al., 1994). EGFR also provides an important link between tobacco smoke, an important risk factor for oral cancer, and increased production of prostaglandin E2 (PGE2), a growth promoting G protein-coupled receptor agonist. Tobacco smoke increases levels of the EGFR ligands, amphiregulin and TGF-α, in oral epithelial cells (Du et al., 2005). Correlated with these *in vitro* findings, the levels of EGFR ligands are increased in the oral mucosa of smokers (Moraitis et al., 2005). This induces EGFR activation and increases levels of cyclooxygenase2 (COX2) and PGE2 leading to transactivation of EGFR, thereby providing a positive feedback loop for tumor cell growth (Pai et al., 2002).

In addition to EGFR, the overexpression of other ErbB family members is also established in HNSCC (Bei et al., 2001; Bei et al., 2004) and have been found to be significantly associated with the presence of lymph node and distance metastases (Xia et al., 1999). Overexpression of ErbB2 has been shown to increase metastatic potential by promoting the EGFR family. In another study, ErbB2 was ranked first among other EGFRs in predicting the outcome of OSCC including histologic grades, nodes and distant metastasis (Xia et al., 1999). The importance of ErbB4 in carcinogenesis has been revealed in papillary thyroid carcinoma (Haugen et al., 1996). The expression levels of ErbB4 in OSCC was significantly associated with distant metastasis, however, there was no significant association of this protein with nodal stage. Therefore, its significance in oral carcinogenesis remains to be elucidated (Xia et al., 1999).

The AKT family of kinases, AKT-1, -2, and -3, a downstream effector of EGFR and PI3K, have been found to play crucial roles in cell proliferation, survival, and glucose metabolism. AKT is also important for epithelial-mesenchymal transition (EMT), a common phenomenon during embryonic development, wound healing, tumor invasion and metastasis

(Kang and Svoboda, 2005). Recently, activation of the PI3K/AKT axis is emerging as an important feature of EMT (Larue and Bellacosa, 2005). By investigating SCC lines, the role of AKT in the biology of human squamous cell carcinoma was elucidated. It was revealed that AKT activation caused EMT characterized by down-regulation of desmoplakin, E-cadherin and beta-catenin and up-regulation of vimentin (Grille et al., 2003). Down-regulation of E-cadherin, in particular, appeared to be the result from up-regulation of the transcription repressors SNAIL and SIP1. In addition, EMT was accompanied by increased *in vivo* cell motility on fibronectin-coated surfaces and increased invasiveness in animals. Recent data revealed that EMT induced by the stromal cell-derived factor-1 (SDF-1)/CXCR4 system might be involved in the lymph node metastasis of OSCC via activation of PI3K/AKT pathway (Onoue et al., 2006). Besides PI3K/AKT pathway, several studies have shown that TGF-beta also mediates EMT (Prime et al., 2004).

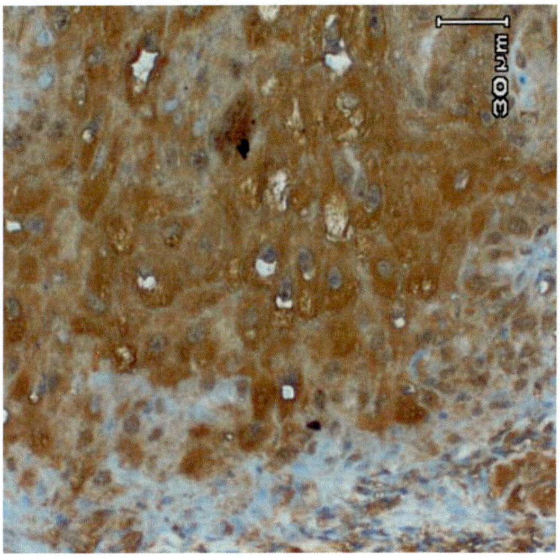

Figure 1. Intense expression of pan-AKT protein (brown staining) at the invasive front of OSCC is shown (Iamaroon and Krisanaprakornkit, unpublished data) (Immunohistochemical technique, original magnification, x200).

Deregulation of the PI3K/AKT signaling pathway also leads to various human cancers including OSCC, glioblastoma, ovarian, breast, pancreatic, and lung cancers (Vivanco and Sawyers, 2002; Bellacosa et al., 2005). Focusing on AKT and its association with OSCC development, AKT kinase was found to be highly expressed in OSCC (Nakayama et al., 2001). Using immunohistochemical technique, the expression of AKT was investigated in OSCC (Iamaroon and Krisanaprakornkit, unpublished data) (Figure 1). The preliminary results showed a strong expression of pan-AKT in OSCC cells. Additionally, the expression of phosphorylated AKT (p-AKT) was found in 34.5% of OSCC (Lim et al., 2005), compared with 26% in prostate cancer (Malik et al., 2002) and 66% in both melanoma (Dhawan et al., 2002) and HNSCC (Gupta et al., 2002). p-AKT expression correlated with lymph node metastasis and TNM stage in patients with OSCC (Lim et al., 2005). In addition, p-AKT was inversely associated with E-cadherin expression. p-AKT appeared to also involve in early carcinogenesis of OSCC as evidenced that 45% of oral preneoplastic lesions expressed p-

AKT (Massarelli et al., 2005). Moreover, p-AKT correlates with the worst outcomes in patients with tongue cancer. Collectively, these findings suggest that p-AKT plays an important role in OSCC carcinogenesis and can be used as a prognostic marker for OSCC.

c-Myc

In 1911, Peyton Rous observed that chicken sarcoma could be transmitted through cell-free extracts from the tumors, suggesting that a virus could be an etiologic agent of these sarcomas (Rous, 1979). Later, Bishop and coworkers studied a specific subgroup of avian retrovirus which induced sarcomas and other tumors in chicken and identified the *v-myc* oncogene (Sheiness and Bishop, 1979). The discovery of a homologous gene termed *c-myc* in chicken supported the view that oncogenic avian retroviruses could capture cellular growth regulatory genes and transmit the activated gene. The finding that human cancers frequently display altered expression of human *c-myc* underscores the importance of this gene in the cause of human cancers (Dang et al., 2005).

The c-Myc oncoprotein belongs to the Myc family of proteins which includes c-, N- and L-Myc. The *c-myc* gene is located on human chromosome 8q24 and has been found to be amplified in several types of cancers (Rodriguez-Pinilla et al., 2006; Furge et al., 2007). The *c-myc* sequence contains several conserved N-terminal transactivation domains, which are also found in N- and L-Myc. The C-terminal region contains a dimerization motif, termed the helix-loop-helix leucine zipper (HLH LZ) which mediates homodimerization and heterodimerization with an obligate partner HLH LZ protein, Max (Luscher and Larsson, 1999). After forming heterodimerization, Myc-Max complexes recognize the E-box sequence CACGTG (as well as related non-canonical sites) and activate transcription of several genes important in cell cycle regulation, metabolism, cell adhesion, and protein systhesis (Blackwood and Eisenman, 1991; Dang et al., 2006). Expression of *c-myc* in the normal cell is tightly regulated by external signals, such as growth factors and extracellular matrix contacts, as well as by internal clocks, such as cell cycle. In resting normal cells, the level of expression of *c-myc* is very low. Upon growth factor stimulation, *c-myc* expression increases dramatically (Kelly et al., 1983). Myc overexpression in cycling cells has been reported to reduce requirements for growth factors, block exit from the cell cycle, accelerate cell division and increase cell size (Sorrentino et al., 1986; Stern et al., 1986; Karn et al., 1989).

When overexpressed, c-Myc is one of the most potent oncogenes. It was found that over 50% of human cancers is associated with the overexpression of *c-myc* gene and is also frequently associated with worse prognosis and more invasive phenotype (Gamberi et al., 1998; Gamberi et al., 1998). c-Myc expression was investigated in oral precancerous and early cancerous lesions using immunohistochemical technique. c-Myc nuclear labeling paralleled the progressive histological changes among various stages of transformation indicating that c-Myc expression correlated with progression of oral carcinogenesis (Eversole and Sapp, 1993). Co-overexpression of p53 and c-Myc proteins was also studied in advanced stages of betel-and tobacco-related OSCC. Utilizing immunohistochemistry, 45.8% and 56.3% of OSCC specimens showed p53 and c-Myc positivity, respectively. In addition, tumors with both p53 and c-Myc positivity were detected in advanced stages of diseases whereas neither p53 nor c-Myc immunoreactivity was found in the earlier stage of OSCC (Baral et al., 1998). *c-Myc* amplification was also discovered in 9% of HNSCC and this frequency is comparable to that reported for other solid tumors (Leonard et al., 1991). When array-based comparative genomic hybridization was used to screen microdissected OSCC for genome wide alterations, c-Myc was also one of most frequent gene that exhibited copy number gain (Chen et al., 2004). Furthermore, in a cellular model to create oral squamous cancer cells using limited sets of genetic alterations frequently observed in human cancers, overexpression of cyclin D1 and p53 inactivation induced immortalization of oral keratinocytes without transformation. However, additional overexpression of EGFR followed by c-Myc could induce colony formation in soft agar, an indication of malignant transformation, in the proviously immortalized cells. These results suggested that overexpression of c-Myc could induce malignant phenotype resembling that discovered in OSCC (Goessel et al., 2005).

Inactivation of Tumor Suppressor Genes

The pRB Pathway

pRB is a tumor suppressor that functions as a regulator of S phase progression by regulating the transcriptional activity of the transcription factor E2F. This transcription factor plays an important role in the temporal expression of S phase genes (Figure 2). Members of the E2F family of transcription factors appear to play a major role in the regulatory circuit in late G1 phase, the so-called “restriction point”. Once bound to the promoter through E2F, the pRB protein can turn off transcription of downstream genes important in S phase progression. Before the cell proceeds into S phase, pRB becomes phosphorylated at multiple sites by cdks and loses its transcriptional repression activity (Mittnacht, 1998). These phosphorylation events also result in dissociation of the E2F-pRB repressor complex, which allows S phase-specific genes to be transcribed resulting in cell cycle progression (Suzuki-Takahashi et al., 1995). In addition to cell cycle control, pRB is also involved in regulating differentiation and apoptosis (Herwig and Strauss, 1997) where it cooperates with another major tumor suppressor, p53.

The biological activity of pRB is found to be regulated by cell cycle dependent phosphorylation and dephosphorylation (Buchkovich et al., 1989). The cyclin D- dependent kinases cdk4 and cdk6 have been implicated as pRB regulators because their kinase activity profiles parallel the major wave of pRB phosphorylation at the G1/S boundary (Matsushime et al., 1994; Meyerson and Harlow, 1994). Cyclin D/cdk4 and cyclin D/cdk6 enzyme complexes can efficiently phosphorylate pRB both *in vitro* and *in vivo* (Kato et al., 1993; Meyerson and Harlow, 1994). The enzymatic activities of these kinase complexes are tightly regulated not only at the level of association with the regulatory subunit, cyclin D, but also by several low molecular weight inhibitory proteins. There are two families of cdk inhibitory proteins (Sherr and Roberts, 1995). One of them is the group of universal cdk-inhibitors comprising $p21^{cip1}$, $p27^{kip1}$ and $p57^{kip2}$. The other family of proteins is called INK4 or inhibitor of cdk4. This group of proteins includes $p16^{ink4A}$, $p15^{ink4B}$, $p18^{ink4C}$ and $p19^{ink4D}$.

While the universal kinase inhibitors bind to cyclin/cdk complexes, the INK4 proteins directly interact with either cdk4 or cdk6 and prevent the formation of enzymatically active cyclin D/cdk4 or cyclin D/cdk6 complexes.

In general, the enzymatic activities of cdks are regulated by several mechanisms: 1) binding to cyclins, 2) binding to inhibitors and 3) phosphorylation of the cdk subunit (Morgan, 1995). The D-type cyclins are the positive regulatory subunits of cdk4 and cdk6 kinases. Members of this cyclin family, consisting of cyclin D1, D2 and D3, are growth factor sensors because they are highly inducible by growth factors and are rapidly degraded when mitogenic factors are withdrawn (Won et al., 1992). The activities of cdk4 and cdk6 are also negatively regulated by their association with inhibitory proteins. The INK4 family of proteins binds to cdk4 or cdk6 and disrupts their interactions with D-type cyclins. The CIP/KIP family of proteins binds to cdk/cyclin complexes and inactivates their kinase activity. These proteins also act as essential assembly factors for cyclin D/cdk4 and cyclin D/cdk6 complexes (Cheng et al., 1999). Hence, the CIP/KIP proteins are potent inhibitors of cyclin E and A-dependent cdk2 activity, but they can act as positive regulators of cyclin D-dependent kinases (Blain et al., 1997).

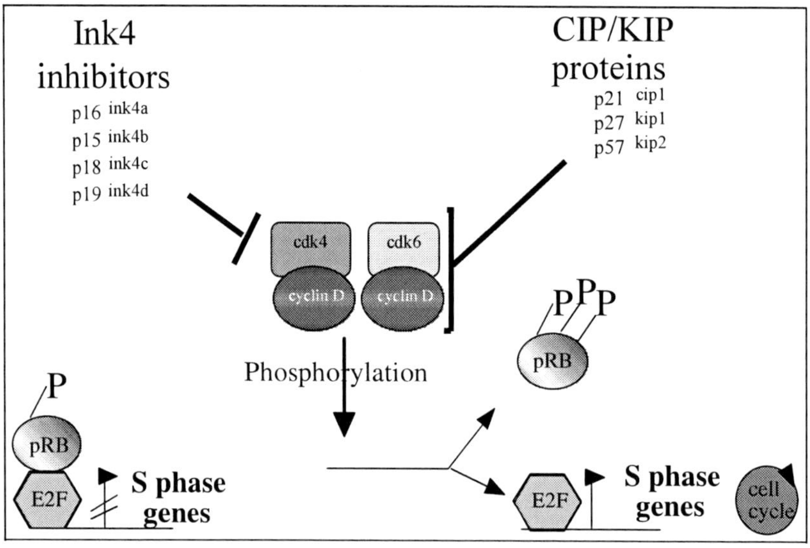

Figure 2. Schematic view of the pRB pathway. Hypophosphorylated pRB binds to E2F to form a transcriptional repressor complex. The kinase complexes cyclin D/cdk4 and cyclin D/cdk6 phosphorylate and inactivate pRB. Hyperphosphorylated, inactive form of pRB releases E2F which now acts as a transcriptional activator for S phase genes and causes cell cycle progession. These kinases are negatively regulated by Ink4 inhibtors, which form a complex with cdk4 or cdk6 and dissociate cdk4 or cdk6 from its regulator, cyclin D. The cip/kip family of proteins also modulates cyclin D/cdk4 and cyclin D/cdk6 activities by accelerating the formation of these complexes.

The pRB Pathway and Oral Cancer

Defects in the pRB pathway have also been delineated in oral carcinogenesis. The pRB tumor suppressor protein controls cell cycle progression and differentiation (Weinberg,

1995). Mutations in the *RB* gene are limited to a specific set of tumor types including retinoblastoma, osteosarcoma, small cell lung carcinoma, bladder and prostate cancers and a small number of breast cancers (Lee et al., 1988) and are not commonly detected in HNSCC (Maestro et al., 1996). However, other components of the pRB pathway such as p16^{ink4A}, cyclin D and cdk6 are frequently abrogated in HNSCC.

As stated previously, the pRB pathway is a key regulatory checkpoint for cells to enter S phase. The pRB protein is active in its hypophosphorylated form and mediates a proliferation block in the G1 phase. After phosphorylation of pRB by cyclin D/cdk4 and cyclin D/cdk6 complexes, the hyperphosphorylated form of pRB dissociates from E2F, allowing cell cycle progression. According to this scenario, mutational inactivation of the pRB protein, aberrant activation of cyclins and cyclin-dependent kinases or inactivation of a kinase inhibitor, are all expected to lead to the deregulation of the pRB pathway. As previously mentioned, mutation of *RB* is limited to a specific set of tumor types (Horowitz et al., 1990). Cyclin D1 amplification has been frequently found in breast cancer (Sicinski et al., 1995). Lack of expression or mutation of p16^{ink4A} has been detected in familial melanoma, HNSCC and other cancers (Wick et al., 1995; Gonzalez et al., 1997). A mutated cdk4 defective in binding to p16^{ink4A} was identified in human melanoma (Wolfel et al., 1995). Furthermore, evidence for cdk6 amplification in gliomas has also been published (Costello et al., 1996), and cdk6 hyperactivity was documented in OSCC lines (Piboonniyom et al., 2002).

p16^{Ink4A} and Oral Carcinogenesis

Several lines of evidence support the notion that p16^{ink4A} possesses a strong growth suppressive activity. As mentioned before, aberrations of p16 ^{ink4A} have been found in several types of cancers (Cairns et al., 1994). Re-expression of endogenous p16 ^{ink4A} in cell lines with promoter methylation by 5-aza-2'-deoxycytidine treatment or re-introduction of p16 ^{ink4A} into cells lacking p16 ^{ink4A} expression induced a senescence-like phenotype (Timmermann et al., 1998). However, re-introduction of p16 ^{ink4A} in human tumor cell lines known to lack functional pRB, such as SAOS2 and a cervical carcinoma cell line, C33A, did not initiate cellular senescence, nor did introduction of p16 ^{ink4A} into immortalized fibroblast from *RB* nullizygous mouse embryos (Medema et al., 1995). Furthermore, the growth suppressive effect of p16 ^{ink4A} was negated when SV40 large T-antigen or E1A, that are known to bind and inactivate pRB, were introduced into cells overexpressing p16 ^{ink4A}. These results indicated that the growth inhibitory effect of p16 ^{ink4A} is dependent on functional pRB (Lukas et al., 1995). In contrast to p16 ^{ink4A}, the introduction of p21^{Cip1} and p27 ^{Kip1} into cells with or without functional pRB can induce growth arrest in G1 phase suggesting that p21^{Cip1} and p27 ^{Kip1} inhibit DNA synthesis by a mechanism independent of pRB function (Waga et al., 1994).

At first, the *INK4A* gene encoding p16 ^{ink4A} was dubbed multiple tumor suppressor gene 1 (*MST1*) because of its frequent deletion or mutation in a wild variety of cancers and cell lines (Pollock et al., 1996). The *INK4A* is inactivated by several distinct events including homozygous gene deletion, point mutation, and promoter hypermethylation (Reed et al., 1996). The *INK4A* gene is localized on chromosome 9p21 which has been reported to be deleted in both premalignant and malignant oral lesions (Lippman and Hong, 2001). Loss of chromosome 9p is thought to be an early event in the development of HNSCC (Papadimitrakopoulou et al., 1997; Papadimitrakopoulou et al., 2001) and loss of heterozygosity (LOH) at 9p21-22 are reported in dysplasia, carcinoma in situ and HNSCC (Ambrosch et al., 2001). Hypermethylation of the promoter region of the *INK4A* gene can also lead to loss of $p16^{ink4A}$ protein expression (Otterson et al., 1995) and was frequently found in OSCC (Piboonniyom et al., 2002). Alteration of $p16^{ink4A}$ was also detected in patients with severe oral epithelial dysplasia. Microscopically confirmed dysplastic oral epithelium and matching normal tissue were laser capture-microdissected. Then the DNA was extracted and subjected to molecular analysis for gene deletion and promoter hypermethylation. The exon 1α of the *INK4A* gene was deleted in 11.5% and hypermethylation was detected in 57.7% (Kresty et al., 2002). The evaluation of the expression of G1/S modulators, cyclin D1, $p16^{ink4A}$ and pRB using immunohistochemical technique has been reported (Soni et al., 2005). The tissue specimens included OSCC, potentially malignant lesions and normal oral tissues. Eighty three percent of potentially malignant lesions and 90% of OSCC showed alteration of at least one of the proteins in the pRB pathway and loss of $p16^{ink4A}$ was found to be the earliest phenomenon of the alterations. This suggested that $p16^{ink4A}$ plays a major role in oral carcinogenesis.

Cyclin D1 and Oral Carcinogenesis

Overexpression of cyclin D1 was observed in OSCC in several studies. Cyclin D1 is a 45-kD protein encoded by the *CCND1* or *PRAD1* gene located on chromosome 11q13 and plays an important role in the regulation of G1-S transition of the cell cycle. This protein are thought to be a growth factor sensors, as D-type cyclins are highly inducible by growth factors and degrade rapidly when mitogenic factors are withdrawn (Matsushime et al., 1994). Overexpression of cyclin D1 leads to shortening of the G1 phase and to less dependency on growth factor, resulting in abnormal cell proliferation that in turn might favor the occurrence of additional genetic lesions (Fracchiolla et al., 1997). A sequential increase in cyclin D1 expression was observed from histologically normal oral tissue to hyperplastic lesions, dysplastic lesions and squamous cell carcinoma (SCC) (Soni et al., 2005). *CCND1* gene was amplified in potentially malignant oral lesions that progressed to invasive carcinoma (Izzo et al., 1998). Cyclin D1 overexpression was also observed in 70.7% of OSCC and 63.3% of verrucous carcinoma (Angadi and Krishnapillai, 2007). In a cellular model for oral-esophageal carcinogenesis, cyclin D1 overexpression and p53 inactivation could induce immortalization in normal human oral keratinocytes (Goessel et al., 2005). However, in some studies, the expression of cyclin D1 was not found to be different in oral hyperplasia and SCCs (Tsuzuki et al., 2003). Moreover, cyclin D1 protein levels was investigated in some OSCC cell lines and it was found that the levels of this protein did not exceed the amount of that expressed in normal oral keratinocytes (Piboonniyom et al., 2002). Taken together, although not in every case, overexpression of cyclin D1 could play some role in oral carcinogenesis.

The p53 Pathway

The p53 gene was first discovered in 1979 in extracts of transformed cells, reacting with antiserum from animals with tumors induced by simian virus 40 (SV40) and was thought to be an oncogene since overexpression of p53 was frequently discovered in malignant neoplasm (Lane and Crawford, 1979; Linzer and Levine, 1979). It was deciphered later that the overexpression of the p53 protein was the mutated and not the wild type protein (Hinds et al., 1989). The p53 protein is a transcription factor which negatively regulates cell cycle progression principally in response to cellular stresses, such as DNA damage, hypoxia, and oncogene activation (Oren, 1999). Activation of signal transduction pathways in stressed cells triggers phosphorylation and acetylation of p53, leading to its stabilization and initiation of a p53-dependent transcriptional program which either inhibits cell proliferation or induces cellular suicide, apoptosis.

One of the important p53 responsive genes is *mdm2* (human *hdm2*), which binds to p53 and represses its transactivation activity (Momand et al., 1992). Mdm2 possesses an E3 ubiquitin ligase activity that targets p53 and induces relocalization of p53 from the cell nucleus to the cytoplasm where p53 undergoes proteasomal degradation (Honda et al., 1997; Roth et al., 1998). This negative feedback loop is thought to be critical in the downregulation of p53 to normal levels after the transient stress induction.

Another crutial transcriptional target of p53 is $p21^{Cip1}$, an inhibitor of cyclin-dependent kinases (el-Deiry et al., 1993; Gu et al., 1993; Harper et al., 1993; Xiong et al., 1993; Noda et al., 1994). The promoter of the *CIP1* gene contains p53 binding sites. During p53-dependent cell cycle arrest, $p21^{Cip1}$ transcription is induced leading to inhibition of cdk activity and obstruction of cell cycle progression. The $p21^{Cip1}$ protein also binds to proliferating cell nuclear antigen (PCNA) and inhibits processivity of DNA replication (Waga et al. , 1994).

Another important regulator of the p53 tumor suppressor pathway is $p19^{ARF}$ (human $p14^{ARF}$). This protein is encoded by an alternative open reading frame that partially overlaps with the *INK4A* gene which encodes an inhibitor of cyclin D/cdk4 and cyclin D/cdk6 kinase activities (Mao et al., 1995; Quelle et al., 1995). Upon upregulation of $p19^{ARF}$, mdm2 activity is antagonized, thus p53 becomes stabilized. A number of studies have revealed direct physical interactions between $p19^{ARF}$, p53 and mdm2. The *ARF* gene is E2F responsive and becomes upregulated when cells receive an aberrant signal that activates E2F transcriptional activity and hence may link the p53 and the pRB pathways (Figure 3).

The p53 Family of Proteins

In 1997, two novel proteins, p63 and p73, were discovered as other members of p53 family of proteins (Kaghad et al., 1997; Schmale and Bamberger, 1997; Yang et al., 1998). Both genes give rise to proteins that have entirely novel functions and p53 related functions. They play important and unique roles in mouse and human development and differentiation. Although these proteins are highly homologous, p63 and p73 knockouts exhibit severe developmental abnormalities without increased cancer susceptibility, whereas this phenomenon is reversed for p53 knockouts (Moll and Slade, 2004). However, p63 knockout mice are born alive but show the most severe developmental phenotype of all p53 family members (Yang et al., 1999). The limbs are absent or truncated owing to a malfunction of the apical ectodermal ridge. They failed to develop stratified epidermis and most epithelial tissues and eventually died from dehydration within hours after birth. This indicated that p63 expression is absolutely essential for limb formation and epidermal morphogenesis (integument and tongue) including the formation of adnexa (teeth, hair, mammary and prostate glands and sweat and lacrimal glands). On the other hand, p73 null mice are born viable, but show a high mortality rate within the first 2 months (Yang et al., 2000). The animal suffered from hydrocephalus, indicative of abnormal cerebrospinal fluid dynamics and other abnormalities in the development of the nervous system.

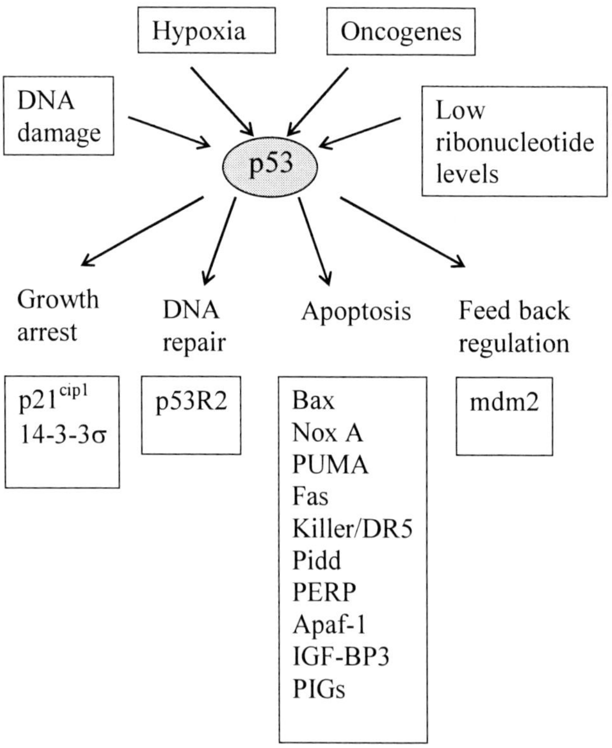

Figure 3. Target genes in cellular response to p53. Cellular stress signals induce accumulation of the p53 protein, which acts as a transcriptional activator for genes promoting cell cycle arrest or apoptosis. A negative feedback loop with mdm2 downregulates p53 levels after induction. The p53 pathway is coupled to the pRB pathway by $p21^{Cip1}$.

Regarding the protein architecture, p53, p63 and p73 consist of a central sequence specific DNA binding domain (DBD), an N-terminal transactivation domain (TA) and a C-terminal oligomerization domain (OD). The highest degree of homology is seen within the DBD. The p63 and p73 share approximately 65% amino acid identity with the DBD of p53. All 3 genes contain a second intronic promoter that generates N-terminally truncated ΔN proteins (Δ133p53, ΔNp63 and ΔNp73). Further ΔN isoforms are generated by alternative splicing events and alternative initiation of translation (Δ40p53, Δex2p73, Δex2/3p73 and ΔN'p73). As the N-terminus is crucial for the transactivation of target genes, transactivating full-length isoforms (FLp53, Tap63 and Tap73) can be distinguished from the transactivation-compromised ΔN isoforms that show anti-apoptotic and dominant–negative properties. Finally, more variation caused by the alternative splicing of C-terminal exons and the use of cryptic splice sites yields a series of different isoforms (α, β, γ, δ, ε, θ, ζ and η) with fundamentally different and still incompletely understood biological functions (Moll and Slade, 2004).

The p53 Family of Proteins and Oral Carcinogenesis

The p53 tumor suppressor protein plays an important role as a gatekeeper that recognizes and refutes the molecular consequences of various forms of cellular insults and malfunctions (Lane, 1992). Mutations in the *p53* gene are frequently found in human cancers (Hollstein et al., 1991). Loss-of-function of p53 corresponds with poor clinical response to radiation or chemotherapy, probably due to loss of induction of programmed cell death (Symonds et al., 1994). The p53 null mice succumb to several types of cancers including malignant lymphoma, sarcoma, and testicular tumors (Donehower et al., 1992). Germline mutations of p53 have been detected in Li-Fraumini syndrome patients who are predisposed to develop multiple types of tumors at an early age (Malkin et al., 1990). Several viral oncoproteins including Adenovirus E1B, SV40 T-antigen and HPV16 E6 also inactivate p53.

Several studies demonstrated that aberrant expression of p53 is associated with progression from hyperkeratosis, epithelial dysplasia to SCC. The immunoreactivity for p53 protein was found in the nuclei of the parabasal layer in hyperplastic and precancerous lesions which increased according to the degree of dysplastic change. Aberration in p53 expression was found in 28% of the benign epithelial hyperplasias, 57% of mild dysplasias, 55% of moderate dysplasias, 71% of severely dysplastic tissues and 76% of SCC (Ichikawa et al., 1997). The proportion of p53 positive tumors found in several studies ranged from 34% to 81% (Brachman et al., 1992; Ahomadegbe et al., 1995; Iamaroon et al., 2004; de Oliveira et al., 2007). The expression of p53 and Ki67, a cell proliferation marker, in OSCC was investigated and a significant correlation between the expression of p53 and Ki67 was observed (Figures 4, 5) (Iamaroon et al., 2004). These findings suggest that p53 mutation leads to increased cell proliferation in OSCC. In one study, the prognostic value of p53 in OSCC was evaluated (de Oliveira et al., 2007). Patients with negative p53 expression had a better prognosis and a significantly reduced number of metastases. In another study of OSCC without initial neck node metastases, negative p53 expression was found to be a significant prognostic factor associated with longer survival (Carlos de Vicente et al., 2004).

The p63 protein may also play a significant role in oral carcinogenesis. The *p63* gene shows structural and functional homology with the p53 and is located in the 3q27-29 chromosome region. The p63 is capable of binding to DNA and transactivate the p53 responsive genes. It was found that expression of p63 protein and mRNA was increased with the severity of oral dysplasia (Chen et al., 2005). Nearly normal expression of p63 could be observed in homogenous leukoplakia and decreased expression was found in nodular leukoplakia and increased significantly in erythroplakia (Kovesi and Szende, 2006). There was also a statistically significant correlation between p63 expression and tumor differentiation. The expression of p63 was amplified in poorly differentiated tumors. When analyzed for prognostic significance, patients with perineural infiltration had poorer survival rates than the group with no perineural infiltration, and patients with increased p63 expression had poorer survival rates than the group with reduced p63 expression. However, the statistical analysis showed no significant correlation between p63 expression, sex, age, tumor size, staging, recurrence, and metastasis (Lo Muzio et al., 2005). This indicated that p63 expression can be used as a prognostic marker for OSCC with more aggressive and invasive phenotype.

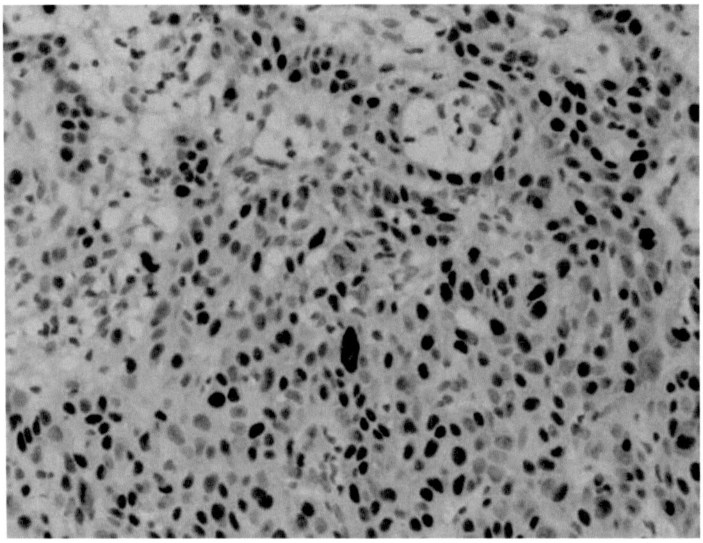

Figure 4. The expression of p53 in the nuclei of OSCC (brown staining) (Iamaroon et al., 2004) (Immunohistochemical technique, original magnification, x200).

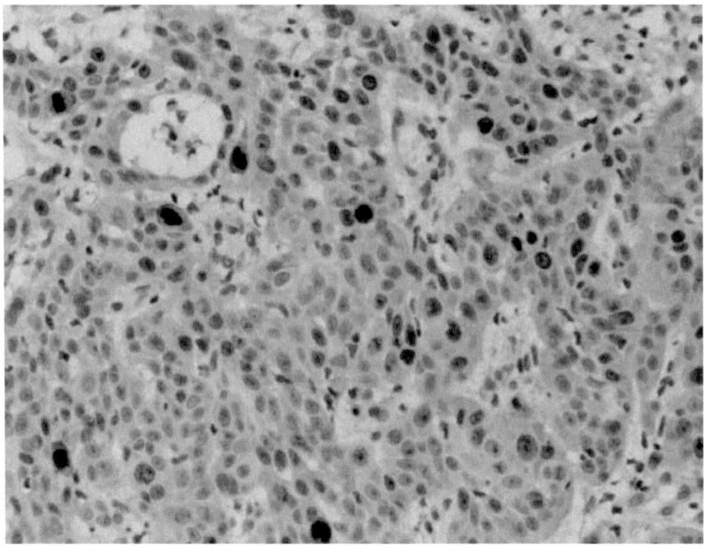

Figure 5. The expression of Ki67 in the nuclei of OSCC (brown staining) (Iamaroon et al., 2004) (Immunohistochemical technique, original magnification, x200).

The *p73* gene maps to chromosome region 1p36.3 which is frequently deleted in a variety of solid tumors (Kaghad et al., 1997). Overexpression of p73 was found in many tumor types, for example, tumors of breast (Zaika et al., 1999), neuroblastoma (Kovalev et al., 1998), lung (Mai et al., 1998) and esophagus (Cai et al., 2000). Regarding the association of p73 and head and neck cancer, early studies aimed to investigate the mutation of *p73* gene since it was extensively found that the mutation of *p53* gene was associated with head and neck tumor. El-Naggar and colleages found 2 missense mutations at codons 469 and 477 and a silent mutation at codon 349 in the C-terminal domain, however, these mutations failed to show any significant functional consequences. They concluded that the mutations of p73 in head and neck tumor are infrequent and p73 may play a minor role in oral carcinogenesis (El-Naggar et al., 2001). This was also supported by another study in that analyses of *p73* gene revealed wild type status and no deletion (Faridoni-Laurens et al., 2001). Nevertheless, in later reports, it was demonstrated that p73 may contribute in head and neck tumorigenesis. Positive staining of p73 proteins was observed in 47% of squamous cell carcinoma of the head and neck whereas only 18% was detected in normal control tissue (Weber et al., 2002). Choi et al. reported an association of p73 expression with distant metastasis of HNSCC (Choi et al., 2002). Moreover, It was demonstrated that p73 expression might be an early event in human oral carcinogenesis since p73 protein levels were significantly elevated in buccal epithelial dysplasia and both protein and mRNA levels were increased in SCC (Chen et al., 2004). Interestingly, p73 expression correlated significantly with cervical lymph node metastasis and patients with epithelial dysplasia with p73 positivity have undergone malignant transformation to squamous cell carcinoma in 2 years (Chen et al., 2004). Taken together, these data suggest that p73 may play some part in the development of head and neck carcinogenesis.

$p21^{Cip1}$ and Oral Carcinogenesis

$p21^{Cip1}$ is the first identified inhibitor of cyclin/cyclin-dependent kinase (CDK) complexes, which regulate transitions between different phases of the cell cycle. $p21^{Cip1}$ appears to be the only inhibitor capable of interacting with essentially all of the CDK complexes. It works as a main downstream effector of the p53 protein, promoting cell cycle arrest in G1 in order to allow for the repair of damaged DNA (el-Deiry et al., 1993; Yeudall and Jakus, 1995; Harada and Ogden, 2000). Several studies reported mutations of $p21^{Cip1}$ gene in human cancers (Bhatia et al., 1995; Gao et al., 1995; Vidal et al., 1995). However, many reports indicated that $p21^{Cip1}$ mutations in human cancer are exceedingly rare (Shiohara et al., 1994; McKenzie et al., 1997). This is in contrast to the aberrations of p53 and $p16^{ink4A}$ in that frequent mutations and deletions of both genes were frequently found in cancers. It has been known that one of the most important functions of $p21^{Cip1}$ is to induce cell cycle arrest; therefore, loss of $p21^{Cip1}$ expression was anticipated as a contribution in carcinogenesis. In oral cancer, loss of $p21^{Cip1}$ was revealed in invasive tumor fronts and such loss was associated with clinicopathological factors of tumor progression and poor prognosis (Goto et al., 2005). Straightforward evidence was from a study that indicated that in patients with OSCC, high $p21^{Cip1}$ expression was associated with increase disease specific survival

(Xie et al., 2002). However, in many cases, $p21^{Cip1}$ expression was concluded to have no prognostic value (Neves Ada et al., 2004). Interestingly, the majority of reports demonstrated that overexpression of $p21^{Cip1}$ was associated with poor outcome and prognosis. $p21^{Cip1}$ was overexpressed in the invasive fronts of lower lip SCC indicating that the presence of $p21^{Cip1}$ is not sufficient to control tumor invasion (Horta et al., 2007). The expression of $p21^{Cip1}$ was associated with tumor size, lymph node involvement, clinical stage and tumor site (Nemes et al., 2005). Furthermore, when $p21^{Cip1}$ was investigated with other proteins such as p53, Ki67 and mdm2, it was found that $p21^{Cip1}$, p53 and Ki67 expression increased with histologic progression (Choi et al., 2003). Combined p53 and $p21^{Cip1}$ positive expression showed a significant association with lymph node metastasis. In survival analysis, tumors with p53/ $p21^{Cip1}$ and $p21^{Cip1}$/p53/mdm2 positivity were associated with poor clinical outcomes (Yanamoto et al., 2002). In summary, it is obvious that $p21^{Cip1}$ not only possesses tumor suppressor activity but also exert oncogenic properties due to the fact that $p21^{Cip1}$ can inhibit apoptosis, inhibit the expression of genes involved in the quality control of mitosis and promote active cyclin-cdk complexes (Roninson, 2002).

$p14^{ARF}$ and Oral Carcinogenesis

The *INK4A/MTS1* tumor suppressor also contains a second "alternative" open reading frame (ARF). It is expressed from a separate promoter and has a unique exon 1β that is then spliced into a different reading frame of exon 2 (Mao et al., 1995; Quelle et al., 1995). The encoded protein, $p14^{ARF}$, is a potent growth suppressor, inhibits mdm2-mediated p53 degradation and has the potential to act as a tumor suppressor (Kamijo et al., 1997; Zhang et al., 1998). Codeletion of *INK4A and ARF* has been demonstrated in a number of tumor types, including those of the head and neck (Sharpless and DePinho, 1999). Concurrent promoter hypermethylation of both genes has been detected and associated with tumor size, lymph node metastasis and stage III/IV advanced OSCC (Ishida et al., 2005). However, in severe oral epithelial dysplasia and in some squamous cell carcinoma cell lines, there is evidence that aberrations of the *INK4A* gene were found to be more frequent than that of *ARF* (Kresty et al., 2002; Piboonniyom et al., 2002).

The TGF-beta Pathway and Oral Carcinogenesis

TGF-beta, a multifunctional growth factor, functions to regulate growth and differentiation of many cell types (Zimmerman and Padgett, 2000). Signaling pathway of TGF-beta in the epithelial cells is very complex. Under normal circumstances, TGF-beta transmits its signal into the cell through the tetrameric cell surface receptors, TGF-beta receptors I and II (Heldin et al., 1997). As a result, the cytoplasmic signaling proteins, Smad2 and Smad3, phosphorylated by the activated TGF-beta receptors I and II, form complexes with Smad4 and translocate into the nucleus, where they function as transcription factors of target genes. Regulation of the TGF-beta signaling transduction pathway is known to be acted by the inhibitory Smad7 (Ito et al., 2001).

The role of TGF-beta in carcinogenesis is rather complex. It is now known that TGF-beta functions as a tumor suppressor early in tumorigenesis when epithelial cell responsiveness to TGF-beta is still relatively normal. Later in the process, paradoxically, TGF-beta becomes to function as an oncogene to promote the progression to aggressive metastatic disease (Moustakas et al., 2002; Prime et al., 2004). It has been shown that the pro-oncogenic functions of TGF-beta are associated with (1) a partial loss of response to the ligand, (2) defects of components of the TGF-beta signal transduction pathway, (3) overexpression and/or activation of the latent complex, (4) epithelial-mesenchymal transition, and (5) recruitment of signaling pathways which act in concert with TGF-beta to facilitate the metastatic phenotype (Prime et al., 2004).

Disruption of the components of TGF-beta signal transduction, namely, the ligand, the receptors, the signal transducers and their transcriptional targets causes a wide variety of human diseases ranging from pulmonary hypertension to malignancies (Attisano and Wrana, 2002). Reduction or loss of TGF-beta receptors and/or downstream signaling molecules, known as Smads, has been observed in various human malignancies including esophageal cancer (Natsugoe et al., 2002), follicular thyroid tumor (West et al., 2000), pancreatic cancer (Schneider and Schmid, 2003), colorectal cancer (Piard et al., 2002) and head and neck cancer (Muro-Cacho et al., 2001). For example, expression of the activated, phosphorylated form of Smad2 (p-Smad2) was found to be lost in approximately 70% of head and neck tumor (Muro-Cacho et al., 2001). A recent investigation revealed a link between a disrupted TGF-beta1-Smad signaling pathway and loss of induction of cell-cycle inhibitory proteins, especially p12cdk2-AP1 in OSCC (Peng et al., 2006). These may lead to the resistance of TGF-beta1 growth-inhibitory effect on OSCC.

Particularly, Smad4, one of the signal transducers in the TGF-beta pathway which acts as a tumor suppressor, has been found to be aberrant in several malignant tumors of the pancreas (Hahn et al., 1996), colorectum (Reinacher-Schick et al., 2004), breast (Pouliot and Labrie, 1999), lung (Nagatake et al., 1996), ovary (Takakura et al., 1999), head and neck (Muro-Cacho et al., 2001; Xie et al., 2003), and esophagus (Natsugoe et al., 2002). Previous studies have shown variable degree of lack of expression of Smad4 in various types of cancer. For example, loss of Smad4 expression has been observed in 23.5-55% of pancreatic adenocarcinoma (Tascilar et al., 2001; Hua et al., 2003), 67.8% of esophageal SCC (Natsugoe et al., 2002), and 22-38.5% of HNSCC (Muro-Cacho et al., 2001; Xie et al., 2003).

Recently, the expression of Smad4 in OSCC has been investigated. It was found that the expression of Smad4 was absent in 40% of OSCC cases compared with only 18% of normal oral mucosa (Figures 6, 7) (Iamaroon et al., 2006). In addition, reduced Smad4 protein levels were clearly shown in all OSCC lines, compared with normal oral keratinocytes by Western blot analysis. These findings indicated that loss of Smad4 expression occurs more frequently in OSCC than in normal oral mucosa and may explain that loss of tumor suppression in the TGF-beta pathway may be involved in carcinogenesis of some OSCC cases.

Activation of Telomerase

Cellular Immortalization

Normal primary cells usually display a restricted replicative life span in cell culture. Almost four decades ago, Hayflick first reported on the *in vitro* growth of human embryonic cells explanted from various tissues. Initially, these cells proliferated for a defined number of generations, but later their mitotic rates were reduced and eventually they underwent replicative senescence (Hayflick, 1968). A maximum of approximately 50 population doublings was achieved with embryonic fibroblasts, whereas cells from differentiated tissue ceased growing after only a few passages. For primary human normal oral keratinocytes, it has been reported that cells cultured from different donors continuously grow until they reach the postmitotic stage at approximately 20-27 population doubling (PD) based on donor age (Kang and Park, 2001). At the end of their life span, most cells displayed the characteristics of terminal differentiation, showing highly enlarged and elongated cytoplasm, and started to round up and detach from the culture dish.

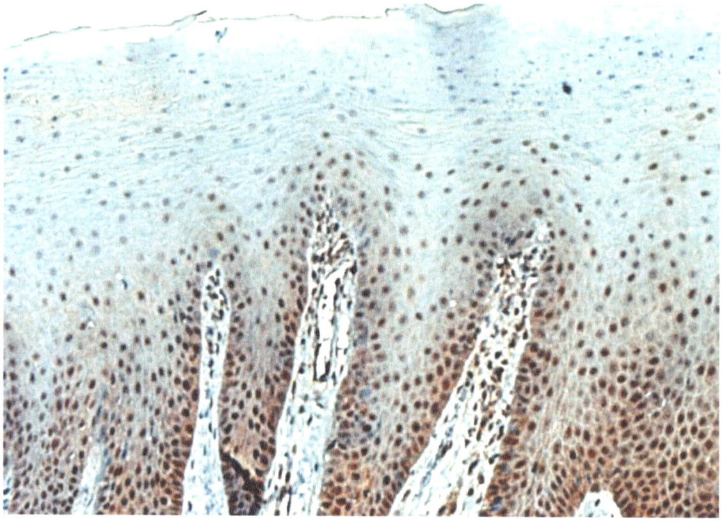

Figure 6. Intense expression of Smad4 in the nuclei of the keratinocytes (brown staining) particularly at the basal and parabasal cell layers (Iamaroon et al., 2006) (Immunohistochemical technique, original magnification, x100).

Genetically determined life span at the single cell level requires two interdependent control systems: one that counts the cell divisions performed and another that irreversibly blocks cell cycle progression. Telomere attrition is responsible for the former while the latter is provided by the action of two main tumor suppressor proteins, p53 and pRB.

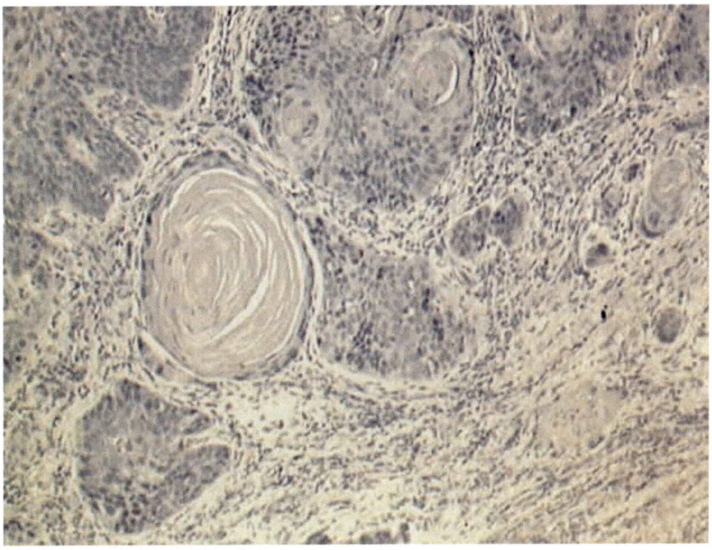

Figure 7. Loss of Smad4 expression in OSCC (Iamaroon et al., 2006) (Immunohistochemical technique, original magnification, x100).

In 1989, Shay and Wright proposed the two-stage model of cellular immortalization (Shay and Wright, 1989; Wright et al., 1989). They stated that aberrant cells must first escape from replicative senescence (M1, mortality stage 1) and enter a period of extended life span. The M1 check point may be regulated by p53, pRb and p16^{ink4A} as well as p21^{Cip1} (Brown et al., 1997; Vaziri et al., 1997). After a finite number of cell doublings during this period, further loss of telomeric sequences and accumulation of chromosome aberrations are observed and eventually, cells encounter an independent second mortality stage (M2), called crisis. During this time, the vast majority of cells will undergo cell death (Guo et al., 1998). Despite the presence of viral oncoproteins that can overcome M1 by inactivating pRB and/or p53, escape from M2 crisis is rare. However, a few surviving cells continue to proliferate beyond crisis and thus, constitute the immortal post-crisis cell population. Analysis of rescued, permanently proliferating cell lines revealed either long or short but stable telomeres (Bryan et al., 1997; Bryan and Cech, 1999) suggesting that retention of telomere length is essential for immortalized cells to by-pass the crisis state.

Telomere Attrition and Telomerase

Eukaryotic chromosomes are capped by hexameric repeat sequences know as telomeres (Allshire et al., 1989). Telomeres are special heterochromatin structures that stabilize and protect chromosomes, prevent fusions and recombination, anchor chromosomes within the nucleus, assist in the replication of linear DNA and also play an important role in chromosome separation during mitosis (Greider, 1996; Kirk et al., 1997).

During DNA replication, DNA polymerase replicates DNA only in the 5'to 3'-direction. Replication is initiated by an 8 to 12-base stretch of RNA hybridized to the template DNA strand. Removal of the terminal RNA primer generates a small gap at the 5' ends of newly replicated strands that cannot be repaired. This phenomenon is called the end-replication problem. Consequently, chromosome ends become shortened and lose at least 50-200 nucleotides during each round of cell division (Kirk et al., 1997). Progressive shortening of the chromosomes in a multi-cellular organism triggers the formation of telomeric fusion between chromosome arms, leading to dicentric chromosomes and chromosomal instability which ultimately signals cell cycle exit resulting in cellular senescence (Allsopp et al., 1995). Telomere shortening is thought to lead to loss of structural integrity of the telemere nucleoprotein, resulting in activation of the p53 and pRb tumor suppressor pathways and cellular senescence (Shay and Wright, 2005).

As previously mentioned, telomere, shortening during cellular replication, limits the replicative life span of most somatic cells. The majority of immortalized and cancer cells that exhibit an unlimited capacity for replication, however, maintain their telomere length through the activation of an enzyme, telomere terminal transferase, or telomerase. This enzyme was first described in ciliated protozoans, *Tetrahymena*, by Greider and Blackburn (1985). Telomerase contains protein and RNA components, both of which are essential for its enzymatic activity which involves adding DNA onto the telomeric region of the chromosome (Morin, 1989; Yu et al., 1990). The RNA component of human telomerase may serve as the template from which telomerase synthesizes the nascent telomeres. Furthermore, the catalytic subunit of telomerase, hTERT, exhibits a reverse transcriptase activity (Morin, 1989; Counter et al., 1997). Most normal human somatic cells have undetectable levels of telomerase activity and do not express hTERT. Since the RNA component of telomerase is present in most cells and tissues, albeit in variable amounts, the expression of hTERT protein may be the major limiting factor for telomerase activity (Kilian et al., 1997; Ulaner et al., 1998). Ectopic expression of hTERT can restore telomerase activity in telomerase-negative cells (Weinrich et al., 1997; Bodnar et al., 1998) and this activity was detected in the vast majority of cancers, including head and neck cancer (Mutirangura et al., 1996).

A strong association exists between high telomerase activity and tumor progression. Detection of telomerase by means of the Telomeric Repeat Amplification Protocol (TRAP) assay or RT-PCR for hTERT expression correlates with the clinical and pathological findings of pre-neoplastic and malignant lesions (Tahara et al., 1995). In a study with proliferative breast lesions, less than 60% of *in situ* carcinomas were telomerase-positive but this percentage increased to 90% in infiltrating breast carcinomas suggesting that reactivation of telomerase is an early event in malignant development (Poremba et al., 1998).

Although there is an association between activated telomerase and cancers, there are some exceptions as a few normal cells, such as germ line cells, activated lymphocytes, and basal cells of stratified epithelium, possess telomerase activity (Hiyama et al., 1995; Yasumoto et al., 1996). Moreover, about 20% of advanced carcinomas lack telomerase activity (Kim et al., 1994; Bryan and Cech, 1999). The observation that some types of tumors retained their telomere length without activation of telomerase led to the hypothesis of alternative telomere lengthening (ALT) which postulates that telomere length can be maintained by a recombination mechanism (Bryan et al., 1997).

Telomerase and Oral Carcinogenesis

It has been reported that expression of the catalytic component of telomerase, hTERT, alone significantly extended the life span of human fibroblasts but was not sufficient to immortalize human epithelial cells (Bodnar et al., 1998). However, inactivation of the pRB/p16 pathway by E7 or downregulation of $p16^{ink4A}$ expression, in combination with telomerase activity leads to efficient immortalization of these cells (Piboonniyom et al., 2003). Therefore, in epithelial cells, two types of aberrations, namely, inactivation of the pRB pathway and enhanced telomerase activity must occur to induce immortalization. We also demonstrated that co-expression of hTERT with HPVE7 and cdk4 induced immortalization in normal oral keratinocytes (NOKs). Induction of hTERT alone into the NOKs also induced immortalization but the $p16^{ink4A}$ protein was found to be down-regulated in the late passages of the immortalized clone. PCR analysis showed no evidence for gross deletions of *INK4A* gene and re-introduction of $p16^{ink4A}$ causes cellular senescence as judged by morphological alterations and expression of senescence-associated β-galactosidase activity suggesting that loss of $p16^{ink4A}$ expression in the hTERT-expressing NOKs may have contributed importantly to inactivation of the pRB pathway during oral cellular immortalization (Piboonniyom et al., 2003).

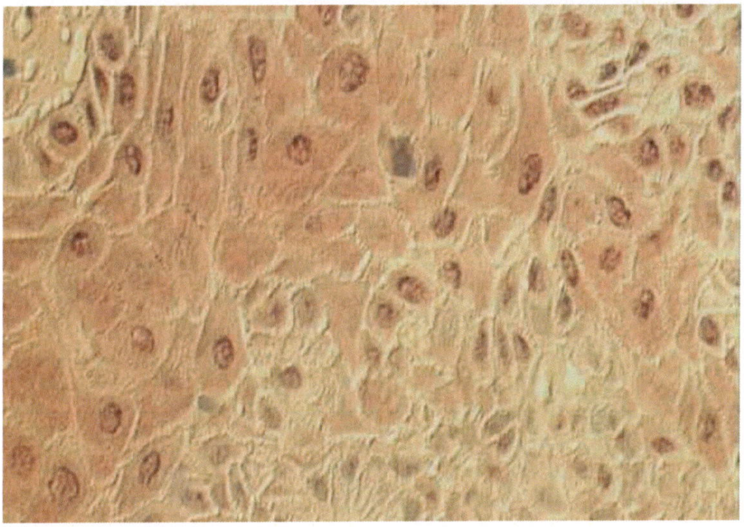

Figure 8. hTERT protein is overexpressed in OSCC (red staining) (Pattamapun and Iamaroon, 2004) (Immunohistochemical technique, original magnification, x400).

It was reported that about 80-90% of squamous cell carcinomas of the head and neck including OSCC were positive for telomerase activity (Kannan et al., 1997). Consistently, we analyzed the expression of hTERT protein in OSCC by immunohistochemical technique and found that 80% of OSCC were positive for hTERT (Figure 8) (Pattamapun and Iamaroon, 2004). This indicates that telomerase plays a central role in telomere maintenance in OSCC. In an investigation using tissue microarray, increased hTERT protein expression was more frequently found in OSCC than in pharyngeal and laryngeal squamous cell carcinimas (PSCC/LSCC). On the contrary, *hTERT* amplifications were less common in OSCC compared with PSCC/LSCC (Freier et al., 2007). The proliferation marker, Ki-67 was also revealed to be significantly higher in OSCC with a high telomerase activity than in those with a low or negative telomerase activity (Liao et al., 2000). There are many reports on telomerase activity and its components as potential clinical diagnostic and prognostic markers in different tumors (Saleh et al., 2007). Using a TRAP assay, telomerase activity has been detected in solid tumors and premalignant lesions, including OSCC (Mutirangura et al., 1996). Although TRAP assay alone may not suffice to detect telomerase activity in some clinical materials, since many factors can interfere with the detection, oral cancer material such as oral rinses may be used in the detection of recurrences and formation of second primary tumors before the symptoms menifest clinically (Mutirangura et al., 1996). An extensive review of telomerase activity and components in tissue samples from patients with different stages of oral cancer has been documented (Sebastian et al., 2005). Although there is no conclusion that telomerase activity correlates with tumor dependent survival or the recurrence of the tumor, recent investigations analyzing telomerase acitivty in primary cancer and lymph node metastasis have shown that in oral cancer, there are more lymph node metastases in telomerase positive cases than in telomerase-negative cases (Koscielny et al., 2004; Liao et al., 2004). There were also only few reports on the correlation of telomerase activity and other tumor marker in oral carcinogenesis, therefore, further investigations on this area should still be of interest.

Tumor Angiogenesis

Angiogenesis or neovascularization is a process for the growth of new blood vessels from pre-existing ones. Physiologically, angiogenesis is found during growth and development, wound healing, and reproduction. Pathologically, angiogenesis plays a critical role in a variety of diseases including solid tumors, psoriasis, rheumatoid arthritis, diabetic retinopathy, and hemangiomas (Hasina and Lingen, 2001; Rundhaug, 2005). It is well accepted that tumor growth is angiogenesis-dependent as emphasized by Folkman and Klagsbrun that every increment of tumor growth requires an increment of vascular growth (Folkman and Klagsbrun, 1987). In the absence of blood supply, a solid tumor can only grow into a mass of approximately 2 mm^3 (Lodish et al., 2000). Once the tumor size increases beyond these critical volumes, oxygen and nutrients have difficulty diffusing into the tumor cells in the center, causing a state of cellular hypoxia. These lead to a "switch-on" of tumor angiogenesis, i.e., the secretion of proangiogenic factors from the tumor cells that can stimulate proliferation of endothelial cells. Endothelial cells, in turns, also produce growth factors and cytokines that stimulate proliferation of tumor cells. Thus, the mechanism of these cellular activations is paracrine, reciprocal and bi-directional. Angiogenesis is a complex process and requires several discrete steps including 1) degradation of the basement membrane surrounding a nearby capillary, 2) migration of endothelial cells lining the capillary into the tumor, 3) division of these endothelial cells, and 4) formation of a new basement membrane around the newly elongated capillary (Lodish et al., 2000).

As the body of knowledge of tumor angiogenesis gained more and more interests, numerous activators involved in angiogenesis have been discovered. These include growth factors, matrix metalloproteinases, oncoproteins, cytokines, endogenous modulators and copper (Table 1) (Rundhaug, 2005). Under normal circumstances, angiogenesis is tightly regulated by several inhibitors including angiopoietin-2, angiostatin, endostatin, vasculostatin, tissue inhibitors of metalloproteinase (TIMPs), and thrombospondin. It could be concluded that angiogenesis occurs as a result of a complex balance of several activators and inhibitors. One then can imagine that the imbalance of the proangiogenic and antiangiogenic factors will lead to a state of human disease.

Table 1. Angiogenic activators and their examples

Angiogenic activators	Examples
Growth factors	Vascular endothelial growth factor (VEGF)
	Acidic and basic fibroblast growth factors (aFGF, bFGF)
	Hepatocyte growth factor (HGF)/scatter factor
	Platelet-derived growth factor (PDGF)
	Angiogenin
	Angiotropin
	Tumor necrosis factor-alpha (TNF-alpha)
Matrix metalloproteinases (MMPs)	Gelatinase A
	Gelatinase B
	Stromelysin
Oncoproteins	c-Myc
	Ras
	c-jun
Cytokines	Interleukin-1 (IL-1)
	IL-6
	IL-8
Endogenous modulators	Alpha(v)beta(3) integrin
	Angiopoietin-1
	Erythropoietin
	Hypoxia
	Nitric oxide synthase
	Prostaglandin E

Angiogenesis and Oral Cancer

Angiogenesis is a key event for growth, invasion and metastasis of OSCC. Previous investigations have shown a significant increase in vascularity during the transition from normal oral mucosa, through hyperkeratosis, differing degrees of dysplasia, to invasive OSCC (Figure 9) (Iamaroon et al., 2003; Johnstone and Logan, 2006). Moreover, a close association between tumor angiogenesis and tumor progression to late stages of OSCC has also been reported (Ascani et al., 2005; Li et al., 2005). A variety of factors have been found to be associated with angiogenesis in OSCC. Particularly, VEGF, a potent proangiogenic factor, acts to induce endothelial proliferation, migration, and specialization in new and developing vascular beds (Johnstone and Logan, 2006). Increased levels of VEGF protein expression have been found in OSCC (Moriyama et al., 1997; Eisma et al., 1999; Bancroft et al., 2001). In a study of 77 patients with oral or oropharyngeal SCC, 41% of these cases were found to be positive for VEGF expression (Smith et al., 2000). In another study of 38 patients with early oral cancer, the tumor-free survival rate of patients with VEGF-positive tumors was significantly poorer than in those with VEGF-negative tumors suggesting that VEGF positivity appeared to be a significant predictor of poor prognosis (Kim et al., 2006). Furthermore, VEGF expression was significantly related with tumor invasion depth. A recent study demonstrated that hypoxia in OSCC was partly responsible for the up-regulation of VEGF and VEGF positivity was correlated with regional lymph node involvement and clinical stage (Shang et al., 2006). Higher expression of VEGF as well as endoglin (CD105) in the tumor bed implicates a more aggressive potential for T1 and T2 tongue cancers, and the expression of CD105 is found to be a useful predictive prognostic factor in early tongue cancer (Chuang et al., 2006). Recently, it has been studied that VEGF-C, a lymphangiogenic growth factor, plays a crucial role in the invasion and metastasis of the cancer cells. In OSCC, high expression of VEGF-C was frequently observed and associated with increased number of lymph vessels and lymphatic invasion (Siriwardena et al., 2007). However, in contrast to the above data, it was shown that there were no significant differences in the staining intensity in the primary OSCC, resection margins, or nodes between cases in which the nodes were involved and in which they were not involved (El-Gazzar et al., 2006). Moreover, there was no correlation between vascularity and VEGF staining. These contradictory data suggest that VEGF may not be the only primary stimulator of angiogenesis in OSCC.

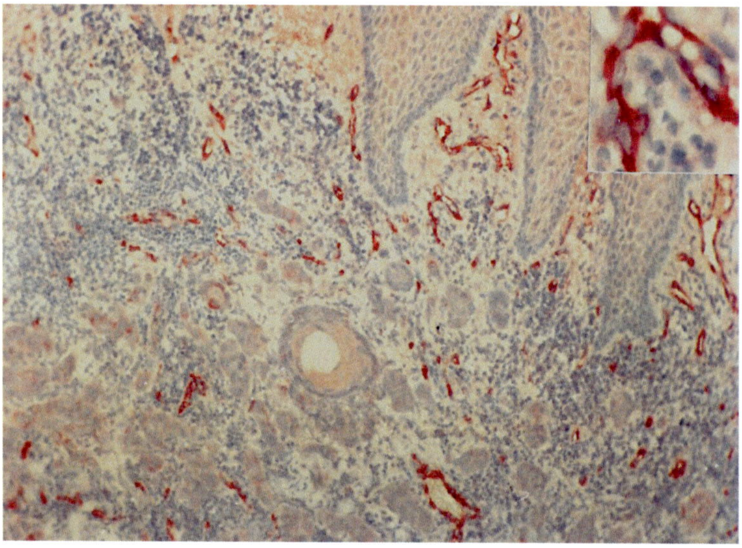

Figure 9. Increased vascularity, stained with anti-von Willebrand factor antibody, is observed in invasive OSCC. High magnification of a capillary is shown in the inset (Modified from Iamaroon et al, 2003) (Immunohistochemical technique, original magnification, x100 and x400).

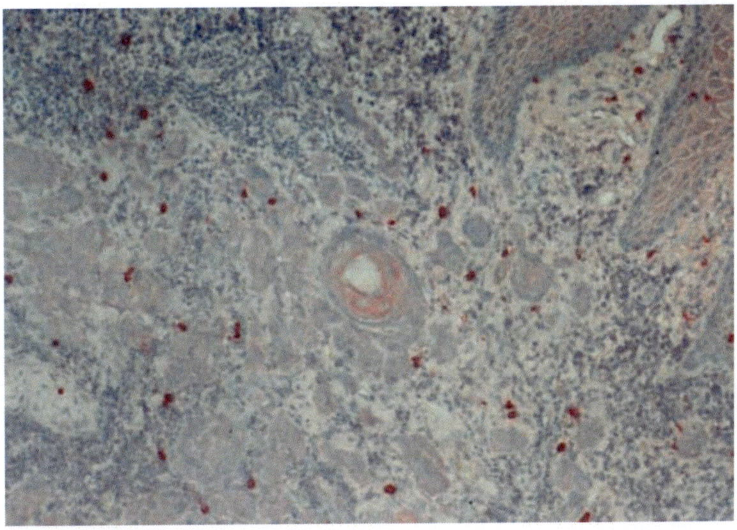

Figure 10. An increase in mast cells, labelled with anti-tryptase antibody (red staining), is shown in invasive OSCC (Modified from Iamaroon et al., 2003) (Immunohistochemical technique, original magnification, x100).

A number of studies have indicated that IL-8 is also a major proangiogenic factor in a variety of malignancies including OSCC (Cohen et al., 1995; Eisma et al., 1999; Bancroft et al., 2001; Lalla et al., 2001). Upregulation of IL-8 was found to be regulated by fibrin present in association with tumor cells in OSCC (Lalla et al., 2001). Coexpression of IL-8 and VEGF was shown to be involved with MEK-MAPK and IKK-NF-kappaB signaling pathways (Eisma et al., 1999; Bancroft et al., 2001). The number of mast cells that expressed tryptase, another proangiogenic factor, was also found to be correlated with microvessel density in OSCC, suggesting a role of tryptase in angiogenesis in OSCC (Figure 10) (Iamaroon et al., 2003).

Angiogenesis is not only important for tumor growth, but also for tumor invasion and metastasis. Various matrix proteases, mentioned above, have been found to be involved in endothelial cell migration and tubule formation as well as tumor cell migration and spreading. Details will be described in the following topics.

Tumor Invasion and Metastasis

Invasion and metastasis are important phenotypes of malignant tumors. The cascade of metastasis can be divided into two phases: (1) invasion of the extracellular matrix (ECM) and (2) vascular dissemination and homing of the tumor cells (Cotran et al., 1999).

The sequential steps of invasion of ECM include detachment of the tumor cells from each other, attachment to matrix components, degradation of ECM, and migration of tumor cells into the underlying tissue. Three classes of proteases involved in tumor invasion have been identified. These include the serine and cysteine proteinases and MMPs. MMP-2 or gelatinase B, a 72-kD type IV collagenase, plays an important role in tumor invasion since it can degrade native type IV collagen resided in epithelial and vascular basement membranes

(Hayashi et al., 1997). Besides this 72-kD type IV collagenase, cathepsin D (a cysteine proteinase) and urokinase-type plasminogen activator (u-PA, a serine proteinase) also help in degrading several ECM molecules including fibronectin, laminin, and protein cores of proteoglycans.

Once tumor cells are circulated in the blood or lymphatic vessels, they tend to aggregate and adhere with platelets. Formation of platelet-tumor aggregates appears to enhance tumor cell survival and implantability (Tuszynski et al., 1997). Formation of secondary deposit of tumors cells is initiated by adhesion of tumors to the endothelium, followed by extravasation of tumor cells through the basement membrane. Molecules involved in these processes include adhesion molecules for example integrins, CD44 and some other proteolytic enzymes, mentioned above. It is generally accepted that fewer than 1 in 10,000 tumor cells, that escape the primary tumor, can survive to colonize another tissue and form a secondary, metastatic tumor (Lodish et al., 2000).

Several MMPs have been involved in tumor progression of OSCC. These MMPs include MMP-2 (Gao et al., 2005; Zhang et al., 2006), MMP-8 (Liu et al., 2007), MMP-9 (Kosunen et al., 2007), MMP-13 (Chiang et al., 2006), membrane type I-MMP (MT1-MMP) (Myoung et al., 2002), and newly identified MMP-28 (Lin et al., 2006). MMP activation, particularly MMP-2 and MMP-9, observed in different cancers, has been shown to be mediated via the transcription factor NF-kappa B. Recent data suggested a regulatory role of NF-kappa B on the activation of MMP-2 and MMP-9 during malignant transformation in the oral mucosa (Bindhu et al., 2006). Previous studies of correlation between MMPs and tumor progression of OSCC have extensively been conducted. The results from a number of studies showed that the expression of some MMPs was correlated with tumor invasion and metastasis. For example, a study of zymographic measurement of the MMP-2 and MMP-9 activities in OSCC specimens revealed that patients with tumors with elevated activity of MMP-2 and MMP-9 had shorter disease-free survival after treatment than patients with tumors exhibiting low MMP activities (Yorioka et al., 2002). Moreover, another study showed that the expression of MMP-2 was found in all cases of OSCC and the expression of MMP-2 at the invasive front was significantly higher than that of MMP-2 at the tumor center. In addition, the expression of MMP2 was found to be related to neck lymph node metastasis (Liu et al., 2004). The expression of MMP-2 and TIMP-2 was related to the differentiation degree of tumor cells, metastatic lymph node status, and stage of OSCC (Gao et al., 2005). The expression of MMP-9 was significantly associated with the differentiation degree of tumor cells and the T stage (de Vicente et al., 2005). Using different methods including immunohistochemistry and film *in situ* zymography as well as conventional zymography to evaluate the expression and gelatinolytic activity of MMP-2 and MMP-9 in freshly frozen OSCC, it was demonstrated that both proforms and activated forms of MMP-2 and MMP-9 were present, and that the activated MMP-2 could be a main enzymatic activity of gelatinolysis (Kato et al., 2005). In addition, interaction of tumor cells and stromal cells seems to play an important role in the invasion and metastasis of OSCC. We have recently investigated the expression of MMP-9 at the invasive front of OSCC by immunohistochemical technique and found that both the malignant epithelial and the stromal cells strongly expressed MMP-9 (Figure 11) (Iamaroon and Krisanaprakornkit, unpublished data). Besides MMP-2 and MMP-9, a marked overexpression of MMP-1, MMP-3, and MT1-

MMP was frequently observed in both invasive and metastatic OSCC cases (Kurahara et al., 1999). The regulation of MMP-8 by betel quid and its effect on OSCC cell migration was analyzed showing that betel quid may accelerate tumor migration by stimulating MMP-8 expression through MEK pathway (Liu et al., 2007). MMP-13 was also found to be overexpressed in OSCC as well as esophageal SCC (Chiang et al., 2006). A study on MMP-28, a newly identified MMP, showed a close correlation between MMP-28 and OSCC and supported the role of MMP-28 in the anchorage-independent growth of OSCC (Lin et al., 2006).

IL-8 is not only important for angiogenesis, but also for tumor invasion and metastasis of OSCC. A study on the role of IL-8 and MMPs for tumorigenesis and metastasis revealed that IL-8 secreted from OSCC may contribute to the invasion of OSCC through the regulation of MMP-7 expression (Watanabe et al., 2002). In addition, IL-6, HGF, and TNF-α can stimulate oral cancer cells to enhanced the secretion of MMP-1 and MMP-9, proteases necessary for tumor invasion and metastasis (Sundelin et al., 2005). A role of claudin-1, a component of tight junctions, for the regulation of invasion activity in OSCC cells was explored. The results suggested that claudin-1 upregulated cancer cell invasion activity through activation of MT1-MMP and MMP-2 leading to an enhanced cleavage of gamma2-chain of laminin-5 (lam-gamma2) (Oku et al., 2006). In a study of the expression of plasminogen activator inhibitor-1 (PAI-1), urokinase receptor (uPAR), and lam-gamma2 in 20 cases of OSCC, PAI-1 was discovered to be a novel potential marker of initial invasion in OSCC, and that the coordinated expression of PAI-1 with uPAR and lam-gamma2 sustained the features of the early invasive cancer cells (Lindberg et al., 2006).

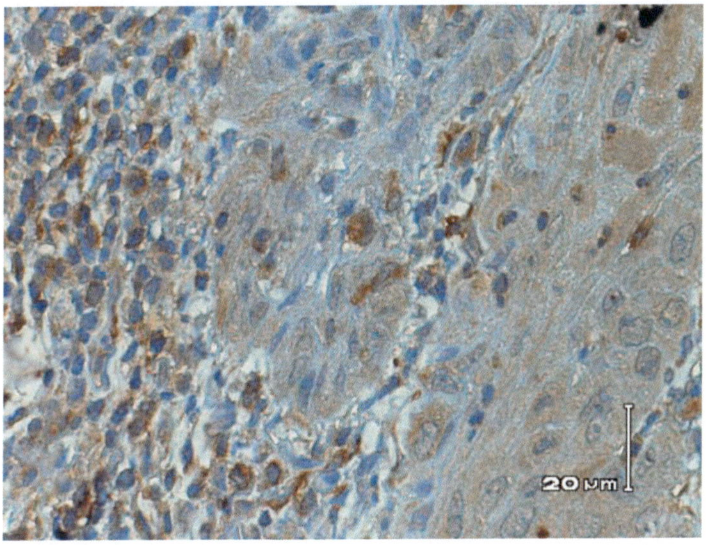

Figure 11. The expression of MMP-9 (brown staining) is demonstrated in the cytoplasm of both malignant epithelial and stromal cells at the invasive front of OSCC (Iamaroon and Krisanaprakornkit, unpublished data) (Immunohistochemical technique, original magnification, x400).

Recent data have shown that the tumor progression of OSCC is associated with a reorganization of ECM especially laminin-5. Increased expression of laminin-5 was found in the areas of direct tumor/stromal interactions (Franz et al., 2007). Stromal laminin-5 deposits revealed a spatial association with TGF-beta1, MT1-MMP, and bone morphogenetic protein-1 (BMP-1). In addition, not only carcinoma cells but also mesenchymal cells were shown to express lam-gamma2 mRNA. Thus, mesenchymal cells also contribute to tumor migration by providing and organizing promigratory lam-gamma2 in the invasive front of OSCC.

Besides MMPs and other proteases, several other molecules have been found to facilitate tumor invasion and metastasis. CD10, in particular, is present in a variety of malignant neoplasms including OSCC. CD10 expression in stromal cells of OSCC appeared to play an important role in tumor invasion, probably facilitating the occurrence of metastases (Piattelli et al., 2006). In addition, OSCC with CD10 positivity was an indicator of worse prognosis.

The relationship between the expression of bFGF and FGFR-1 in cancer cells and fibroblasts at the invasive front of OSCC, and the pathologic and clinical characteristics were also evaluated (Hase et al., 2006). The expression of bFGF and FGFR-1 in cancer cells were observed in all cases, whereas, detection of these molecules was observed in fibroblasts in only 67% of the cases. The expression of bFGF and FGFR-1 in fibroblasts at the invasive front appeared to link to the mode of invasion and prognosis in OSCC. FGFR-2 and FGFR-3 seemed to play an important role in the initial stages of oral cancer progression since a significant elevation of both FGFR-2 and FGFR-3 was observed during the stages of dysplasia and early invasion, while at the later stages, the expression of FGFR-2 and FGFR-3 was decreased (Vairaktaris et al., 2006).

Integrins, cell surface receptors for adhesive glycoproteins, are found on most cells where they mediate cell adhesion through cell-ECM interations. The alpha(v)beta(6) integrin, in particular, is epithelial-specific and binds to fibronectin, vitronectin, tenascin, and the latency associated peptide of TGF-beta (Thomas et al., 2006). It is known that alpha(v)beta(6) integrins are not expressed constitutively by normal keratinocytes but is up-regulated during wound healing and oral carcinogenesis. Interestingly, alpha(v)beta(6) integrins have been shown to modulate tumor invasion, inhibit apoptosis, regulate protease expression, and activate TGF-beta1. Alpha(v)beta(6) integrins up-regulate MMP-3 and MMP-9 expression in OSCC cells but down-regulate MMP-13 expression at both mRNA and protein levels (Ylipalosaari et al., 2005).

In summary, invasion and metastasis are crutial phenomenons in oral carcinogenesis. The process of tumor cell invasion is complex. Several factors are implicated in these mechanisms and the potential to inhibit or interfere with any or all of these processes may provide the basis of new treatments for oral cancer growth, invasion and metastasis.

Molecular Markers

The progression from premalignant to malignant lesions is usually accompanied by the accumulation of genetic alterations leading to altered expression patterns and modifications in protein structure and function. Changes that occur solely or more commonly in cancer cells compared with their corresponding normal tissue can be detected by biopsy or in body fluids, and used as molecular markers for cancer. Moreover, since the ability to predict the malignant potential of the premalignant lesions based on pathological findings is very limited, molocular marker representing molecular alterations may be promising in improving the ability to determine the true cancer risk of these lesions. Molecular markers are expected to become essential in the diagnosis and management of patients with oral cancer. They will guide future study and clinical care and will finally lead to new intervention directed at the molecular changes of cancer. Use of molecular markers allows earlier diagnosis and staging of tissue change, before changes in cell morphology occur and before changes become clinically visible. Some examples of molecular marker which are now being used in the clinical practice include prostate-specific antigen (PSA) for prostate cancer and carcinoembryonic antigen (CEA) for colorectal cancer. However, the reliability of these markers is still in question since the elevation of these proteins does not necessary correlate with clinical manifestation (Kalish and McKinlay, 1999). There are only a few molecular markers that are available at present for determining treatment response. In breast cancer, the cancer cells may overexpress high levels of the tyrosine receptor kinase ErbB2 (Her2/neu) and are more likely to respond to trastuzumab, an antibody that targets receptor tyrosine kinase (Pietras et al., 1995).

Three main types of molecules can be used as molecular markers, namely DNA, RNA and protein. DNA is a very stable molecule and can be used in the detection from tumors and body fluids. The earlier genetic analyses were initially carried out on biopsy samples, but the discovery of free DNA in plasma created an area in screening for cancer (Sidransky, 2002). Moreover, other body fluids such as saliva, urine and stools can also be used in the detection of DNA as tumor markers. There are many techniques for DNA analysis. Loss of heterozygosity (LOH) and microsatellite instability are common techniques utilized. Usually, all cells are composed of two copies of autosomal genes, one from the mother and the other from the father. An LOH in a cell represents the loss of one parent's contribution to part of the cell's genome. It often indicates the presence of tumor suppressor gene in the lost region. Often, the remaining copy of the tumor suppressor gene had been inactivated by a point mutation. If a cell develops a mutation in one allele of a tumor suppressor gene, loss of the remaining wild type allele can initiate tumorigenesis. LOH is a hallmark of cancer and can be examined by various PCR-based approaches.

LOH on many chromosomes, in particular, chromosomes 3, 9, 11 and 17 was reported in head and neck cancer (Scully et al., 2000). LOH has been seen at 3p14 and at 9p in severely dysplastic lesions and carcinoma in situ (van der Riet et al., 1994; Mao et al., 1996; Lydiatt et al., 1998). LOH has been identified at 3p in 52% of oral carcinomas (Maestro et al., 1993). In HNSCC, LOH at this region was identified to be strongly associated with the prognosis and correlated with nodal metastases (Field et al., 1995). Several tumor suppressor genes in these 3p regions have been proposed to be involved in oral carcinogenesis. These include the fragile histidine triad (FHIT), retinoic acid receptor-β (RAR-β), aminoacylase1 (ACY1), Acylpeptidase hydrolase (APEH), and protein tyrosine phosphatase gamma (PTP-γ) (Scully et al., 2000). LOH on several regions of 9P was reported, however, most studies revealed that the *INK4A* gene which encodes $p16^{ink4A}$ plays a significant role in oral carcinogenesis. This locus also encodes another protein, the $p14^{ARF}$. The $p16^{ink4A}$, as stated earlier, plays a major role in controlling the pRB pathway and the $p14^{ARF}$ mediates the control of the p53 pathway. The *p53* gene situates on chromosome 17p13 and LOH of this region has been discovered in 50-55% in HNSCC (Nawroz et al., 1994; Califano et al., 1996; Huang et al., 1999). LOH at

11q has also been reported in over 60% HNSCC (Ah-See et al., 1994), 50% of oral cancers (Califano et al., 1996; Uzawa et al., 1996) and rearrangements at this region have also been described (Zaslav et al., 1991).

Microsatellite DNA markers are also used as a tool to detect LOH in primary cancer. Because cancer cells are generally unstable, microsatellite are often expanded or deleted in cancer cells. This characteristic, namely microsatellite instability, is another valuable clonal marker of cancer (Mao et al., 1994). Analysis of a panel of 23 microsatellite markers detected microsatellite instability in exfoliated oral mucosal cells. LOH or microsatellite instability of at least one marker was detected in 86% of primary tumors, and identical alterations were found in the saliva samples in 79% of cases (Spafford et al., 2001). In another study, 29% of HNSCC patients were found to have one or more microsatellite alteration(s) in serum that precisely matched that in the primary tumors (Nawroz et al., 1996). This indicates that LOH and microsatellite instability can be used as molecular markers. In addition, serum and exfoliated cell from the oral cavity can also be used as sources for molecular marker analyses.

Another encouraging type of marker is based on detecting hypermethylation of promoter regions of cancer-associated genes. Many types of cancer cells, including oral cancer, have been shown to use this mechanism to inactivate tumor suppressor genes. To detect hypermethylation in a specific promoter region, the DNA is usually treated with bisulphite, which converts unmethylated cytosine to uracil. If the cytosine is methylated, then it is protected and not converted. Then 2 sets of primers, one of which is specific for unmethylated DNA and the other for methylated DNA will be used for PCR analysis. This approach has been used to detect cancer cells in the saliva of patients with oral cancer (Rosas et al., 2001). In our report, we analyzed a region of the *INK4A* promoter that contains CpG islands that are targets for DNA methylation which may lead to the decreased expression of the *INK4A* gene. The results showed that some OSCC cell lines contained unmethylated promoter sequences while in one cell line, *INK4A* promoter methylation was detected. These results correlate well with the protein expression in each cell line in that the ones without promoter methylation expressed high levels of $p16^{ink4A}$ whereas, lack of $p16^{ink4A}$ protein expression was denoted in a cell line with hypermethylation (Piboonniyom et al., 2002).

The method of laser capture microdissection (LCM) has made the study of cancer biology more precise since this procedure enables only cancer cell population to be procured from human tissue sections (Emmert-Buck et al., 1996; Patel et al., 2001). Using this approach, one can now successfully use DNA extracted from microdissected tissue to identify LOH, mutational changes, etc. Combine this technology with array technology, enormous numbers of genes including unknown genes associated with oral cancer can be identified. The ability to investigate from 1000 up to 40,000 genes simultaneously using microarray technology has significantly changed our approach to the analysis of expression profiles. Microarray technology also permits the assessment of clusters of genes that are coordinately expressed to generate fingerprints of biologic states. One way to use microarray is to compare tumor and normal tissues. The basic principle underlying microarray technology is that complementary nucleic acids will hybridize. Hybridization provides exquisite selectivity of complementary stranded nucleic acids, with high sensitivity and specificity. In the traditional techniques in which radioactive labeling materials are usually utilized, the simultaneous hybridization of test and reference samples is impossible. In microarray-based technology, the solid surface contains hundreds to thousands of immobilized DNA spots which can be simultaneously hybridized with two samples labeled with different color of fluorescent dyes. After hybridization, the fluorescent signals of two probes bind to individual spots and can be detected with a confocal laser scanner. The separately scanned images from each of the two probes are then combined, and then the expression ratios of two probes are calculated. Based on these systematic procedures, microarray makes possible large-scale gene expression montoring in a parallel fashion (Iida and Nishimura, 2002).

Regarding the materials used, there are 2 main types of microarray, namely the glass slide microarray and the fitter or membrane array. Microarrays can also be separated into 2 different formats depending on the target nucleic acid components, which are the oligonucleotide array and the cDNA microarray. The oligonucleotide array consists of less than 25 bp in length oligonucleotide (Shoemaker et al., 1996; Lipshutz et al., 1999). In contrast, the cDNA microarray is fabricated by the printing of cloned and amplified cDNA onto the solid surface. Since cDNA microarray possesses longer nucleotide sequences, the specificity in the detection is higher.

To investigate gene expression profiles at different stages of tumor progression in HNSCC, a combination of LCM and cDNA array was utilized by cDNA membrane arrays from Clontech (BD Biosiences, Palo Alto, CA, USA). When compared to normal tissues, a consistent decrease in expression of differentiation markers such as cytokeratins, and an increase in the expression of a number of signal transduction and cell cycle regulatory molecules, as well as growth and angiogenic factors and tissue degrading proteases were demonstrated (Leethanakul et al., 2000). Unexpectedly, genes involved in the wnt (wingless) and notch signaling pathway were found to be highly represented in tumor tissue. Thus, these findings support an unexpected role for the wnt and notch signaling system in squamous cell carcinogenesis.

Another study using LCM was conducted on isolated paired normal and malignant epithelium from five snap frozen biopsy specimens taken from patients with head and neck and oral cancer (Alevizos et al., 2001). Using microarrays from Affymetrix (Santa Clara, CA, USA), it was revealed that among the 404 probe sets, 211 were up-regulated and 193 were down-regulated in the tumor tissues. Many genes in the metastatic and invasion pathways, oncogenes and tumor suppressor gene and differentiation markers were found to be altered. Interestingly, genes which were down-regulated were important enzymes in the xenobiotic metabolic pathway including COX vb, GST-II, ADH7, COX C VIII, ALDH8, EPH2 and ALDH10 implicated that the control of metabolic pathway is important in oral carcinogenesis.

To investigate different expression of genes in normal, premalignant and malignant lesions of oropharynx and oral tissues, oligonucleotide arrays representing approximately 7000 human genes were analysed (Mendez et al., 2002). Unsupervised hierarchical clustering analysis showed that oral carcinoma samples were grouped into one cluster, whereas the normal control samples were clustered separately, indicating that OSCC can be easily distinguished from normal tissue based on their expression signatures. Many up-regulated genes in the OSCC were up-regulated in the premalignant lesions. However, the pattern of down-regulated group of genes in the premalignant lesions was similar to that of normal tissues. Interestingly, OSCC tumors of the same clinical stage and grade revealed discrepancies in their gene expression profiles, suggesting that the grading system may not be used for the prognosis of the tumors.

Typically, 50% of patients with OSCC have detectable lymph node involvement at presentation. Only 25-40% of patients with lymph node metastasis at presentation will achieve 5-year survival, compared to approximately 90% of patients without metastasis (Greenberg et al., 2003). An expression profile for diagnosis of lymph node metastases from primary HNSCC was investigated using DNA microarray (Roepman et al., 2005). The predictor, established with an 82-tumor training set, outperforms current clinical diagnosis when independently validated. Many of the predictor genes, for example, *COL5A1*, *COL5A3*, *NCOR2*, *PLAU* and *SPOCK* have previously been implicated in metastasis. Interestingly, more than half of the predictor genes have not been directly associated with tumorigenesis or metastasis before. Additionally, other genes encoding extracellular matrix components, genes involved in cell adhesion, cell death genes, cell growth and maintenance genes and genes encoding hydrolyzing activities were also found to be predictive genes for lymph node metastasis.

During the past decade, the emphasis in oncology has been focused on the incorporation of genomics tool into oncology research. The National Cancer Institute (NCI) has also started the Cancer Genome Anatomy Project (CGAP) and the head and neck CGAP was established as a cooperative effort between the National Institute of Dental and Craniofacial Research (NIDCR) and the NCI CGAP. The CGAP has identified 1445 genes, of which 195 have only been identified in oral cancer or adjacent normal oral tissue (Shillitoe et al., 2000). By combining the results of all approaches including CGAP, microarray technology, laser capture microdissection and the general literature, a total of 1891 genes have been associated with oral cancer (Levine and Steffen, 2001). Future trend in oral cancer research based on the high-troughput techniques, such as microarray, will provide important clues to the understanding of the various gene networks contributed in oral carcinogenesis and will guide researcher to find target genes for possible efficient therapy.

Although genomics has been the recent trend, attention has turned to proteomics for the next wave of innovation. This approach is important, because although certain genes have been transcribed, many proteins are not present and post-translational protein modifications cannot be detected from genomic information. Traditionally, proteomic approaches have involved analysis of two-dimentional gels that separate proteins on the basis of size and charge which will be then subjected to mass spectrometry for protein identification. Recently, investigators compared the proteomic profile of cancer cells with normal cells, and identify unique proteins in the serum of patients with prostate and ovarian cancers (Bichsel et al., 2001; Paweletz et al., 2001). LCM, protein biochips, and isotope-coded affinity tag peptide (ICAT) labeling are among the technologies that are currently having an important impact on cancer research (Jain, 2002). Nowadays, electrospray (ESI), matrix-assisted laser desorption/ionization time-of-flight mass spectrometry (MALDI-TOF MS) and a new protein analysis system, based on the surface enhanced laser desorption/ionization (SELDI) has been recently applied for the separation, detection, and analysis of multiple protiens in very small amount of cancer tissues (Kolch et al., 2005).

Proteomic analyses of oral cancer cells and tissue have emerged. To identify tumor-associated proteins as biomarkers, a two-dimentional polyacrylamide gel electrophorysis and MALDI-TOF MS were utilized. Comparison of the portein expression profiles of OSCC cell lines and normal oral keratinocytes identified six proteins with markedly different expression levels. Down-regulation of 1D-myo-inositol 1,4,5-triphosphate 3-kinase A (ITPKA), a protien important in cellular signalling, was significantly revealed. Western blot analysis and real-time quantitative reverse transcriptase-polymerase chain reaction also showed relavant data to that of proteomics (Kato et al., 2006). In another study, comparing proteomic profiling between human oral normal keratinocytes (HNOKs) and OSCC-derived cell lines (HSC-2 and HSC-3) using fluorescent two-dimentional difference in-gel electrophorysis, 22 proteins were identified as differentially expressed between the HNOKs and OSCC cells. Nine proteins were up-regulated and 13 were down-regulated. Some of the examples of the proteins which could be potentially used as markers included the cancer-related proteins; annexin A1, heat shock protein 27, lamin A/C, interleukin 1 receptor antagonist, serine proteinase inhibitor clade B5, stathmin 1, and superoxide dismutase 2 (Koike et al., 2005). Proteomics and real-time quantitative RT-PCR were also used to analyse overexpressed proteins in 10 OSCC patients. Forty-one proteins were identified as commonly overexpressed in OSCC tissues. In OSCC tissues, alphaB-crystallin, tropomyosin 2, myosin light chain 1, heat shock protein 27 (HSP27), stratifin, thioredoxin-dependent peroxide reductase, flavin reductase, vimentin, rho GDP-dissociation inhibitor 2 (rho GDI-2), glutathione S-transferase Pi (GST-pi) and superoxide dismutase [Mn] (MnSOD) were significantly overexpressed. In real-time quantitative RT-PCR analysis, the gene expressions of alphaB-crystallin, HSP27 and MnSOD were also increased in the cancer tissues, consistent with proteomic results (Lo et al., 2007). These data suggest that identification of particular proteins could be used as diagnostic markers for OSCC.

Advanced Treatment

Although enormous advances have been made in understanding the molecular pathogenesis of oral cancer, three types of treatment namely, surgery, chemotherapy and radiation therapy are still the major types of treatment for oral cancer. At present, other areas of reasearch for head and neck cancer treatment have been focused on the finding of new anticancer agents and gene therapy.

New Anticancer Agents for the Treatment of Head and Neck Cancer

Many anticancer agents are still in development but according to clinical trials, these agents are either toxic to the patients or some side effects are intoralatable. However, there is an attempt to develop therapeutic agents that targets specific molecules or pathways found to be aberrated in oral cancer.

The most widely studied anticancer agents for head and neck cancer are molecules that target EGFR. There are 2 major classes of anti-ErbB therapeutics: ectodomain-binding antibodies and small molecule tyrosine kinase inhibitors (TKIs). The first EGFR-specific monoclonal antibodies (mABs) were isolated using partially purified receptor and A431-EGFR-overexpressing cancer cells (Schreiber et al., 1981; Sato et al., 1983). The development of humanized monoclonal antibodies against the extracellular domain of the receptor is based on antireceptor strategy. Monoclonal antibodies such as cetuximab, compete for the binding of receptor ligands and can induce EGFR downregulation from the tumor cell surface (Arteaga and Baselga, 2003). Cetuximab is a chimeric human: murine derivative of mAB225 and is a potent inhibitor of cancer cells that have autocrine EGFR activation and human tumor xenografts that overexpress the receptor (Goldstein et al., 1995). The small molecules, such as gefitinib and erlotinib compete with ATP in the tyrosine-kinase domain leading to abrogation of catalytic activity of the receptor, autophosphorylation, and its engagement with signal transducers (Arteaga and Baselga, 2003).

The use of EGFR as a target of head and neck cancer treatment has been investigated extensively in preclinical studies. Both the EGFR tyrosine kinase inhibitors and monoclonal antibodies inhibit the proliferation of head and neck cancer cells in a dose-dependent manner (Magne et al., 2002; Di Gennaro et al., 2003; Matheny et al., 2003). Treatment of OSCC cell lines with mAb 225 (cetuximab) induced G1 growth arrest leading to inhibition of proliferation of the cancer cells. G1 arrest was accompanied by a decrease in cdk2, cdk4 and cdk6 associated histone H1 kinase activities and increase in the expression levels of cell cycle inhibitors $p27^{Kip1}$ and $p15^{ink4B}$ (Kiyota et al., 2002). Antitumor activity of EGFR tyrosine kinase inhibitors combined with cytotoxic agents was also elucidated (Pollack et al., 1999; Magne et al., 2002). Combination of EGFR inhibitor, CP-358,77 with cisplatin produced a significant response above that of cisplatin alone with no detectable effects on body weight or lethal toxicity (Pollack et al., 1999). Enhancement of radiosensitivity in head and neck cancer cells by ZD1839 (Iressa or gifitinib) was also demonstrated in 5 HNSCC cell lines (Shintani et al., 2003). EGFR expression levels (EGFR number/cell) correlated with increased tumor resistance to radiation. Following exposure of the HNSCC cells to Iressa and radiation, greater than additive growth inhibitory effects were observed. Several investigators have also reported that cetuximab enhanced the efficacy of irradiation, with synergistic interaction in some studies (Bonner et al., 2000; Bonner et al., 2004).

Several clinical trials have been conducted to investigate the effect of EGFR inhibitor alone or in combination with chemotherapy and radiation therapy in the treatment of HNSCC. In phase I clinical trial of gifitinib, the common adverse effects were reversible skin rash and diarrhea (Baselga et al., 2002; Herbst et al., 2002; Ranson et al., 2002). The result also indicated that 250 and 500 mg of gifitinib should be used in clinical study. In a phase II clincial trial, patients with recurrence or metastatic HNSCC were treated with 500 mg/day of gifitinib. The control rate of 53.2% was found in these patients, with 10.6% of patial response and 42.6% with stable disease or minor response (Cohen et al., 2003). The median time to progression and median survival were 3.4 months and 8.1 months, respectively, with 1-year survival rate of 29%. Development of skin toxicity was found to be strong predictors of response progression and survival. Erlotinib (Tarceva) is also another small molecule tyrosine kinase inhibitor which acts as reversible EGFR-specific inhibitor in the same fashion as gefitinib. In a phase I study of erlotinib, 40 patients (3 with HNSCC) received once-daily erlotinib. Diarrhea and skin rash were the most common toxicities and the dose determined for phase II trial was 150 mg/day (Hidalgo et al., 2001). A multicenter phase II trial of erlotinib in patients with recurrent and/or metastatic HNSCC indicated that the majority of patients (87%) had tumors that demonstrated strong EGFR staining intensity. Out of 115 patients, 5 patients achieved partial responses. Disease stabilization was maintained in 44 patients (38.3%) for a median duration of 16.1 weeks. The median progression-free survival for the entire study population was 9.6 weeks, and the median overall survival was 6.0 months. Rash and diarrhea were the most common drug-related toxicities, encountered in 79% and 37% of patients, respectively, though the severity was mild to moderate in most cases. Further evaluation of these agents in the treatment of HNSCC is still warranted (Soulieres et al., 2004).

The use of cetuximab, a chimeric EGFR monoclonal antibody, in clinical trial was also investigated in the treatment of HNSCC. In a preliminary study of radiotherapy plus cetuximab in patients with locoregionally advanced head and neck cancer, the regimen was well tolerated, and all the patients who could be assessed had a complete or partial regression (Robert et al., 2001). In a phase II clinical trial, patients with locoregional advanced head and neck cancer were randomly assigned to treatment with high-dose radiotherapy alone or high-dose rediotherapy with weekly cetuximab at an initial dose of 400 mg per square meter of body-surface area, followed by 250 mg per square meter for the duration of radiotherapy. It was found that treatment with high-dose radiotherapy plus cetuximab improved locoregional control and reduced mortality without increasing common toxic side effects (Bonner et al., 2006). Therefore, this molecule should be further investigated for the treatment of head and neck cancer as a radiosensitizer.

Another molecular target for oral cancer is the cdk. Cyclin D1 is proto-oncogene that regulates G1 to S progression through the cell cycle. The protein forms complexes with cdks and mediates progression by phosphorylating the pRB gene product. In preclinical testing, the cdk inhibitor, flavopiridol, repressed the transcription of cyclin D1, induced cell-cycle arrest at the transitions between the G2 and M phases and between G1 and S phases, and induces p53-independent apoptosis (Patel et al., 1998). E7070 is a synthetic sulfonamide that targets the G1 phase of the cell cycle, inducing inhibition of cdk phosphorylation leading to blockade in G1/S transition. A phase II study of E7070, administered at the dose of 700 mg/m^2 every 3 weeks in patients with recurrent and metastatic HNSCC has shown no objective responses, however, pharmacodynamic data showed that cdk activity could be inhibited in the tumor cells (Haddad et al., 2004).

In an attempt to inhibit growth, invasion and metastasis in OSCC, a number of investigations have been studied on the blocking of angiogenesis by various inhibitors. Using an orthotopic nude mouse model, the tyrosine kinase inhibitor PTK787 combined with CPT-11, a semisynthetic camptothecin analogue was found to block the VEGF receptor signaling pathway and inhibit the tumor growth and angiogenesis of OSCC (Yazici et al., 2005). This indicated that targeting VEGF receptor tyrosine kinase activity can be an effective therapeutic approach in OSCC. Another recent study showed that a selective antigelatinolytic peptide, CTT1, an inhibitor of MMP-2 and MMP-9, could be useful to diminish the invasion and angiogenesis of human tongue carcinomas (Heikkila et al., 2006). In addition, vesnarinone, a synthesized positive oral inotropic agent, was reported to be able to suppress angiogenesis and growth of OSCC cells by inhibiting the expression of VEGF and IL-8 involved in blockade of NF-kappB activity (Harada et al., 2005). Genistein, a soybean product known to be an effective natural anti-angiogenic agent, showed some anti-cancer effects in OSCC particularly down-regulation of VEGF, reduction of gelatinolytic activity and reduction of *in vitro* invasion of tumor cells through the artificial basement membrane (Myoung et al., 2003).

TNP-470, sigma-(chloro-acethyl-carbamoyl) fumagillol, a synthetic analogue of fumagillin, has also been studied as an angiogenesis inhibitor. Combination treatment of TNP-470 and anti-IL-8 antibody significantly reduced the proliferation of KB cells, one of the human head and neck carcinoma cell lines that produce IL-8 (Kawano et al., 2001). In addition, the effects of TNP-470 on human OSCC cell lines with combining radiation therapy in the nude mice were studied and the results suggested that TNP-470 significantly enhanced the effect of radiation on the cells with high neovascularization (Shintani et al., 2006). Endostatin, an endogenous antiangiogenic factor, was found to inhibit lymphangiogenesis and lymph node metastasis by suppressing the production of VEGF-C in human OSCC cells (Fukumoto et al., 2005). Retinoic acid was reported to effectively suppress head and neck SCC in mice as well as prevent metastases (Strauss et al., 2005).

Since the expression of COX-2 in tumors is associated with enhanced angiogenesis, suppression of host immunity, and tumor invasion, COX-2 inhibitors have gained interests from many investigators especially in the aspect of suppression of epithelial cancers including cancers of the upper aerodigestive tract (Mohan and Epstein, 2003). In a study, NS-398, a selective COX-2 inhibitor and COX-2 antisense oligonucleotide (COX-2 AS) were found to inhibit the invasiveness of OSCC cells via down-regulation of MMP-2 and CD44 (Kinugasa et al., 2004). Using OSCC cell lines, modified to express varying levels of alpha(v)beta(6), the effect of COX-2 inhibition on cell invasion was investigated. It was found that NS398 inhibited specifically alpha(v)beta(6)-dependent, but not alpha(v)beta(6)-independent OSCC invasion *in vitro* and *in vivo*, and this effect was modulated through PGE2-dependent activation of Rac-1. Celecoxib, another selective COX-2 inhibitor, was shown to suppress proliferation and invasiveness in OSCC (Kwak et al., 2007). Celecoxib also reduced both MMP-2 and MMP-9 enzyme activity. Silibinin, an anti-metastatic agent, showed a marked inhibition of invasion and motility of SCC-4 tongue cancer cells as well as reduced expression of MMP-2 and u-PA and enhanced expression of TIMP-2 and plasminogen activator inhibitor-1 (PAI-1) (Chen et al., 2006). ZD1839 (Iressa), a quinazoline derivative that selectively inhibits the EGFR tyrosine kinase activity, has been clinically used for cancer patients. A recent *in vitro* study indicated that the inhibition of proliferation and invasion/migration in OSCC cell lines by ZD1839 resulted in an anticancer effect via multiple cellular and molecular mechanisms, and suggested that ZD1839 may be useful in inhibiting and/or preventing metastasis (Lee et al., 2007).

Gene Therapy for Head and Neck Cancer

Gene therapy can be defined as gene transfer for the purpose of treating human disease (Cusack and Tanabe, 1998). There are several strategies of gene therapy in the treatment of cancer. These include 1) addition of a tumor suppressor gene (gene addition therapy) 2) deletion of a defective tumor gene (gene excision therapy) 3) down-regulation of the expression of genes that stimulate tumor growth (antisense RNA) 4) enhancement of immune surveillance (immunotherapy) 5) activation of prodrugs that have a chemotherapeutic effect ("suicide" gene therapy) 6) introduction of viruses that destroy tumor cells as part of the replication cycle 7) delivery of drug resistance gene(s) to normal tissue for protection from chemotherapy and 8) introduction of genes to inhibit tumor angiogenesis (Xi and Grandis, 2003). The effectiveness of gene therapy in the treatment of cancer is not only dependent on the genes introduced but also the delivery system utilized. Two main delivery systems namely non-viral and viral systems are presently used for gene therapy. Regarding non-viral systems for gene therapy, liposome-mediated gene transfer has been used in several preclinical studies. However, disadvantages of this system are the limitation of transfection efficiency. Thus further development is required for this system for gene therapy application.

Viruses commonly used encompass retroviruses, adenoviruses and herpesviruses. Retroviruses are different from other viruses in that they are RNA viruses that undergo reverse transcription after infecting a cell and their genomes are randomly and stably integrated into the host genome. The limitation of the use of retroviruses in gene therapy is that they can infect only actively dividing cells hence infection efficiency is seemingly low in some types of cells. Adenoviruses are DNA viruses that usually infect most types of cells regardless of there position in the cell cycle. The DNA of adenovirus, however, does not integrate into the host genome, thus requires multiple administrations. Herpesviruses are double-stranded DNA viruses which can remain latent in tissues and can be reactivated at the original site of infection. They also exert high gene transfer efficiency and low immunogenicity, therefore can be used in the treatment several types of cancer. Herpes simplex virus type 1 has emerged as the leading candidate oncolytic virus with several clinical trials either completed or underway for patients with malignant glioma (Markert et al., 2006).

Several studies have documented the application of gene therapy in the treatment of head and neck cancers. As stated earlier, $p16^{ink4A}$ was frequently inactivated in oral premalignant and malignant lesions. Introduction of $p16^{ink4A}$ into OSCC cell lines using retroviruses or adenoviruses induced G1 cell cycle arrest (Rocco et al., 1998; Piboonniyom et al., 2003). Aberrations of the p53 gene are also commonly documented in head and neck cancer. Several strategies for cancer gene therapy based on wild-type p53 administration have been extensively evaluated both in preclinical and clinical models. Introducing wild-type p53 using recombinant adenoviral vector, Ad5CMV-p53 in HNSCC cell lines successfully attenuated their replication and tumor growth (Liu et al., 1994). Albeit with disappointment in treating ovarian cancer with p53 gene therapy (Zeimet and Marth, 2003), encouraging results were retreived for phase II and III clinical trials on 135 patients with late-stage HNSCC. In this study, 135 patients were treated with a combination of recombinant adenovirus-p53 (Genedicine) administration and radiotherapy (Pearson et al., 2004). The results showed 64% of patients with complete regression and 32% with partial regression without serious side effects. Furthermore, clinical trials of p53 gene replacement have provided useful information of the design of future gene therapy strategies (Moon et al., 2003). According to these results, p53 gene therapy could be a potential treatment in combination with conventional therapy in the treatment of head and neck cancer.

Another novel approach of gene therapy that has been extensively investigated in clinical studies for SCC involves a vector that selectively replicates within and lyses tumor cells. McCormick at Onyx Pharmaceuticals introduced the hypothesis that an adenovirus deleted of the E1B region could only replicate and generate cellular lysis in cells lacking functional p53 (McCormick, 2000). Accordingly, the ONYX-015 reagent has been developed for clincial applications (Bischoff et al., 1996). A potential advantage of this viral therapy is that infected cells will provide neighboring cancer cells with high titers of new virus particles when their lysis occurs. Animal study with ONYX-015 suggested that the efficacy of the virus is significantly augmented with the administration of standard chemotherapeutic agents (McCormick, 2003). In a Phase II clinical trial of a combination of intra-tumoral ONYX-015 injection with cisplatin and 5-fluorouracil in patients with HNSCC, there were substantial objective responses. By six months, none of the tumors that responded to the therapy has progressed, in contrast to tumors treated with chemotherapy alone (Khuri et al., 2000). Although not commercially available in the United State at present, the ONYX-015 (with some modification), by the name of H101 received commercial approval in China and now being further investigated (Yu and Fang, 2007). The results of large clinical trial in China wait to be seen in the near future.

References

Ahomadegbe, JC; Barrois, M; Fogel, S; Le Bihan, ML; Douc-Rasy, S; Duvillard, P, et al. High incidence of p53 alterations (mutation, deletion, overexpression) in head and neck primary tumors and metastases; absence of correlation with clinical outcome. Frequent protein overexpression in normal epithelium and in early non-invasive lesions. *Oncogene* 1995;10(6):1217-27.

Ah-See, KW; Cooke, TG; Pickford, IR; Soutar, D; Balmain, A. An allelotype of squamous carcinoma of the head and neck using microsatellite markers. *Cancer Res* 1994;54(7):1617-21.

Alevizos, I; Mahadevappa, M; Zhang, X; Ohyama, H; Kohno, Y; Posner, M, et al. Oral cancer *in vivo* gene expression profiling assisted by laser capture microdissection and microarray analysis. *Oncogene* 2001;20(43):6196-204.

Allshire, RC; Dempster, M; Hastie, ND. Human telomeres contain at least three types of G-rich repeat distributed non-randomly. *Nucleic Acids Res* 1989;17(12):4611-27.

Allsopp, RC; Chang, E; Kashefi-Aazam, M; Rogaev, EI; Piatyszek, MA; Shay, JW, et al. Telomere shortening is associated with cell division *in vitro* and *in vivo*. *Exp Cell Res* 1995;220(1):194-200.

Ambrosch, P; Schlott, T; Hilmes, D; Ruschenburg, I. p16 alterations and retinoblastoma protein expression in squamous cell carcinoma and neighboring dysplasia from the upper aerodigestive tract. *Virchows Arch* 2001;438(4):343-9.

Angadi, PV; Krishnapillai, R. Cyclin D1 expression in oral squamous cell carcinoma and verrucous carcinoma: correlation with histological differentiation. *Oral Surg Oral Med Oral Pathol Oral Radiol Endod* 2007;103(3):e30-5.

Arteaga, CL; Baselga, J. Clinical trial design and end points for epidermal growth factor receptor-targeted therapies: implications for drug development and practice. *Clin Cancer Res* 2003;9(5):1579-89.

Ascani, G; Balercia, P; Messi, M; Lupi, L; Goteri, G; Filosa, A, et al. Angiogenesis in oral squamous cell carcinoma. *Acta Otorhinolaryngol Ital* 2005;25(1):13-7.

Attisano, L; Wrana, JL. Signal transduction by the TGF-beta superfamily. *Science* 2002;296(5573):1646-7.

Bancroft, CC; Chen, Z; Dong, G; Sunwoo, JB; Yeh, N; Park, C, et al. Coexpression of proangiogenic factors IL-8 and VEGF by human head and neck squamous cell carcinoma involves coactivation by MEK-MAPK and IKK-NF-kappaB signal pathways. *Clin Cancer Res* 2001;7(2):435-42.

Baral, R; Patnaik, S; Das, BR. Co-overexpression of p53 and c-myc proteins linked with advanced stages of betel- and tobacco-related oral squamous cell carcinomas from eastern India. *Eur J Oral Sci* 1998;106(5):907-13.

Bargmann, CI; Hung, MC; Weinberg, RA. The neu oncogene encodes an epidermal growth factor receptor-related protein. *Nature* 1986;319(6050):226-30.

Baselga, J; Rischin, D; Ranson, M; Calvert, H; Raymond, E; Kieback, DG, et al. Phase I safety, pharmacokinetic, and pharmacodynamic trial of ZD1839, a selective oral epidermal growth factor receptor tyrosine kinase inhibitor, in patients with five selected solid tumor types. *J Clin Oncol* 2002;20(21):4292-302.

Bei, R; Budillon, A; Masuelli, L; Cereda, V; Vitolo, D; Di Gennaro, E, et al. Frequent overexpression of multiple ErbB receptors by head and neck squamous cell carcinoma contrasts with rare antibody immunity in patients. *J Pathol* 2004;204(3):317-25.

Bei, R; Pompa, G; Vitolo, D; Moriconi, E; Ciocci, L; Quaranta, M, et al. Co-localization of multiple ErbB receptors in stratified epithelium of oral squamous cell carcinoma. *J Pathol* 2001;195(3):343-8.

Bellacosa, A; Kumar, CC; Di Cristofano, A; Testa, JR. Activation of AKT kinases in cancer: implications for therapeutic targeting. *Adv Cancer Res* 2005;94:29-86.

Bhatia, K; Fan, S; Spangler, G; Weintraub, M; O'Connor, PM; Judde, JG, et al. A mutant p21 cyclin-dependent kinase inhibitor isolated from a Burkitt's lymphoma. *Cancer Res* 1995;55(7):1431-5.

Bichsel, VE; Liotta, LA; Petricoin, EF, 3rd. Cancer proteomics: from biomarker discovery to signal pathway profiling. *Cancer J* 2001;7(1):69-78.

Bindhu, OS; Ramadas, K; Sebastian, P; Pillai, MR. High expression levels of nuclear factor kappa B and gelatinases in the tumorigenesis of oral squamous cell carcinoma. *Head Neck* 2006;28(10):916-25.

Bischoff, JR; Kirn, DH; Williams, A; Heise, C; Horn, S; Muna, M, et al. An adenovirus mutant that replicates selectively in p53-deficient human tumor cells. *Science* 1996;274(5286):373-6.

Bjornsti, MA; Houghton, PJ. The TOR pathway: a target for cancer therapy. *Nat Rev Cancer* 2004;4(5):335-48.

Blackwood, EM; Eisenman, RN. Max: a helix-loop-helix zipper protein that forms a sequence-specific DNA-binding complex with Myc. *Science* 1991;251(4998):1211-7.

Blain, SW; Montalvo, E; Massague, J. Differential interaction of the cyclin-dependent kinase (Cdk) inhibitor p27Kip1 with cyclin A-Cdk2 and cyclin D2-Cdk4. *J Biol Chem* 1997;272(41):25863-72.

Bodnar, AG; Ouellette, M; Frolkis, M; Holt, SE; Chiu, CP; Morin, GB, et al. Extension of life-span by introduction of telomerase into normal human cells. *Science* 1998;279(5349):349-52.

Bonner, JA; Buchsbaum, DJ; Russo, SM; Fiveash, JB; Trummell, HQ; Curiel, DT, et al. Anti-EGFR-mediated radiosensitization as a result of augmented EGFR expression. *Int J Radiat Oncol Biol Phys* 2004;59(2 Suppl):2-10.

Bonner, JA; Harari, PM; Giralt, J; Azarnia, N; Shin, DM; Cohen, RB, et al. Radiotherapy plus cetuximab for squamous-cell carcinoma of the head and neck. *N Engl J Med* 2006;354(6):567-78.

Bonner, JA; Raisch, KP; Trummell, HQ; Robert, F; Meredith, RF; Spencer, SA, et al. Enhanced apoptosis with combination C225/radiation treatment serves as the impetus for clinical investigation in head and neck cancers. *J Clin Oncol* 2000;18(21 Suppl):47S-53S.

Brachman, DG; Graves, D; Vokes, E; Beckett, M; Haraf, D; Montag, A, et al. Occurrence of p53 gene deletions and human papilloma virus infection in human head and neck cancer. *Cancer Res* 1992;52(17):4832-6.

Brown, JP; Wei, W; Sedivy, JM. Bypass of senescence after disruption of p21CIP1/WAF1 gene in normal diploid human fibroblasts. *Science* 1997;277(5327):831-4.

Bryan, TM; Cech, TR. Telomerase and the maintenance of chromosome ends. *Curr Opin Cell Biol* 1999;11(3):318-24.

Bryan, TM; Englezou, A; Dalla-Pozza, L; Dunham, MA; Reddel, RR. Evidence for an alternative mechanism for maintaining telomere length in human tumors and tumor-derived cell lines. *Nat Med* 1997;3(11):1271-4.

Buchkovich, K; Duffy, LA; Harlow, E. The retinoblastoma protein is phosphorylated during specific phases of the cell cycle. *Cell* 1989;58(6):1097-105.

Cai, YC; Yang, GY; Nie, Y; Wang, LD; Zhao, X; Song, YL, et al. Molecular alterations of p73 in human esophageal squamous cell carcinomas: loss of heterozygosity occurs frequently; loss of imprinting and elevation of p73 expression may be related to defective p53. *Carcinogenesis* 2000;21(4):683-9.

Cairns, P; Mao, L; Merlo, A; Lee, DJ; Schwab, D; Eby, Y, et al. Rates of p16 (MTS1) mutations in primary tumors with 9p loss. *Science* 1994;265(5170):415-7.

Califano, J; van der Riet, P; Westra, W; Nawroz, H; Clayman, G; Piantadosi, S, et al. Genetic progression model for head and neck cancer: implications for field cancerization. *Cancer Res* 1996;56(11):2488-92.

Callender, T; el-Naggar, AK; Lee, MS; Frankenthaler, R; Luna, MA; Batsakis, JG. PRAD-1 (CCND1)/cyclin D1 oncogene amplification in primary head and neck squamous cell carcinoma. *Cancer* 1994;74(1):152-8.

Carlos de Vicente, J; Junquera Gutierrez, LM; Zapatero, AH; Fresno Forcelledo, MF; Hernandez-Vallejo, G; Lopez Arranz, JS. Prognostic significance of p53 expression in oral squamous cell carcinoma without neck node metastases. *Head Neck* 2004;26(1):22-30.

Chen, P; Xie, H; Wells, A. Mitogenic signaling from the egf receptor is attenuated by a phospholipase C-gamma/protein kinase C feedback mechanism. *Mol Biol Cell* 1996;7(6):871-81.

Chen, PN; Hsieh, YS; Chiang, CL; Chiou, HL; Yang, SF; Chu, SC. Silibinin inhibits invasion of oral cancer cells by suppressing the MAPK pathway. *J Dent Res* 2006;85(3):220-5.

Chen, YJ; Lin, SC; Kao, T; Chang, CS; Hong, PS; Shieh, TM, et al. Genome-wide profiling of oral squamous cell carcinoma. *J Pathol* 2004;204(3):326-32.

Chen, YK; Hsue, SS; Lin, LM. Expression of p63 protein and mRNA in oral epithelial dysplasia. *J Oral Pathol Med* 2005;34(4):232-9.

Chen, YK; Hsue, SS; Lin, LM. p73 expression for human buccal epithelial dysplasia and squamous cell carcinoma: does it correlate with nodal status of carcinoma and is there a relationship with malignant change of epithelial dysplasia? *Head Neck* 2004;26(11):945-52.

Cheng, M; Olivier, P; Diehl, JA; Fero, M; Roussel, MF; Roberts, JM, et al. The p21(Cip1) and p27(Kip1) CDK 'inhibitors' are essential activators of cyclin D-dependent kinases in murine fibroblasts. *Embo J* 1999;18(6):1571-83.

Chiang, WC; Wong, YK; Lin, SC; Chang, KW; Liu, CJ. Increase of MMP-13 expression in multi-stage oral carcinogenesis and epigallocatechin-3-gallate suppress MMP-13 expression. *Oral Dis* 2006;12(1):27-33.

Choi, HR; Batsakis, JG; Zhan, F; Sturgis, E; Luna, MA; El-Naggar, AK. Differential expression of p53 gene family members p63 and p73 in head and neck squamous tumorigenesis. *Hum Pathol* 2002;33(2):158-64.

Choi, HR; Tucker, SA; Huang, Z; Gillenwater, AM; Luna, MA; Batsakis, JG, et al. Differential expressions of cyclin-dependent kinase inhibitors (p27 and p21) and their relation to p53 and Ki-67 in oral squamous tumorigenesis. *Int J Oncol* 2003;22(2):409-14.

Chuang, HC; Su, CY; Huang, HY; Chien, CY; Chen, CM; Huang, CC. High expression of CD105 as a prognostic predictor of early tongue cancer. *Laryngoscope* 2006;116(7):1175-9.

Cohen, EE; Rosen, F; Stadler, WM; Recant, W; Stenson, K; Huo, D, et al. Phase II trial of ZD1839 in recurrent or metastatic squamous cell carcinoma of the head and neck. *J Clin Oncol* 2003;21(10):1980-7.

Cohen, T; Gitay-Goren, H; Sharon, R; Shibuya, M; Halaban, R; Levi, BZ, et al. VEGF121, a vascular endothelial growth factor (VEGF) isoform lacking heparin binding ability, requires cell-surface heparan sulfates for efficient binding to the VEGF receptors of human melanoma cells. *J Biol Chem* 1995;270(19):11322-6.

Costello, JF; Berger, MS; Huang, HS; Cavenee, WK. Silencing of p16/CDKN2 expression in human gliomas by methylation and chromatin condensation. *Cancer Res* 1996;56(10):2405-10.

Cotran RS, Kumar V, Collins T. Robbins Pathologic Basis of Disease. 6th Edition. Philadelphia: Saunders, 1999.

Counter, CM; Meyerson, M; Eaton, EN; Weinberg, RA. The catalytic subunit of yeast telomerase. *Proc Natl Acad Sci U S A* 1997;94(17):9202-7.

Culouscou, JM; Plowman, GD; Carlton, GW; Green, JM; Shoyab, M. Characterization of a breast cancer cell differentiation factor that specifically activates the HER4/p180erbB4 receptor. *J Biol Chem* 1993;268(25):18407-10.

Cusack, JC, Jr.; Tanabe, KK. Cancer gene therapy. *Surg Oncol Clin N Am* 1998;7(3):421-69.

Dang, CV; O'Donnell K, A; Juopperi, T. The great MYC escape in tumorigenesis. *Cancer Cell* 2005;8(3):177-8.

Dang, CV; O'Donnell, KA; Zeller, KI; Nguyen, T; Osthus, RC; Li, F. The c-Myc target gene network. *Semin Cancer Biol* 2006;16(4):253-64.

de Oliveira, LR; Ribeiro-Silva, A; Zucoloto, S. Prognostic impact of p53 and p63 immunoexpression in oral squamous cell carcinoma. *J Oral Pathol Med* 2007;36(4):191-7.

de Vicente, JC; Fresno, MF; Villalain, L; Vega, JA; Hernandez Vallejo, G. Expression and clinical significance of matrix metalloproteinase-2 and matrix metalloproteinase-9 in oral squamous cell carcinoma. *Oral Oncol* 2005;41(3):283-93.

Dhawan, P; Singh, AB; Ellis, DL; Richmond, A. Constitutive activation of Akt/protein kinase B in melanoma leads to up-regulation of nuclear factor-kappaB and tumor progression. *Cancer Res* 2002;62(24):7335-42.

Di Gennaro, E; Barbarino, M; Bruzzese, F; De Lorenzo, S; Caraglia, M; Abbruzzese, A, et al. Critical role of both p27KIP1 and p21CIP1/WAF1 in the antiproliferative effect of ZD1839 ('Iressa'), an epidermal growth factor receptor tyrosine kinase inhibitor, in head and neck squamous carcinoma cells. *J Cell Physiol* 2003;195(1):139-50.

Donehower, LA; Harvey, M; Slagle, BL; McArthur, MJ; Montgomery, CA, Jr.; Butel, JS, et al. Mice deficient for p53 are developmentally normal but susceptible to spontaneous tumours. *Nature* 1992;356(6366):215-21.

Du, B; Altorki, NK; Kopelovich, L; Subbaramaiah, K; Dannenberg, AJ. Tobacco smoke stimulates the transcription of amphiregulin in human oral epithelial cells: evidence of a cyclic AMP-responsive element binding protein-dependent mechanism. *Cancer Res* 2005;65(13):5982-8.

Eisma, RJ; Spiro, JD; Kreutzer, DL. Role of angiogenic factors: coexpression of interleukin-8 and vascular endothelial growth factor in patients with head and neck squamous carcinoma. *Laryngoscope* 1999;109(5):687-93.

el-Deiry, WS; Tokino, T; Velculescu, VE; Levy, DB; Parsons, R; Trent, JM, et al. WAF1, a potential mediator of p53 tumor suppression. *Cell* 1993;75(4):817-25.

El-Gazzar, R; Macluskey, M; Williams, H; Ogden, GR. Vascularity and expression of vascular endothelial growth factor in oral squamous cell carcinoma, resection margins, and nodal metastases. *Br J Oral Maxillofac Surg* 2006;44(3):193-7.

El-Naggar, AK; Lai, S; Clayman, GL; Mims, B; Lippman, SM; Coombes, M, et al. p73 gene alterations and expression in primary oral and laryngeal squamous carcinomas. *Carcinogenesis* 2001;22(5):729-35.

Emmert-Buck, MR; Bonner, RF; Smith, PD; Chuaqui, RF; Zhuang, Z; Goldstein, SR, et al. Laser capture microdissection. *Science* 1996;274(5289):998-1001.

Eversole, LR; Sapp, JP. c-myc oncoprotein expression in oral precancerous and early cancerous lesions. *Eur J Cancer B Oral Oncol* 1993;29B(2):131-5.

Faridoni-Laurens, L; Bosq, J; Janot, F; Vayssade, M; Le Bihan, ML; Kaghad, M, et al. P73 expression in basal layers of head and neck squamous epithelium: a role in differentiation and carcinogenesis in concert with p53 and p63? *Oncogene* 2001;20(38):5302-12.

Fedi, P; Pierce, JH; di Fiore, PP; Kraus, MH. Efficient coupling with phosphatidylinositol 3-kinase, but not phospholipase C gamma or GTPase-activating protein, distinguishes ErbB-3 signaling from that of other ErbB/EGFR family members. *Mol Cell Biol* 1994;14(1):492-500.

Field, JK; Kiaris, H; Risk, JM; Tsiriyotis, C; Adamson, R; Zoumpourlis, V, et al. Allelotype of squamous cell carcinoma of the head and neck: fractional allele loss correlates with survival. *Br J Cancer* 1995;72(5):1180-8.

Folkman, J; Klagsbrun, M. Angiogenic factors. *Science* 1987;235(4787):442-7.

Fracchiolla, NS; Pruneri, G; Pignataro, L; Carboni, N; Capaccio, P; Boletini, A, et al. Molecular and immunohistochemical analysis of the bcl-1/cyclin D1 gene in laryngeal squamous cell carcinomas: correlation of protein expression with lymph node metastases and advanced clinical stage. *Cancer* 1997;79(6):1114-21.

Franz, M; Richter, P; Geyer, C; Hansen, T; Acuna, LD; Hyckel, P, et al. Mesenchymal cells contribute to the synthesis and deposition of the laminin-5 gamma2 chain in the invasive front of oral squamous cell carcinoma. *J Mol Histol* 2007;38(3):183-90.

Freier, K; Pungs, S; Flechtenmacher, C; Bosch, FX; Lichter, P; Joos, S, et al. Frequent high telomerase reverse transcriptase expression in primary oral squamous cell carcinoma. *J Oral Pathol Med* 2007;36(5):267-72.

Fukumoto, S; Morifuji, M; Katakura, Y; Ohishi, M; Nakamura, S. Endostatin inhibits lymph node metastasis by a down-regulation of the vascular endothelial growth factor C expression in tumor cells. *Clin Exp Metastasis* 2005;22(1):31-8.

Furge, KA; Chen, J; Koeman, J; Swiatek, P; Dykema, K; Lucin, K, et al. Detection of DNA copy number changes and oncogenic signaling abnormalities from gene expression data reveals MYC activation in high-grade papillary renal cell carcinoma. *Cancer Res* 2007;67(7):3171-6.

Gamberi, G; Benassi, MS; Bohling, T; Ragazzini, P; Molendini, L; Sollazzo, MR, et al. Prognostic relevance of C-myc gene expression in giant-cell tumor of bone. *J Orthop Res* 1998;16(1):1-7.

Gamberi, G; Benassi, MS; Bohling, T; Ragazzini, P; Molendini, L; Sollazzo, MR, et al. C-myc and c-fos in human osteosarcoma: prognostic value of mRNA and protein expression. *Oncology* 1998;55(6):556-63.

Gao, X; Chen, YQ; Wu, N; Grignon, DJ; Sakr, W; Porter, AT, et al. Somatic mutations of the WAF1/CIP1 gene in primary prostate cancer. *Oncogene* 1995;11(7):1395-8.

Gao, ZB; Duan, YQ; Zhang, L; Chen, DW; Ding, PT. Expression of matrix metalloproteinase 2 and its tissue inhibitor in oral squamous cell carcinoma. *Int J Mol Med* 2005;16(4):599-603.

Garcia, R; Bowman, TL; Niu, G; Yu, H; Minton, S; Muro-Cacho, CA, et al. Constitutive activation of Stat3 by the Src and JAK tyrosine kinases participates in growth regulation of human breast carcinoma cells. *Oncogene* 2001;20(20):2499-513.

Goessel, G; Quante, M; Hahn, WC; Harada, H; Heeg, S; Suliman, Y, et al. Creating oral squamous cancer cells: a cellular model of oral-esophageal carcinogenesis. *Proc Natl Acad Sci U S A* 2005;102(43):15599-604.

Goldstein, NI; Prewett, M; Zuklys, K; Rockwell, P; Mendelsohn, J. Biological efficacy of a chimeric antibody to the epidermal growth factor receptor in a human tumor xenograft model. *Clin Cancer Res* 1995;1(11):1311-8.

Gonzalez, MV; Pello, MF; Lopez-Larrea, C; Suarez, C; Menendez, MJ; Coto, E. Deletion and methylation of the tumour suppressor gene p16/CDKN2 in primary head and neck squamous cell carcinoma. *J Clin Pathol* 1997;50(6):509-12.

Goto, M; Tsukamoto, T; Inada, K; Mizoshita, T; Ogawa, T; Terada, A, et al. Loss of p21WAF1/CIP1 expression in invasive fronts of oral tongue squamous cell carcinomas is correlated with tumor progression and poor prognosis. *Oncol Rep* 2005;14(4):837-46.

Grandis, JR; Tweardy, DJ. Elevated levels of transforming growth factor alpha and epidermal growth factor receptor messenger RNA are early markers of carcinogenesis in head and neck cancer. *Cancer Res* 1993;53(15):3579-84.

Greenberg, JS; Fowler, R; Gomez, J; Mo, V; Roberts, D; El Naggar, AK, et al. Extent of extracapsular spread: a critical prognosticator in oral tongue cancer. *Cancer* 2003;97(6):1464-70.

Greider, CW. Telomere length regulation. *Annu Rev Biochem* 1996;65:337-65.

Greider, CW; Blackburn, EH. Identification of a specific telomere terminal transferase activity in Tetrahymena extracts. *Cell* 1985;43(2 Pt 1):405-13.

Grille, SJ; Bellacosa, A; Upson, J; Klein-Szanto, AJ; van Roy, F; Lee-Kwon, W, et al. The protein kinase Akt induces epithelial mesenchymal transition and promotes enhanced motility and invasiveness of squamous cell carcinoma lines. *Cancer Res* 2003;63(9):2172-8.

Gu, Y; Turck, CW; Morgan, DO. Inhibition of CDK2 activity *in vivo* by an associated 20K regulatory subunit. *Nature* 1993;366(6456):707-10.

Guo, W; Kang, MK; Kim, HJ; Park, NH. Immortalization of human oral keratinocytes is associated with elevation of telomerase activity and shortening of telomere length. *Oncol Rep* 1998;5(4):799-804.

Gupta, AK; McKenna, WG; Weber, CN; Feldman, MD; Goldsmith, JD; Mick, R, et al. Local recurrence in head and neck cancer: relationship to radiation resistance and signal transduction. *Clin Cancer Res* 2002;8(3):885-92.

Haddad, RI; Weinstein, LJ; Wieczorek, TJ; Bhattacharya, N; Raftopoulos, H; Oster, MW, et al. A phase II clinical and pharmacodynamic study of E7070 in patients with metastatic, recurrent, or refractory squamous cell carcinoma of the head and neck: modulation of retinoblastoma protein phosphorylation by a novel chloroindolyl sulfonamide cell cycle inhibitor. *Clin Cancer Res* 2004;10(14):4680-7.

Hahn, SA; Schutte, M; Hoque, AT; Moskaluk, CA; da Costa, LT; Rozenblum, E, et al. DPC4, a candidate tumor suppressor gene at human chromosome 18q21.1. *Science* 1996;271(5247):350-3.

Hanahan, D; Weinberg, RA. The hallmarks of cancer. *Cell* 2000;100(1):57-70.

Harada, K; Ogden, GR. An overview of the cell cycle arrest protein, p21(WAF1). *Oral Oncol* 2000;36(1):3-7.

Harada, K; Supriatno; Yoshida, H; Sato, M. Vesnarinone inhibits angiogenesis and tumorigenicity of human oral squamous cell carcinoma cells by suppressing the expression of vascular endothelial growth factor and interleukin-8. *Int J Oncol* 2005;27(6):1489-97.

Harper, JW; Adami, GR; Wei, N; Keyomarsi, K; Elledge, SJ. The p21 Cdk-interacting protein Cip1 is a potent inhibitor of G1 cyclin-dependent kinases. *Cell* 1993;75(4):805-16.

Hase, T; Kawashiri, S; Tanaka, A; Nozaki, S; Noguchi, N; Kato, K, et al. Correlation of basic fibroblast growth factor expression with the invasion and the prognosis of oral squamous cell carcinoma. *J Oral Pathol Med* 2006;35(3):136-9.

Hasina, R; Lingen, MW. Angiogenesis in oral cancer. *J Dent Educ* 2001;65(11):1282-90.

Haugen, DR; Akslen, LA; Varhaug, JE; Lillehaug, JR. Expression of c-erbB-3 and c-erbB-4 proteins in papillary thyroid carcinomas. *Cancer Res* 1996;56(6):1184-8.

Hayashi, T; Fleming, MV; Stetler-Stevenson, WG; Liotta, LA; Moss, J; Ferrans, VJ, et al. Immunohistochemical study of matrix metalloproteinases (MMPs) and their tissue inhibitors (TIMPs) in pulmonary lymphangioleiomyomatosis (LAM). *Hum Pathol* 1997;28(9):1071-8.

Hayflick, L. Human cells and aging. *Sci Am* 1968;218(3):32-7.

Heikkila, P; Suojanen, J; Pirila, E; Vaananen, A; Koivunen, E; Sorsa, T, et al. Human tongue carcinoma growth is inhibited by selective antigelatinolytic peptides. *Int J Cancer* 2006;118(9):2202-9.

Heldin, CH; Miyazono, K; ten Dijke, P. TGF-beta signalling from cell membrane to nucleus through SMAD proteins. *Nature* 1997;390(6659):465-71.

Herbst, RS; Maddox, AM; Rothenberg, ML; Small, EJ; Rubin, EH; Baselga, J, et al. Selective oral epidermal growth factor receptor tyrosine kinase inhibitor ZD1839 is generally well-tolerated and has activity in non-small-cell lung cancer and other solid tumors: results of a phase I trial. *J Clin Oncol* 2002;20(18):3815-25.

Herwig, S; Strauss, M. The retinoblastoma protein: a master regulator of cell cycle, differentiation and apoptosis. *Eur J Biochem* 1997;246(3):581-601.

Hidalgo, M; Siu, LL; Nemunaitis, J; Rizzo, J; Hammond, LA; Takimoto, C, et al. Phase I and pharmacologic study of OSI-774, an epidermal growth factor receptor tyrosine kinase inhibitor, in patients with advanced solid malignancies. *J Clin Oncol* 2001;19(13):3267-79.

Hinds, P; Finlay, C; Levine, AJ. Mutation is required to activate the p53 gene for cooperation with the ras oncogene and transformation. *J Virol* 1989;63(2):739-46.

Hiyama, K; Hirai, Y; Kyoizumi, S; Akiyama, M; Hiyama, E; Piatyszek, MA, et al. Activation of telomerase in human lymphocytes and hematopoietic progenitor cells. *J Immunol* 1995;155(8):3711-5.

Hollstein, M; Sidransky, D; Vogelstein, B; Harris, CC. p53 mutations in human cancers. *Science* 1991;253(5015):49-53.

Honda, R; Tanaka, H; Yasuda, H. Oncoprotein MDM2 is a ubiquitin ligase E3 for tumor suppressor p53. *FEBS Lett* 1997;420(1):25-7.

Horowitz, JM; Park, SH; Bogenmann, E; Cheng, JC; Yandell, DW; Kaye, FJ, et al. Frequent inactivation of the retinoblastoma anti-oncogene is restricted to a subset of human tumor cells. *Proc Natl Acad Sci U S A* 1990;87(7):2775-9.

Horta, MC; de Assis, LA; de Souza, AF; de Araujo, VC; Gomez, RS; Aguiar, MC. p53 and p21WAF1/CIP1 overexpression at the invasive front of lower lip squamous cell carcinoma. *J Oral Pathol Med* 2007;36(2):88-92.

Hua, Z; Zhang, YC; Hu, XM; Jia, ZG. Loss of DPC4 expression and its correlation with clinicopathological parameters in pancreatic carcinoma. *World J Gastroenterol* 2003;9(12):2764-7.

Huang, MF; Chang, YC; Liao, PS; Huang, TH; Tsay, CH; Chou, MY. Loss of heterozygosity of p53 gene of oral cancer detected by exfoliative cytology. *Oral Oncol* 1999;35(3):296-301.

Hynes, NE; Lane, HA. ERBB receptors and cancer: the complexity of targeted inhibitors. *Nat Rev Cancer* 2005;5(5):341-54.

Iamaroon, A; Khemaleelakul, U; Pongsiriwet, S; Pintong, J. Co-expression of p53 and Ki67 and lack of EBV expression in oral squamous cell carcinoma. *J Oral Pathol Med* 2004;33(1):30-6.

Iamaroon, A; Pattamapun, K; Piboonniyom, SO. Aberrant expression of Smad4, a TGF-beta signaling molecule, in oral squamous cell carcinoma. *J Oral Sci* 2006;48(3):105-9.

Iamaroon, A; Pattanaporn, K; Pongsiriwet, S; Wanachantararak, S; Prapayasatok, S; Jittidecharaks, S, et al. Analysis of 587 cases of oral squamous cell carcinoma in northern Thailand with a focus on young people. *Int J Oral Maxillofac Surg* 2004;33(1):84-8.

Iamaroon, A; Pongsiriwet, S; Jittidecharaks, S; Pattanaporn, K; Prapayasatok, S; Wanachantararak, S. Increase of mast cells and tumor angiogenesis in oral squamous cell carcinoma. *J Oral Pathol Med* 2003;32(4):195-9.

Ichikawa, M; Ishii, K; Nakajima, T; Mogi, K. The overexpression of p53 and proliferative activity in precancerous and cancerous lesions of oral squamous epithelium. *J Exp Clin Cancer Res* 1997;16(2):141-6.

Iida, K; Nishimura, I. Gene expression profiling by DNA microarray technology. *Crit Rev Oral Biol Med* 2002;13(1):35-50.

Ishida, E; Nakamura, M; Ikuta, M; Shimada, K; Matsuyoshi, S; Kirita, T, et al. Promotor hypermethylation of p14ARF is a key alteration for progression of oral squamous cell carcinoma. *Oral Oncol* 2005;41(6):614-22.

Ishizawar, R; Parsons, SJ. c-Src and cooperating partners in human cancer. *Cancer Cell* 2004;6(3):209-14.

Ito, Y; Zhao, J; Mogharei, A; Shuler, CF; Weinstein, M; Deng, C, et al. Antagonistic effects of Smad2 versus Smad7 are sensitive to their expression level during tooth development. *J Biol Chem* 2001;276(47):44163-72.

Izzo, JG; Papadimitrakopoulou, VA; Li, XQ; Ibarguen, H; Lee, JS; Ro, JY, et al. Dysregulated cyclin D1 expression early in head and neck tumorigenesis: *in vivo* evidence for an association with subsequent gene amplification. *Oncogene* 1998;17(18):2313-22.

Jain, KK. Personalized medicine. *Curr Opin Mol Ther* 2002;4(6):548-58.

Jefferies, S; Foulkes, WD. Genetic mechanisms in squamous cell carcinoma of the head and neck. *Oral Oncol* 2001;37(2):115-26.

Johnstone, S; Logan, RM. The role of vascular endothelial growth factor (VEGF) in oral dysplasia and oral squamous cell carcinoma. *Oral Oncol* 2006;42(4):337-42.

Kaghad, M; Bonnet, H; Yang, A; Creancier, L; Biscan, JC; Valent, A, et al. Monoallelically expressed gene related to p53 at 1p36, a region frequently deleted in neuroblastoma and other human cancers. *Cell* 1997;90(4):809-19.

Kalish, LA; McKinlay, JB. Serum prostate-specific antigen levels (PSA) in men without clinical evidence of prostate cancer: age-specific reference ranges for total PSA, free PSA, and percent free PSA. *Urology* 1999;54(6):1022-7.

Kalyankrishna, S; Grandis, JR. Epidermal growth factor receptor biology in head and neck cancer. *J Clin Oncol* 2006;24(17):2666-72.

Kamijo, T; Zindy, F; Roussel, MF; Quelle, DE; Downing, JR; Ashmun, RA, et al. Tumor suppression at the mouse INK4a locus mediated by the alternative reading frame product p19ARF. *Cell* 1997;91(5):649-59.

Kang, MK; Park, NH. Conversion of normal to malignant phenotype: telomere shortening, telomerase activation, and genomic instability during immortalization of human oral keratinocytes. *Crit Rev Oral Biol Med* 2001;12(1):38-54.

Kang, P; Svoboda, KK. Epithelial-mesenchymal transformation during craniofacial development. *J Dent Res* 2005;84(8):678-90.

Kannan, S; Tahara, H; Yokozaki, H; Mathew, B; Nalinakumari, KR; Nair, MK, et al. Telomerase activity in premalignant and malignant lesions of human oral mucosa. *Cancer Epidemiol Biomarkers Prev* 1997;6(6):413-20.

Karn, J; Watson, JV; Lowe, AD; Green, SM; Vedeckis, W. Regulation of cell cycle duration by c-myc levels. *Oncogene* 1989;4(6):773-87.

Kato, H; Uzawa, K; Onda, T; Kato, Y; Saito, K; Nakashima, D, et al. Down-regulation of 1D-myo-inositol 1,4,5-trisphosphate 3-kinase A protein expression in oral squamous cell carcinoma. *Int J Oncol* 2006;28(4):873-81.

Kato, J; Matsushime, H; Hiebert, SW; Ewen, ME; Sherr, CJ. Direct binding of cyclin D to the retinoblastoma gene product (pRb) and pRb phosphorylation by the cyclin D-dependent kinase CDK4. *Genes Dev* 1993;7(3):331-42.

Kato, K; Hara, A; Kuno, T; Kitaori, N; Huilan, Z; Mori, H, et al. Matrix metalloproteinases 2 and 9 in oral squamous cell carcinomas: manifestation and localization of their activity. *J Cancer Res Clin Oncol* 2005;131(6):340-6.

Kawano, T; Yanoma, S; Nishimura, G; Tsukuda, M. The inhibitory effects of TNP470 on tumour growth of head and neck carcinoma cell producing interleukin-8. *J Laryngol Otol* 2001;115(10):802-7.

Kelly, K; Cochran, BH; Stiles, CD; Leder, P. Cell-specific regulation of the c-myc gene by lymphocyte mitogens and platelet-derived growth factor. *Cell* 1983;35(3 Pt 2):603-10.

Khuri, FR; Nemunaitis, J; Ganly, I; Arseneau, J; Tannock, IF; Romel, L, et al. a controlled trial of intratumoral ONYX-015, a selectively-replicating adenovirus, in combination with cisplatin and 5-fluorouracil in patients with recurrent head and neck cancer. *Nat Med* 2000;6(8):879-85.

Kilian, A; Bowtell, DD; Abud, HE; Hime, GR; Venter, DJ; Keese, PK, et al. Isolation of a candidate human telomerase catalytic subunit gene, which reveals complex splicing patterns in different cell types. *Hum Mol Genet* 1997;6(12):2011-9.

Kim, NW; Piatyszek, MA; Prowse, KR; Harley, CB; West, MD; Ho, PL, et al. Specific association of human telomerase activity with immortal cells and cancer. *Science* 1994;266(5193):2011-5.

Kim, SH; Cho, NH; Kim, K; Lee, JS; Koo, BS; Kim, JH, et al. Correlations of oral tongue cancer invasion with matrix metalloproteinases (MMPs) and vascular endothelial growth factor (VEGF) expression. *J Surg Oncol* 2006;93(4):330-7.

Kinugasa, Y; Hatori, M; Ito, H; Kurihara, Y; Ito, D; Nagumo, M. Inhibition of cyclooxygenase-2 suppresses invasiveness of oral squamous cell carcinoma cell lines via down-regulation of matrix metalloproteinase-2 and CD44. *Clin Exp Metastasis* 2004;21(8):737-45.

Kirk, KE; Harmon, BP; Reichardt, IK; Sedat, JW; Blackburn, EH. Block in anaphase chromosome separation caused by a telomerase template mutation. *Science* 1997;275(5305):1478-81.

Kiyota, A; Shintani, S; Mihara, M; Nakahara, Y; Ueyama, Y; Matsumura, T, et al. Anti-epidermal growth factor receptor monoclonal antibody 225 upregulates p27(KIP1) and p15(INK4B) and induces G1 arrest in oral squamous carcinoma cell lines. *Oncology* 2002;63(1):92-8.

Koike, H; Uzawa, K; Nakashima, D; Shimada, K; Kato, Y; Higo, M, et al. Identification of differentially expressed proteins in oral squamous cell carcinoma using a global proteomic approach. *Int J Oncol* 2005;27(1):59-67.

Kolch, W; Mischak, H; Pitt, AR. The molecular make-up of a tumour: proteomics in cancer research. *Clin Sci (Lond)* 2005;108(5):369-83.

Koscielny, S; Eggeling, F; Dahse, R; Fiedler, W. The influence of reactivation of the telomerase in tumour tissue on the prognosis of squamous cell carcinomas in the head and neck. *J Oral Pathol Med* 2004;33(9):538-42.

Kosunen, A; Pirinen, R; Ropponen, K; Pukkila, M; Kellokoski, J; Virtaniemi, J, et al. CD44 expression and its relationship with MMP-9, clinicopathological factors and survival in oral squamous cell carcinoma. *Oral Oncol* 2007;43(1):51-9.

Kovalev, S; Marchenko, N; Swendeman, S; LaQuaglia, M; Moll, UM. Expression level, allelic origin, and mutation analysis of the p73 gene in neuroblastoma tumors and cell lines. *Cell Growth Differ* 1998;9(11):897-903.

Kovesi, G; Szende, B. Prognostic value of cyclin D1, p27, and p63 in oral leukoplakia. *J Oral Pathol Med* 2006;35(5):274-7.

Kraus, MH; Fedi, P; Starks, V; Muraro, R; Aaronson, SA. Demonstration of ligand-dependent signaling by the erbB-3 tyrosine kinase and its constitutive activation in human breast tumor cells. *Proc Natl Acad Sci U S A* 1993;90(7):2900-4.

Kresty, LA; Mallery, SR; Knobloch, TJ; Song, H; Lloyd, M; Casto, BC, et al. Alterations of p16(INK4a) and p14(ARF) in patients with severe oral epithelial dysplasia. *Cancer Res* 2002;62(18):5295-300.

Kurahara, S; Shinohara, M; Ikebe, T; Nakamura, S; Beppu, M; Hiraki, A, et al. Expression of MMPS, MT-MMP, and TIMPs in squamous cell carcinoma of the oral cavity: correlations with tumor invasion and metastasis. *Head Neck* 1999;21(7):627-38.

Kwak, YE; Jeon, NK; Kim, J; Lee, EJ. The cyclooxygenase-2 selective inhibitor celecoxib suppresses proliferation and invasiveness in the human oral squamous carcinoma. *Ann N Y Acad Sci* 2007;1095:99-112.

Laimer, K; Spizzo, G; Gastl, G; Obrist, P; Brunhuber, T; Fong, D, et al. High EGFR expression predicts poor prognosis in patients with squamous cell carcinoma of the oral cavity and oropharynx: a TMA-based immunohistochemical analysis. *Oral Oncol* 2007;43(2):193-8.

Lalla, RV; Goralnick, SJ; Tanzer, ML; Kreutzer, DL. Fibrin induces IL-8 expression from human oral squamous cell carcinoma cells. *Oral Oncol* 2001;37(3):234-42.

Lane, DP. Cancer. p53, guardian of the genome. *Nature* 1992;358(6381):15-6.

Lane, DP; Crawford, LV. T antigen is bound to a host protein in SV40-transformed cells. *Nature* 1979;278(5701):261-3.

Larue, L; Bellacosa, A. Epithelial-mesenchymal transition in development and cancer: role of phosphatidylinositol 3' kinase/AKT pathways. *Oncogene* 2005;24(50):7443-54.

Lee, EJ; Whang, JH; Jeon, NK; Kim, J. The epidermal growth factor receptor tyrosine kinase inhibitor ZD1839 (Iressa) suppresses proliferation and invasion of human oral squamous carcinoma cells via p53 independent and MMP, uPAR dependent mechanism. *Ann N Y Acad Sci* 2007;1095:113-28.

Lee, WH; Bookstein, R; Lee, EY. Studies on the human retinoblastoma susceptibility gene. *J Cell Biochem* 1988;38(3):213-27.

Leethanakul, C; Patel, V; Gillespie, J; Pallente, M; Ensley, JF; Koontongkaew, S, et al. Distinct pattern of expression of differentiation and growth-related genes in squamous cell carcinomas of the head and neck revealed by the use of laser capture microdissection and cDNA arrays. *Oncogene* 2000;19(28):3220-4.

Leonard, JH; Kearsley, JH; Chenevix-Trench, G; Hayward, NK. Analysis of gene amplification in head-and-neck squamous-cell carcinoma. *Int J Cancer* 1991;48(4):511-5.

Levine, AE; Steffen, DL. OrCGDB: a database of genes involved in oral cancer. *Nucleic Acids Res* 2001;29(1):300-2.

Li, C; Shintani, S; Terakado, N; Klosek, SK; Ishikawa, T; Nakashiro, K, et al. Microvessel density and expression of vascular endothelial growth factor, basic fibroblast growth factor, and platelet-derived endothelial growth factor in oral squamous cell carcinomas. *Int J Oral Maxillofac Surg* 2005;34(5):559-65.

Liao, CT; Tung-Chieh Chang, J; Wang, HM; Chen, IH; Lin, CY; Chen, TM, et al. Telomerase as an independent prognostic factor in head and neck squamous cell carcinoma. *Head Neck* 2004;26(6):504-12.

Liao, J; Mitsuyasu, T; Yamane, K; Ohishi, M. Telomerase activity in oral and maxillofacial tumors. *Oral Oncol* 2000;36(4):347-52.

Lim, J; Kim, JH; Paeng, JY; Kim, MJ; Hong, SD; Lee, JI, et al. Prognostic value of activated Akt expression in oral squamous cell carcinoma. *J Clin Pathol* 2005;58(11):1199-205.

Lin, MH; Liu, SY; Su, HJ; Liu, YC. Functional role of matrix metalloproteinase-28 in the oral squamous cell carcinoma. *Oral Oncol* 2006;42(9):907-13.

Lindberg, P; Larsson, A; Nielsen, BS. Expression of plasminogen activator inhibitor-1, urokinase receptor and laminin gamma-2 chain is an early coordinated event in incipient oral squamous cell carcinoma. *Int J Cancer* 2006;118(12):2948-56.

Linzer, DI; Levine, AJ. Characterization of a 54K dalton cellular SV40 tumor antigen present in SV40-transformed cells and uninfected embryonal carcinoma cells. *Cell* 1979;17(1):43-52.

Lippman, SM; Hong, WK. Molecular markers of the risk of oral cancer. *N Engl J Med* 2001;344(17):1323-6.

Lipshutz, RJ; Fodor, SP; Gingeras, TR; Lockhart, DJ. High density synthetic oligonucleotide arrays. *Nat Genet* 1999;21(1 Suppl):20-4.

Liu, LK; Li, YN; Jiang, HB; He, ZX; Yi, XZ. [The correlation between neck lymphy node metastasis and matrixmetalloproteinase-2 expression at the invasive tumor front of oral squamous cell carcinomas]. *Hua Xi Kou Qiang Yi Xue Za Zhi* 2004;22(2):106-8.

Liu, SY; Liu, YC; Huang, WT; Huang, GC; Chen, TC; Lin, MH. Up-regulation of matrix metalloproteinase-8 by betel quid extract and arecoline and its role in 2D motility. *Oral Oncol* 2007.

Liu, TJ; Zhang, WW; Taylor, DL; Roth, JA; Goepfert, H; Clayman, GL. Growth suppression of human head and neck cancer cells by the introduction of a wild-type p53 gene via a recombinant adenovirus. *Cancer Res* 1994;54(14):3662-7.

Lo Muzio, L; Santarelli, A; Caltabiano, R; Rubini, C; Pieramici, T; Trevisiol, L, et al. p63 overexpression associates with poor prognosis in head and neck squamous cell carcinoma. *Hum Pathol* 2005;36(2):187-94.

Lo, WY; Tsai, MH; Tsai, Y; Hua, CH; Tsai, FJ; Huang, SY, et al. Identification of over-expressed proteins in oral squamous cell carcinoma (OSCC) patients by clinical proteomic analysis. *Clin Chim Acta* 2007;376(1-2):101-7.

Lodish, H; Berk, A; Zipursky, SL; Matsudaira, P; Baltimore, D; Darnell, J. Molecular Cell Biology. 4th Edition. New York: W.H. Freeman and Company, 2000.

Lorimer, IA. Mutant epidermal growth factor receptors as targets for cancer therapy. *Curr Cancer Drug Targets* 2002;2(2):91-102.

Lukas, J; Parry, D; Aagaard, L; Mann, DJ; Bartkova, J; Strauss, M, et al. Retinoblastoma-protein-dependent cell-cycle inhibition by the tumour suppressor p16. *Nature* 1995;375(6531):503-6.

Luscher, B; Larsson, LG. The basic region/helix-loop-helix/leucine zipper domain of Myc proto-oncoproteins: function and regulation. *Oncogene* 1999;18(19):2955-66.

Lydiatt, WM; Anderson, PE; Bazzana, T; Casale, M; Hughes, CJ; Huvos, AG, et al. Molecular support for field cancerization in the head and neck. *Cancer* 1998;82(7):1376-80.

Maestro, R; Gasparotto, D; Vukosavljevic, T; Barzan, L; Sulfaro, S; Boiocchi, M. Three discrete regions of deletion at 3p in head and neck cancers. *Cancer Res* 1993;53(23):5775-9.

Maestro, R; Piccinin, S; Doglioni, C; Gasparotto, D; Vukosavljevic, T; Sulfaro, S, et al. Chromosome 13q deletion mapping in head and neck squamous cell carcinomas:

identification of two distinct regions of preferential loss. *Cancer Res* 1996;56(5):1146-50.

Magne, N; Fischel, JL; Dubreuil, A; Formento, P; Marcie, S; Lagrange, JL, et al. Sequence-dependent effects of ZD1839 ('Iressa') in combination with cytotoxic treatment in human head and neck cancer. *Br J Cancer* 2002;86(5):819-27.

Magne, N; Fischel, JL; Dubreuil, A; Formento, P; Poupon, MF; Laurent-Puig, P, et al. Influence of epidermal growth factor receptor (EGFR), p53 and intrinsic MAP kinase pathway status of tumour cells on the antiproliferative effect of ZD1839 ("Iressa"). *Br J Cancer* 2002;86(9):1518-23.

Mai, M; Yokomizo, A; Qian, C; Yang, P; Tindall, DJ; Smith, DI, et al. Activation of p73 silent allele in lung cancer. *Cancer Res* 1998;58(11):2347-9.

Malik, SN; Brattain, M; Ghosh, PM; Troyer, DA; Prihoda, T; Bedolla, R, et al. Immunohistochemical demonstration of phospho-Akt in high Gleason grade prostate cancer. *Clin Cancer Res* 2002;8(4):1168-71.

Malkin, D; Li, FP; Strong, LC; Fraumeni, JF, Jr.; Nelson, CE; Kim, DH, et al. Germ line p53 mutations in a familial syndrome of breast cancer, sarcomas, and other neoplasms. *Science* 1990;250(4985):1233-8.

Mao, L; Lee, DJ; Tockman, MS; Erozan, YS; Askin, F; Sidransky, D. Microsatellite alterations as clonal markers for the detection of human cancer. *Proc Natl Acad Sci U S A* 1994;91(21):9871-5.

Mao, L; Lee, JS; Fan, YH; Ro, JY; Batsakis, JG; Lippman, S, et al. Frequent microsatellite alterations at chromosomes 9p21 and 3p14 in oral premalignant lesions and their value in cancer risk assessment. *Nat Med* 1996;2(6):682-5.

Mao, L; Merlo, A; Bedi, G; Shapiro, GI; Edwards, CD; Rollins, BJ, et al. A novel p16INK4A transcript. *Cancer Res* 1995;55(14):2995-7.

Markert, JM; Parker, JN; Buchsbaum, DJ; Grizzle, WE; Gillespie, GY; Whitley, RJ. Oncolytic HSV-1 for the treatment of brain tumours. *Herpes* 2006;13(3):66-71.

Massarelli, E; Liu, DD; Lee, JJ; El-Naggar, AK; Lo Muzio, L; Staibano, S, et al. Akt activation correlates with adverse outcome in tongue cancer. *Cancer* 2005;104(11):2430-6.

Matheny, KE; Barbieri, CE; Sniezek, JC; Arteaga, CL; Pietenpol, JA. Inhibition of epidermal growth factor receptor signaling decreases p63 expression in head and neck squamous carcinoma cells. *Laryngoscope* 2003;113(6):936-9.

Matsushime, H; Quelle, DE; Shurtleff, SA; Shibuya, M; Sherr, CJ; Kato, JY. D-type cyclin-dependent kinase activity in mammalian cells. *Mol Cell Biol* 1994;14(3):2066-76.

McCormick, F. Cancer-specific viruses and the development of ONYX-015. *Cancer Biol Ther* 2003;2(4 Suppl 1):S157-60.

McCormick, F. Interactions between adenovirus proteins and the p53 pathway: the development of ONYX-015. *Semin Cancer Biol* 2000;10(6):453-9.

McKenzie, KE; Siva, A; Maier, S; Runnebaum, IB; Seshadri, R; Sukumar, S. Altered WAF1 genes do not play a role in abnormal cell cycle regulation in breast cancers lacking p53 mutations. *Clin Cancer Res* 1997;3(9):1669-73.

Medema, RH; Herrera, RE; Lam, F; Weinberg, RA. Growth suppression by p16ink4 requires functional retinoblastoma protein. *Proc Natl Acad Sci U S A* 1995;92(14):6289-93.

Mendez, MA; Hodar, C; Vulpe, C; Gonzalez, M; Cambiazo, V. Discriminant analysis to evaluate clustering of gene expression data. *FEBS Lett* 2002;522(1-3):24-8.

Meyerson, M; Harlow, E. Identification of G1 kinase activity for cdk6, a novel cyclin D partner. *Mol Cell Biol* 1994;14(3):2077-86.

Mittnacht, S. Control of pRB phosphorylation. *Curr Opin Genet Dev* 1998;8(1):21-7.

Mohan, S; Epstein, JB. Carcinogenesis and cyclooxygenase: the potential role of COX-2 inhibition in upper aerodigestive tract cancer. *Oral Oncol* 2003;39(6):537-46.

Moll, UM; Slade, N. p63 and p73: roles in development and tumor formation. *Mol Cancer Res* 2004;2(7):371-86.

Momand, J; Zambetti, GP; Olson, DC; George, D; Levine, AJ. The mdm-2 oncogene product forms a complex with the p53 protein and inhibits p53-mediated transactivation. *Cell* 1992;69(7):1237-45.

Moon, C; Oh, Y; Roth, JA. Current status of gene therapy for lung cancer and head and neck cancer. *Clin Cancer Res* 2003;9(14):5055-67.

Moraitis, D; Du, B; De Lorenzo, MS; Boyle, JO; Weksler, BB; Cohen, EG, et al. Levels of cyclooxygenase-2 are increased in the oral mucosa of smokers: evidence for the role of epidermal growth factor receptor and its ligands. *Cancer Res* 2005;65(2):664-70.

Morgan, DO. Principles of CDK regulation. *Nature* 1995;374(6518):131-4.

Morin, GB. The human telomere terminal transferase enzyme is a ribonucleoprotein that synthesizes TTAGGG repeats. *Cell* 1989;59(3):521-9.

Moriyama, M; Kumagai, S; Kawashiri, S; Kojima, K; Kakihara, K; Yamamoto, E. Immunohistochemical study of tumour angiogenesis in oral squamous cell carcinoma. *Oral Oncol* 1997;33(5):369-74.

Moustakas, A; Pardali, K; Gaal, A; Heldin, CH. Mechanisms of TGF-beta signaling in regulation of cell growth and differentiation. *Immunol Lett* 2002;82(1-2):85-91.

Muro-Cacho, CA; Rosario-Ortiz, K; Livingston, S; Munoz-Antonia, T. Defective transforming growth factor beta signaling pathway in head and neck squamous cell carcinoma as evidenced by the lack of expression of activated Smad2. *Clin Cancer Res* 2001;7(6):1618-26.

Mutirangura, A; Supiyaphun, P; Trirekapan, S; Sriuranpong, V; Sakuntabhai, A; Yenrudi, S, et al. Telomerase activity in oral leukoplakia and head and neck squamous cell carcinoma. *Cancer Res* 1996;56(15):3530-3.

Myoung, H; Hong, SP; Yun, PY; Lee, JH; Kim, MJ. Anti-cancer effect of genistein in oral squamous cell carcinoma with respect to angiogenesis and *in vitro* invasion. *Cancer Sci* 2003;94(2):215-20.

Myoung, H; Kim, MJ; Hong, SD; Lee, JI; Lim, CY; Hong, SP. Expression of membrane type I-matrix metalloproteinase in oral squamous cell carcinoma. *Cancer Lett* 2002;185(2):201-9.

Nagatake, M; Takagi, Y; Osada, H; Uchida, K; Mitsudomi, T; Saji, S, et al. Somatic *in vivo* alterations of the DPC4 gene at 18q21 in human lung cancers. *Cancer Res* 1996;56(12):2718-20.

Nakayama, H; Ikebe, T; Beppu, M; Shirasuna, K. High expression levels of nuclear factor kappaB, IkappaB kinase alpha and Akt kinase in squamous cell carcinoma of the oral cavity. *Cancer* 2001;92(12):3037-44.

Natsugoe, S; Xiangming, C; Matsumoto, M; Okumura, H; Nakashima, S; Sakita, H, et al. Smad4 and transforming growth factor beta1 expression in patients with squamous cell carcinoma of the esophagus. *Clin Cancer Res* 2002;8(6):1838-42.

Nawroz, H; Koch, W; Anker, P; Stroun, M; Sidransky, D. Microsatellite alterations in serum DNA of head and neck cancer patients. *Nat Med* 1996;2(9):1035-7.

Nawroz, H; van der Riet, P; Hruban, RH; Koch, W; Ruppert, JM; Sidransky, D. Allelotype of head and neck squamous cell carcinoma. *Cancer Res* 1994;54(5):1152-5.

Nemes, JA; Nemes, Z; Marton, IJ. p21WAF1/CIP1 expression is a marker of poor prognosis in oral squamous cell carcinoma. *J Oral Pathol Med* 2005;34(5):274-9.

Neves Ada, C; Mesquita, RA; Novelli, MD; Toddai, E; De Sousa, SO. Comparison between immunohistochemical expression of cyclin D1 and p21 and histological malignancy graduation of oral squamous cell carcinomas. *Braz Dent J* 2004;15(2):93-8.

Noda, A; Ning, Y; Venable, SF; Pereira-Smith, OM; Smith, JR. Cloning of senescent cell-derived inhibitors of DNA synthesis using an expression screen. *Exp Cell Res* 1994;211(1):90-8.

Oku, N; Sasabe, E; Ueta, E; Yamamoto, T; Osaki, T. Tight junction protein claudin-1 enhances the invasive activity of oral squamous cell carcinoma cells by promoting cleavage of laminin-5 gamma2 chain via matrix metalloproteinase (MMP)-2 and membrane-type MMP-1. *Cancer Res* 2006;66(10):5251-7.

Onoue, T; Uchida, D; Begum, NM; Tomizuka, Y; Yoshida, H; Sato, M. Epithelial-mesenchymal transition induced by the stromal cell-derived factor-1/CXCR4 system in oral squamous cell carcinoma cells. *Int J Oncol* 2006;29(5):1133-8.

Oren, M. Regulation of the p53 tumor suppressor protein. *J Biol Chem* 1999;274(51):36031-4.

Otterson, GA; Khleif, SN; Chen, W; Coxon, AB; Kaye, FJ. CDKN2 gene silencing in lung cancer by DNA hypermethylation and kinetics of p16INK4 protein induction by 5-aza 2'deoxycytidine. *Oncogene* 1995;11(6):1211-6.

Pai, R; Soreghan, B; Szabo, IL; Pavelka, M; Baatar, D; Tarnawski, AS. Prostaglandin E2 transactivates EGF receptor: a novel mechanism for promoting colon cancer growth and gastrointestinal hypertrophy. *Nat Med* 2002;8(3):289-93.

Papadimitrakopoulou, V; Izzo, J; Lippman, SM; Lee, JS; Fan, YH; Clayman, G, et al. Frequent inactivation of p16INK4a in oral premalignant lesions. *Oncogene* 1997;14(15):1799-803.

Papadimitrakopoulou, VA; Izzo, J; Mao, L; Keck, J; Hamilton, D; Shin, DM, et al. Cyclin D1 and p16 alterations in advanced premalignant lesions of the upper aerodigestive tract: role in response to chemoprevention and cancer development. *Clin Cancer Res* 2001;7(10):3127-34.

Parkin, DM; Pisani, P; Ferlay, J. Estimates of the worldwide incidence of eighteen major cancers in 1985. *Int J Cancer* 1993;54(4):594-606.

Patel, V; Leethanakul, C; Gutkind, JS. New approaches to the understanding of the molecular basis of oral cancer. *Crit Rev Oral Biol Med* 2001;12(1):55-63.

Patel, V; Senderowicz, AM; Pinto, D, Jr.; Igishi, T; Raffeld, M; Quintanilla-Martinez, L, et al. Flavopiridol, a novel cyclin-dependent kinase inhibitor, suppresses the growth of head and neck squamous cell carcinomas by inducing apoptosis. *J Clin Invest* 1998;102(9):1674-81.

Pattamapun, K; Iamaroon, A. Overexpression of IPO-38 and telomerase in oral squamous cell carcinoma. *J Dent Res* 2004;83(Spec Iss A):4045.

Paweletz, CP; Liotta, LA; Petricoin, EF, 3rd. New technologies for biomarker analysis of prostate cancer progression: Laser capture microdissection and tissue proteomics. *Urology* 2001;57(4 Suppl 1):160-3.

Pearson, S; Jia, H; Kandachi, K. China approves first gene therapy. *Nat Biotechnol* 2004;22(1):3-4.

Peng, H; Shintani, S; Kim, Y; Wong, DT. Loss of p12CDK2-AP1 expression in human oral squamous cell carcinoma with disrupted transforming growth factor-beta-Smad signaling pathway. *Neoplasia* 2006;8(12):1028-36.

Piard, F; Chapusot, C; Ecarnot-Laubriet, A; Ponnelle, T; Martin, L. Molecular markers of heterogeneity in colorectal cancers and adenomas. *Eur J Cancer Prev* 2002;11(1):85-97.

Piattelli, A; Fioroni, M; Iezzi, G; Perrotti, V; Stellini, E; Piattelli, M, et al. CD10 expression in stromal cells of oral cavity squamous cell carcinoma: a clinic and pathologic correlation. *Oral Dis* 2006;12(3):301-4.

Piboonniyom, SO; Duensing, S; Swilling, NW; Hasskarl, J; Hinds, PW; Munger, K. Abrogation of the retinoblastoma tumor suppressor checkpoint during keratinocyte immortalization is not sufficient for induction of centrosome-mediated genomic instability. *Cancer Res* 2003;63(2):476-83.

Piboonniyom, SO; Timmermann, S; Hinds, P; Munger, K. Aberrations in the MTS1 tumor suppressor locus in oral squamous cell carcinoma lines preferentially affect the INK4A gene and result in increased cdk6 activity. *Oral Oncol* 2002;38(2):179-86.

Pietras, RJ; Arboleda, J; Reese, DM; Wongvipat, N; Pegram, MD; Ramos, L, et al. HER-2 tyrosine kinase pathway targets estrogen receptor and promotes hormone-independent growth in human breast cancer cells. *Oncogene* 1995;10(12):2435-46.

Plowman, GD; Whitney, GS; Neubauer, MG; Green, JM; McDonald, VL; Todaro, GJ, et al. Molecular cloning and expression of an additional epidermal growth factor receptor-related gene. *Proc Natl Acad Sci U S A* 1990;87(13):4905-9.

Pollack, VA; Savage, DM; Baker, DA; Tsaparikos, KE; Sloan, DE; Moyer, JD, et al. Inhibition of epidermal growth factor receptor-associated tyrosine phosphorylation in human carcinomas with CP-358,774: dynamics of receptor inhibition in situ and antitumor effects in athymic mice. *J Pharmacol Exp Ther* 1999;291(2):739-48.

Pollock, PM; Pearson, JV; Hayward, NK. Compilation of somatic mutations of the CDKN2 gene in human cancers: non-random distribution of base substitutions. *Genes Chromosomes Cancer* 1996;15(2):77-88.

Poremba, C; Bocker, W; Willenbring, H; Schafer, KL; Otterbach, F; Burger, H, et al. Telomerase activity in human proliferative breast lesions. *Int J Oncol* 1998;12(3):641-8.

Pouliot, F; Labrie, C. Expression profile of agonistic Smads in human breast cancer cells: absence of regulation by estrogens. *Int J Cancer* 1999;81(1):98-103.

Prime, SS; Davies, M; Pring, M; Paterson, IC. The role of TGF-beta in epithelial malignancy and its relevance to the pathogenesis of oral cancer (part II). *Crit Rev Oral Biol Med* 2004;15(6):337-47.

Quelle, DE; Zindy, F; Ashmun, RA; Sherr, CJ. Alternative reading frames of the INK4a tumor suppressor gene encode two unrelated proteins capable of inducing cell cycle arrest. *Cell* 1995;83(6):993-1000.

Ranson, M; Hammond, LA; Ferry, D; Kris, M; Tullo, A; Murray, PI, et al. ZD1839, a selective oral epidermal growth factor receptor-tyrosine kinase inhibitor, is well tolerated and active in patients with solid, malignant tumors: results of a phase I trial. *J Clin Oncol* 2002;20(9):2240-50.

Reed, AL; Califano, J; Cairns, P; Westra, WH; Jones, RM; Koch, W, et al. High frequency of p16 (CDKN2/MTS-1/INK4A) inactivation in head and neck squamous cell carcinoma. *Cancer Res* 1996;56(16):3630-3.

Reinacher-Schick, A; Baldus, SE; Romdhana, B; Landsberg, S; Zapatka, M; Monig, SP, et al. Loss of Smad4 correlates with loss of the invasion suppressor E-cadherin in advanced colorectal carcinomas. *J Pathol* 2004;202(4):412-20.

Robert, F; Ezekiel, MP; Spencer, SA; Meredith, RF; Bonner, JA; Khazaeli, MB, et al. Phase I study of anti--epidermal growth factor receptor antibody cetuximab in combination with radiation therapy in patients with advanced head and neck cancer. *J Clin Oncol* 2001;19(13):3234-43.

Rocco, JW; Li, D; Liggett, WH, Jr.; Duan, L; Saunders, JK, Jr.; Sidransky, D, et al. p16INK4A adenovirus-mediated gene therapy for human head and neck squamous cell cancer. *Clin Cancer Res* 1998;4(7):1697-704.

Rodriguez-Pinilla, SM; Jones, RL; Lambros, MB; Arriola, E; Savage, K; James, M, et al. MYC amplification in breast cancer: a chromogenic in situ hybridisation study. *J Clin Pathol* 2006.

Roepman, P; Wessels, LF; Kettelarij, N; Kemmeren, P; Miles, AJ; Lijnzaad, P, et al. An expression profile for diagnosis of lymph node metastases from primary head and neck squamous cell carcinomas. *Nat Genet* 2005;37(2):182-6.

Roninson, IB. Oncogenic functions of tumour suppressor p21(Waf1/Cip1/Sdi1): association with cell senescence and tumour-promoting activities of stromal fibroblasts. *Cancer Lett* 2002;179(1):1-14.

Rosas, SL; Koch, W; da Costa Carvalho, MG; Wu, L; Califano, J; Westra, W, et al. Promoter hypermethylation patterns of p16, O6-methylguanine-DNA-methyltransferase, and death-associated protein kinase in tumors and saliva of head and neck cancer patients. *Cancer Res* 2001;61(3):939-42.

Roth, J; Dobbelstein, M; Freedman, DA; Shenk, T; Levine, AJ. Nucleo-cytoplasmic shuttling of the hdm2 oncoprotein regulates the levels of the p53 protein via a pathway used by the human immunodeficiency virus rev protein. *Embo J* 1998;17(2):554-64.

Rous, P. A transmissible avian neoplasm. (Sarcoma of the common fowl) by Peyton Rous, M.D., Experimental Medicine for Sept. 1, 1910, vol. 12, pp.696-705. *J Exp Med* 1979;150(4):738-53.

Rubin Grandis, J; Melhem, MF; Gooding, WE; Day, R; Holst, VA; Wagener, MM, et al. Levels of TGF-alpha and EGFR protein in head and neck squamous cell carcinoma and patient survival. *J Natl Cancer Inst* 1998;90(11):824-32.

Rundhaug, JE. Matrix metalloproteinases and angiogenesis. *J Cell Mol Med* 2005;9(2):267-85.

Saleh, S; King-Yin Lam, A; Gertraud Buettner, P; Glasby, M; Raasch, B; Ho, YH. Telomerase activity of basal cell carcinoma in patients living in North Queensland, Australia. *Hum Pathol* 2007.

Sato, JD; Kawamoto, T; Le, AD; Mendelsohn, J; Polikoff, J; Sato, GH. Biological effects *in vitro* of monoclonal antibodies to human epidermal growth factor receptors. *Mol Biol Med* 1983;1(5):511-29.

Schechter, AL; Hung, MC; Vaidyanathan, L; Weinberg, RA; Yang-Feng, TL; Francke, U, et al. The neu gene: an erbB-homologous gene distinct from and unlinked to the gene encoding the EGF receptor. *Science* 1985;229(4717):976-8.

Schmale, H; Bamberger, C. A novel protein with strong homology to the tumor suppressor p53. *Oncogene* 1997;15(11):1363-7.

Schneider, G; Schmid, RM. Genetic alterations in pancreatic carcinoma. *Mol Cancer* 2003;2:15.

Schreiber, AB; Lax, I; Yarden, Y; Eshhar, Z; Schlessinger, J. Monoclonal antibodies against receptor for epidermal growth factor induce early and delayed effects of epidermal growth factor. *Proc Natl Acad Sci U S A* 1981;78(12):7535-9.

Scully, C; Field, JK; Tanzawa, H. Genetic aberrations in oral or head and neck squamous cell carcinoma 2: chromosomal aberrations. *Oral Oncol* 2000;36(4):311-27.

Scully, C; Field, JK; Tanzawa, H. Genetic aberrations in oral or head and neck squamous cell carcinoma (SCCHN): 1. Carcinogen metabolism, DNA repair and cell cycle control. *Oral Oncol* 2000;36(3):256-63.

Sebastian, S; Grammatica, L; Paradiso, A. Telomeres, telomerase and oral cancer (Review). *Int J Oncol* 2005;27(6):1583-96.

Shang, ZJ; Li, ZB; Li, JR. VEGF is up-regulated by hypoxic stimulation and related to tumour angiogenesis and severity of disease in oral squamous cell carcinoma: *in vitro* and *in vivo* studies. *Int J Oral Maxillofac Surg* 2006;35(6):533-8.

Sharpless, NE; DePinho, RA. The INK4A/ARF locus and its two gene products. *Curr Opin Genet Dev* 1999;9(1):22-30.

Shay, JW; Wright, WE. Quantitation of the frequency of immortalization of normal human diploid fibroblasts by SV40 large T-antigen. *Exp Cell Res* 1989;184(1):109-18.

Shay, JW; Wright, WE. Senescence and immortalization: role of telomeres and telomerase. *Carcinogenesis* 2005;26(5):867-74.

Sheiness, D; Bishop, JM. DNA and RNA from uninfected vertebrate cells contain nucleotide sequences related to the putative transforming gene of avian myelocytomatosis virus. *J Virol* 1979;31(2):514-21.

Sherr, CJ; Roberts, JM. Inhibitors of mammalian G1 cyclin-dependent kinases. *Genes Dev* 1995;9(10):1149-63.

Shillitoe, EJ; May, M; Patel, V; Lethanakul, C; Ensley, JF; Strausberg, RL, et al. Genome-wide analysis of oral cancer--early results from the Cancer Genome Anatomy Project. *Oral Oncol* 2000;36(1):8-16.

Shin, DM; Ro, JY; Hong, WK; Hittelman, WN. Dysregulation of epidermal growth factor receptor expression in premalignant lesions during head and neck tumorigenesis. *Cancer Res* 1994;54(12):3153-9.

Shintani, S; Kiyota, A; Mihara, M; Sumida, T; Kayahara, H; Nakashiro, K, et al. Enhancement of radiosensitivity in head and neck cancer cells by ZD1839 ('IRESSA'), a selective epidermal growth factor receptor tyrosine kinase inhibitor. *Am J Clin Oncol* 2003;26(5):e150-6.

Shintani, S; Li, C; Mihara, M; Klosek, SK; Terakado, N; Hino, S, et al. Anti-tumor effect of radiation response by combined treatment with angiogenesis inhibitor, TNP-470, in oral squamous cell carcinoma. *Oral Oncol* 2006;42(1):66-72.

Shiohara, M; el-Dciry, WS; Wada, M; Nakamaki, T; Takeuchi, S; Yang, R, et al. Absence of WAF1 mutations in a variety of human malignancies. *Blood* 1994;84(11):3781-4.

Shoemaker, DD; Lashkari, DA; Morris, D; Mittmann, M; Davis, RW. Quantitative phenotypic analysis of yeast deletion mutants using a highly parallel molecular bar-coding strategy. *Nat Genet* 1996;14(4):450-6.

Sicinski, P; Donaher, JL; Parker, SB; Li, T; Fazeli, A; Gardner, H, et al. Cyclin D1 provides a link between development and oncogenesis in the retina and breast. *Cell* 1995;82(4):621-30.

Sidransky, D. Emerging molecular markers of cancer. *Nat Rev Cancer* 2002;2(3):210-9.

Sini, P; Wyder, L; Schnell, C; O'Reilly, T; Littlewood, A; Brandt, R, et al. The antitumor and antiangiogenic activity of vascular endothelial growth factor receptor inhibition is potentiated by ErbB1 blockade. *Clin Cancer Res* 2005;11(12):4521-32.

Siriwardena, B; Kudo, Y; Ogawa, I; Udagama, K; Tilakaratne, WM; Takata, T. VEGF-C is associated with lymphatic status and invasion in oral cancer. *J Clin Pathol* 2007.

Smith, BD; Smith, GL; Carter, D; Sasaki, CT; Haffty, BG. Prognostic significance of vascular endothelial growth factor protein levels in oral and oropharyngeal squamous cell carcinoma. *J Clin Oncol* 2000;18(10):2046-52.

Soni, S; Kaur, J; Kumar, A; Chakravarti, N; Mathur, M; Bahadur, S, et al. Alterations of rb pathway components are frequent events in patients with oral epithelial dysplasia and predict clinical outcome in patients with squamous cell carcinoma. *Oncology* 2005;68(4-6):314-25.

Sorrentino, V; Drozdoff, V; McKinney, MD; Zeitz, L; Fleissner, E. Potentiation of growth factor activity by exogenous c-myc expression. *Proc Natl Acad Sci U S A* 1986;83(21):8167-71.

Soulieres, D; Senzer, NN; Vokes, EE; Hidalgo, M; Agarwala, SS; Siu, LL. Multicenter phase II study of erlotinib, an oral epidermal growth factor receptor tyrosine kinase inhibitor, in patients with recurrent or metastatic squamous cell cancer of the head and neck. *J Clin Oncol* 2004;22(1):77-85.

Spafford, MF; Koch, WM; Reed, AL; Califano, JA; Xu, LH; Eisenberger, CF, et al. Detection of head and neck squamous cell carcinoma among exfoliated oral mucosal cells by microsatellite analysis. *Clin Cancer Res* 2001;7(3):607-12.

Stanton, P; Richards, S; Reeves, J; Nikolic, M; Edington, K; Clark, L, et al. Epidermal growth factor receptor expression by human squamous cell carcinomas of the head and neck, cell lines and xenografts. *Br J Cancer* 1994;70(3):427-33.

Stern, DF; Roberts, AB; Roche, NS; Sporn, MB; Weinberg, RA. Differential responsiveness of myc- and ras-transfected cells to growth factors: selective stimulation of myc-transfected cells by epidermal growth factor. *Mol Cell Biol* 1986;6(3):870-7.

Strauss, L; Volland, D; Guerrero, A; Reichert, T. [Antiangiogenic and anti-immunosuppressive therapeutic strategies in human head and neck squamous cell carcinoma (HNSCC)]. *Mund Kiefer Gesichtschir* 2005;9(5):273-81.

Sundelin, K; Roberg, K; Grenman, R; Hakansson, L. Effects of cytokines on matrix metalloproteinase expression in oral squamous cell carcinoma *in vitro*. *Acta Otolaryngol* 2005;125(7):765-73.

Suzuki-Takahashi, I; Kitagawa, M; Saijo, M; Higashi, H; Ogino, H; Matsumoto, H, et al. The interactions of E2F with pRB and with p107 are regulated via the phosphorylation of pRB and p107 by a cyclin-dependent kinase. *Oncogene* 1995;10(9):1691-8.

Symonds, H; Krall, L; Remington, L; Saenz Robles, M; Jacks, T; Van Dyke, T. p53-dependent apoptosis *in vivo*: impact of p53 inactivation on tumorigenesis. *Cold Spring Harb Symp Quant Biol* 1994;59:247-57.

Tahara, H; Kuniyasu, H; Yokozaki, H; Yasui, W; Shay, JW; Ide, T, et al. Telomerase activity in preneoplastic and neoplastic gastric and colorectal lesions. *Clin Cancer Res* 1995;1(11):1245-51.

Takakura, S; Okamoto, A; Saito, M; Yasuhara, T; Shinozaki, H; Isonishi, S, et al. Allelic imbalance in chromosome band 18q21 and SMAD4 mutations in ovarian cancers. *Genes Chromosomes Cancer* 1999;24(3):264-71.

Tascilar, M; Skinner, HG; Rosty, C; Sohn, T; Wilentz, RE; Offerhaus, GJ, et al. The SMAD4 protein and prognosis of pancreatic ductal adenocarcinoma. *Clin Cancer Res* 2001;7(12):4115-21.

Thomas, GJ; Nystrom, ML; Marshall, JF. Alphavbeta6 integrin in wound healing and cancer of the oral cavity. *J Oral Pathol Med* 2006;35(1):1-10.

Timmermann, S; Hinds, PW; Munger, K. Re-expression of endogenous p16ink4a in oral squamous cell carcinoma lines by 5-aza-2'-deoxycytidine treatment induces a senescence-like state. *Oncogene* 1998;17(26):3445-53.

Tsuzuki, H; Fujieda, S; Sunaga, H; Narita, N; Tokuriki, M; Saito, H. Expression of p27 and apoptosis in oral leukoplakia. *Anticancer Res* 2003;23(2B):1265-70.

Tuszynski, GP; Wang, TN; Berger, D. Adhesive proteins and the hematogenous spread of cancer. *Acta Haematol* 1997;97(1-2):29-39.

Ulaner, GA; Hu, JF; Vu, TH; Giudice, LC; Hoffman, AR. Telomerase activity in human development is regulated by human telomerase reverse transcriptase (hTERT) transcription and by alternate splicing of hTERT transcripts. *Cancer Res* 1998;58(18):4168-72.

Uzawa, K; Suzuki, H; Komiya, A; Nakanishi, H; Ogawara, K; Tanzawa, H, et al. Evidence for two distinct tumor-suppressor gene loci on the long arm of chromosome 11 in human oral cancer. *Int J Cancer* 1996;67(4):510-4.

Vairaktaris, E; Ragos, V; Yapijakis, C; Derka, S; Vassiliou, S; Nkenke, E, et al. FGFR-2 and -3 play an important role in initial stages of oral oncogenesis. *Anticancer Res* 2006;26(6B):4217-21.

van der Riet, P; Nawroz, H; Hruban, RH; Corio, R; Tokino, K; Koch, W, et al. Frequent loss of chromosome 9p21-22 early in head and neck cancer progression. *Cancer Res* 1994;54(5):1156-8.

Vaziri, H; West, MD; Allsopp, RC; Davison, TS; Wu, YS; Arrowsmith, CH, et al. ATM-dependent telomere loss in aging human diploid fibroblasts and DNA damage lead to the post-translational activation of p53 protein involving poly(ADP-ribose) polymerase. *Embo J* 1997;16(19):6018-33.

Vidal, MJ; Loganzo, F, Jr.; de Oliveira, AR; Hayward, NK; Albino, AP. Mutations and defective expression of the WAF1 p21 tumour-suppressor gene in malignant melanomas. *Melanoma Res* 1995;5(4):243-50.

Vivanco, I; Sawyers, CL. The phosphatidylinositol 3-Kinase AKT pathway in human cancer. *Nat Rev Cancer* 2002;2(7):489-501.

Waga, S; Hannon, GJ; Beach, D; Stillman, B. The p21 inhibitor of cyclin-dependent kinases controls DNA replication by interaction with PCNA. *Nature* 1994;369(6481):574-8.

Watanabe, H; Iwase, M; Ohashi, M; Nagumo, M. Role of interleukin-8 secreted from human oral squamous cell carcinoma cell lines. *Oral Oncol* 2002;38(7):670-9.

Weber, A; Bellmann, U; Bootz, F; Wittekind, C; Tannapfel, A. Expression of p53 and its homologues in primary and recurrent squamous cell carcinomas of the head and neck. *Int J Cancer* 2002;99(1):22-8.

Weinberg, RA. The retinoblastoma protein and cell cycle control. *Cell* 1995;81(3):323-30.

Weinrich, SL; Pruzan, R; Ma, L; Ouellette, M; Tesmer, VM; Holt, SE, et al. Reconstitution of human telomerase with the template RNA component hTR and the catalytic protein subunit hTRT. *Nat Genet* 1997;17(4):498-502.

West, J; Munoz-Antonia, T; Johnson, JG; Klotch, D; Muro-Cacho, CA. Transforming growth factor-beta type II receptors and smad proteins in follicular thyroid tumors. *Laryngoscope* 2000;110(8):1323-7.

Wick, ST; Dubay, MM; Imanil, I; Brizuela, L. Biochemical and mutagenic analysis of the melanoma tumor suppressor gene product/p16. *Oncogene* 1995;11(10):2013-9.

Williams, HK. Molecular pathogenesis of oral squamous carcinoma. *Mol Pathol* 2000;53(4):165-72.

Wolfel, T; Hauer, M; Schneider, J; Serrano, M; Wolfel, C; Klehmann-Hieb, E, et al. A p16INK4a-insensitive CDK4 mutant targeted by cytolytic T lymphocytes in a human melanoma. *Science* 1995;269(5228):1281-4.

Won, KA; Xiong, Y; Beach, D; Gilman, MZ. Growth-regulated expression of D-type cyclin genes in human diploid fibroblasts. *Proc Natl Acad Sci U S A* 1992;89(20):9910-4.

Wright, WE; Pereira-Smith, OM; Shay, JW. Reversible cellular senescence: implications for immortalization of normal human diploid fibroblasts. *Mol Cell Biol* 1989;9(7):3088-92.

Xi, S; Grandis, JR. Gene therapy for the treatment of oral squamous cell carcinoma. *J Dent Res* 2003;82(1):11-6.

Xia, W; Lau, YK; Zhang, HZ; Xiao, FY; Johnston, DA; Liu, AR, et al. Combination of EGFR, HER-2/neu, and HER-3 is a stronger predictor for the outcome of oral squamous cell carcinoma than any individual family members. *Clin Cancer Res* 1999;5(12):4164-74.

Xie, W; Bharathy, S; Kim, D; Haffty, BG; Rimm, DL; Reiss, M. Frequent alterations of Smad signaling in human head and neck squamous cell carcinomas: a tissue microarray analysis. *Oncol Res* 2003;14(2):61-73.

Xie, X; Clausen, OP; Boysen, M. Prognostic significance of p21WAF1/CIP1 expression in tongue squamous cell carcinomas. *Arch Otolaryngol Head Neck Surg* 2002;128(8):897-902.

Xie, Y; Pendergast, AM; Hung, MC. Dominant-negative mutants of Grb2 induced reversal of the transformed phenotypes caused by the point mutation-activated rat HER-2/Neu. *J Biol Chem* 1995;270(51):30717-24.

Xiong, Y; Hannon, GJ; Zhang, H; Casso, D; Kobayashi, R; Beach, D. p21 is a universal inhibitor of cyclin kinases. *Nature* 1993;366(6456):701-4.

Yanamoto, S; Kawasaki, G; Yoshitomi, I; Mizuno, A. p53, mdm2, and p21 expression in oral squamous cell carcinomas: relationship with clinicopathologic factors. *Oral Surg Oral Med Oral Pathol Oral Radiol Endod* 2002;94(5):593-600.

Yang, A; Kaghad, M; Wang, Y; Gillett, E; Fleming, MD; Dotsch, V, et al. p63, a p53 homolog at 3q27-29, encodes multiple products with transactivating, death-inducing, and dominant-negative activities. *Mol Cell* 1998;2(3):305-16.

Yang, A; Schweitzer, R; Sun, D; Kaghad, M; Walker, N; Bronson, RT, et al. p63 is essential for regenerative proliferation in limb, craniofacial and epithelial development. *Nature* 1999;398(6729):714-8.

Yang, A; Walker, N; Bronson, R; Kaghad, M; Oosterwegel, M; Bonnin, J, et al. p73-deficient mice have neurological, pheromonal and inflammatory defects but lack spontaneous tumours. *Nature* 2000;404(6773):99-103.

Yarden, Y. The EGFR family and its ligands in human cancer. signalling mechanisms and therapeutic opportunities. *Eur J Cancer* 2001;37 Suppl 4:S3-8.

Yasumoto, S; Kunimura, C; Kikuchi, K; Tahara, H; Ohji, H; Yamamoto, H, et al. Telomerase activity in normal human epithelial cells. *Oncogene* 1996;13(2):433-9.

Yazici, YD; Kim, S; Jasser, SA; Wang, Z; Carter, KB, Jr.; Bucana, CD, et al. Antivascular therapy of oral tongue squamous cell carcinoma with PTK787. *Laryngoscope* 2005;115(12):2249-55.

Yeudall, WA; Jakus, J. Cyclin kinase inhibitors add a new dimension to cell cycle control. *Eur J Cancer B Oral Oncol* 1995;31B(5):291-8.

Ylipalosaari, M; Thomas, GJ; Nystrom, M; Salhimi, S; Marshall, JF; Huotari, V, et al. Alpha v beta 6 integrin down-regulates the MMP-13 expression in oral squamous cell carcinoma cells. *Exp Cell Res* 2005;309(2):273-83.

Yorioka, CW; Coletta, RD; Alves, F; Nishimoto, IN; Kowalski, LP; Graner, E. Matrix metalloproteinase-2 and -9 activities correlate with the disease-free survival of oral squamous cell carcinoma patients. *Int J Oncol* 2002;20(1):189-94.

Yu, GL; Bradley, JD; Attardi, LD; Blackburn, EH. *In vivo* alteration of telomere sequences and senescence caused by mutated Tetrahymena telomerase RNAs. *Nature* 1990;344(6262):126-32.

Yu, W; Fang, H. Clinical trials with oncolytic adenovirus in China. *Curr Cancer Drug Targets* 2007;7(2):141-8.

Zaika, AI; Kovalev, S; Marchenko, ND; Moll, UM. Overexpression of the wild type p73 gene in breast cancer tissues and cell lines. *Cancer Res* 1999;59(13):3257-63.

Zaslav, AL; Stamberg, J; Steinberg, BM; Lin, YJ; Abramson, A. Cytogenetic analysis of head and neck carcinomas. *Cancer Genet Cytogenet* 1991;56(2):181-7.

Zeimet, AG; Marth, C. Why did p53 gene therapy fail in ovarian cancer? *Lancet Oncol* 2003;4(7):415-22.

Zhang, Y; Wang, C; Mizukami, H; Itoh, H; Kusama, M; Ozawa, K, et al. Increased expression and activation of matrix metalloproteinase-2 (MMP-2) in O-1N: hamster oral squamous cell carcinoma with high potential lymph node metastasis. *J Exp Clin Cancer Res* 2006;25(3):417-23.

Zhang, Y; Xiong, Y; Yarbrough, WG. ARF promotes MDM2 degradation and stabilizes p53: ARF-INK4a locus deletion impairs both the Rb and p53 tumor suppression pathways. *Cell* 1998;92(6):725-34.

Zimmerman, CM; Padgett, RW. Transforming growth factor beta signaling mediators and modulators. *Gene* 2000;249(1-2):17-30.

In: Cancer Research Perspectives
Editor: Larissa S. Pereira, pp. 73-103

ISBN 978-1-60021-980-1

Chapter II

Passive Smoking and Cancer Risk in Companion Animals: Sentinels for Health Effects in Humans

Audra L. Gollenberg and Elizabeth R. Bertone-Johnson

Department of Public Health, School of Public Health and Health Sciences, University of Massachusetts, Amherst, MA (AG, ERBJ), USA;

Department of Clinical Sciences, Cummings School of Veterinary Medicine, Tufts University, North Grafton, MA (ERBJ), USA.

Abstract

From the first use of canaries in coal mines a century ago, companion animals have been useful sentinels for risk associated with environmental exposures they share with humans. There has been a great deal of inconsistency in results from studies of passive smoking and cancer in humans, due largely to misclassification of exposure levels and confounding by other factors. Evaluations of how passive smoking relates to cancers in companion animals may potentially clarify these relationships in humans.

Similarities in cancer incidence and biology make dogs and cats appropriate models for the etiology of a variety of human cancers, including breast, testes, bladder, lung, nasal/sinus, bone and lymphatic cancers. Because dogs and cats have shorter life spans, the effects of passive smoking on cancer development can be assessed more quickly than in most human studies. In humans, associations between passive smoking and cancer may be confounded by factors such as alcohol intake and occupational exposures, but because these are not relevant to pets the likelihood of confounding is greatly reduced.

Pets living in smoking households undoubtedly receive a substantial exposure dose, which may be more consistent and easily measured than in humans. Recent data suggest that dogs and cats absorb and metabolize nicotine after household exposure, and demonstrate urinary cotinine levels that increase linearly with exposure. In addition to inhalation and trans-dermal exposure, oral grooming leads to oral ingestion of particulates; therefore pets may serve as models for both adults and young children, who may be exposed through these multiple routes.

In dogs, household passive smoking exposure has been associated with increased risks of lung and nasal/sinus cancers. In one study dogs living with smokers had a 60% greater risk of lung cancer than unexposed dogs. Passive smoking also appears related to cancer incidence in cats. In a recent study, cats exposed to household passive smoking had a significant 2-fold increase in risk of malignant lymphoma. Passive smoking may also increase risk of oral cancer, perhaps by altering expression of p53.

In summary, epidemiologic studies of companion animals can make a unique and valuable contribution to knowledge of the relationship between passive smoking and cancer in humans. Though this field is still in its adolescence, provocative results from early investigations suggest that cancer risk increased with both the duration and quantity of exposure. Additional studies of the health effects of passive smoking in animal populations are clearly warranted.

INTRODUCTION

From the first use of canaries in coal mines a century ago, companion animals have been useful sentinels for risk associated with environmental exposures they share with humans. In recent years, companion animals have been used in epidemiologic studies of the health effects of environmental contaminants to identify risk of disease of relevance to both animal and human populations. Specifically, several studies have evaluated the relationship between companion animals' exposure to environmental tobacco smoke (ETS) and risk of spontaneously-occurring cancers. There has been a great deal of inconsistency in results from studies of ETS exposure and cancer in humans, due largely to misclassification of exposure levels and confounding by other factors. Evaluations of how ETS exposure relates to cancers in companion animals may potentially clarify these relationships in humans. This chapter presents rationale for studying ETS exposure in companion animals, discusses how results from these studies may be relevant to understand how passive smoking may contribute to cancer in humans, and reviews results from recent studies of ETS exposure and a variety of cancers in cats and dogs.

FUNDAMENTALS OF COMPANION ANIMAL EPIDEMIOLOGY

A growing number of studies in recent years have applied methods used in epidemiologic investigations of cancer in humans to populations of companion animals [1-5]. The basic premise of these studies is that domestic animals that live in households with humans have similar levels of exposure to environmental hazards as their human owners, and therefore may serve as sentinels of environmental cancer risk [6-9]. To date, subjects have largely been limited to pet dogs and cats, though birds, ferrets, rodents and other animals may also be appropriate subjects for many situations.

High rates of pet ownership in the United States provide ample numbers of subjects for epidemiologic studies. According to the American Pet Products Manufacturers Association

(AAPMA) 2003-2004 National Pet Owner's Survey, there are approximately 65 million owned dogs and 77.6 million owned cats in the United States, with 60% of households having at least one dog or cat [10]. The average amount spent on veterinary bills in the past 12 months was $263 for dog owners and $113 for cat owners, an indication of many owners' substantial commitment to their pets' health. The close relationship that many owners have with their pets translates to a high willingness to participate in research studies that will further understanding of animal health. For example, in a recent study conducted by our research group, approximately 42% of dog owners contacted by mail and invited to join a long-term study of canine health agreed to participate [11]. Other studies by our group and other investigators have observed high participation rates [3,12-14].

The majority of studies of the association between ETS exposure and the risk of cancer in companion animals conducted to date have been case-control studies. In case-control studies, a case group of subjects with a disease is identified along with a comparison group of control participants who are free from the disease under study. Case and control participants are commonly identified and recruited through veterinary teaching hospitals where cancer diagnoses are verified through biopsy confirmation and cancer subtype documentation is rigorous [2]. Large tertiary care veterinary hospitals that treat large numbers of cancer patients also provide an efficient means of identifying a sufficient number of study participants for statistically powerful epidemiologic studies even if the cancer type is rare. For both cases and controls, the level of exposure to ETS is then assessed, often through questionnaires completed by each subject's human owner. To evaluate whether a relationship exists between an environmental factor such as ETS exposure and the development of cancer, the odds of being exposed in cases is compared to odds of exposure in control animals through the calculation of an odds ratio (OR). When the disease under study is rare, the OR is an estimate of relative risk (RR), the standard measure of association used in epidemiology. RR values greater than 1.0 indicate an increased risk of disease in those who are exposed as compared to those who are not, while an RR less than 1.0 indicates a decreased risk of disease. A RR of 1.0 indicates that the risk factor under study is not related to the risk of disease.

In addition to case-control studies, a limited number of prospective cohort studies have been conducted in companion animals, mostly in specialized populations such as military working dogs [15]. In cohort studies, exposure to an environmental factor such as ETS is measured in a defined population, known as a 'cohort.' The population is then followed forward in time to document the incidence of disease. To evaluate the relationship between ETS and disease, the disease incidence in exposed individuals is then compared to the disease incidence in unexposed individuals to calculate the RR.

Benefits of Companion Animal Epidemiology

Epidemiologic studies conducted in companion animals provide another means of examining associations between ETS and cancers in humans for which results are inconsistent or controversial. Although a limited number of studies have been conducted to date, the association between ETS exposure and the risk of various types of cancer has been studied in companion animals and provides useful information for extrapolating findings to human populations.

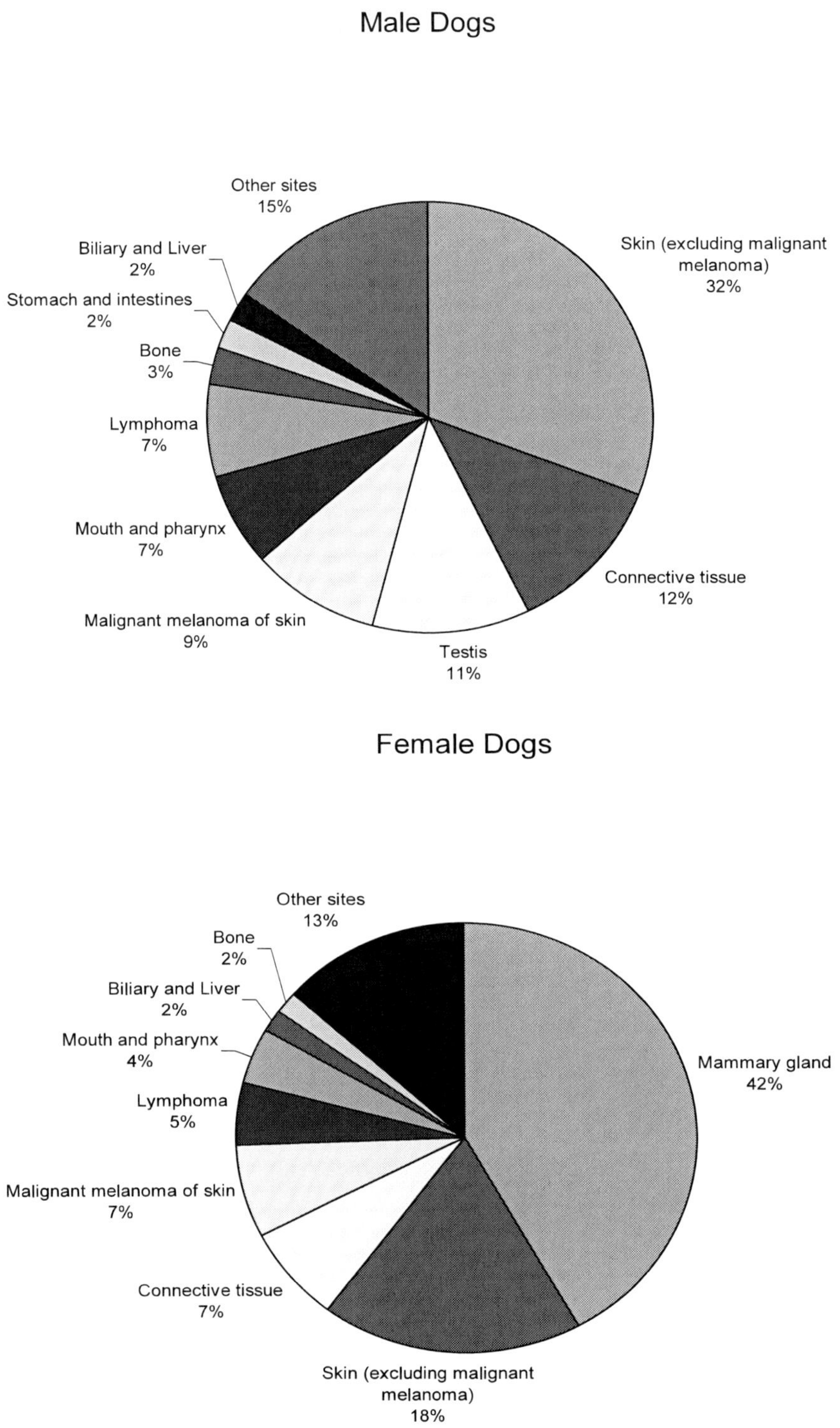

Figure 1. Continued

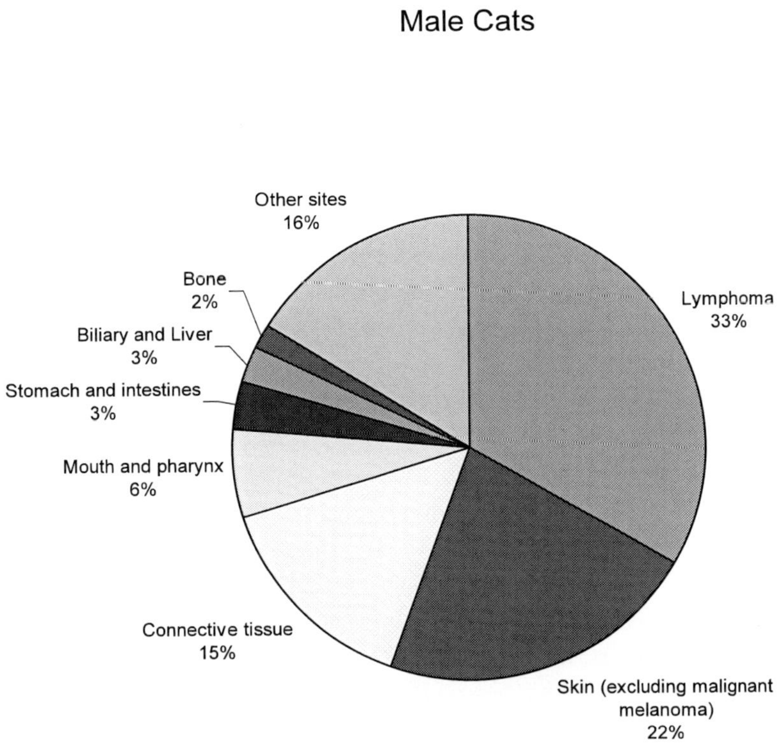

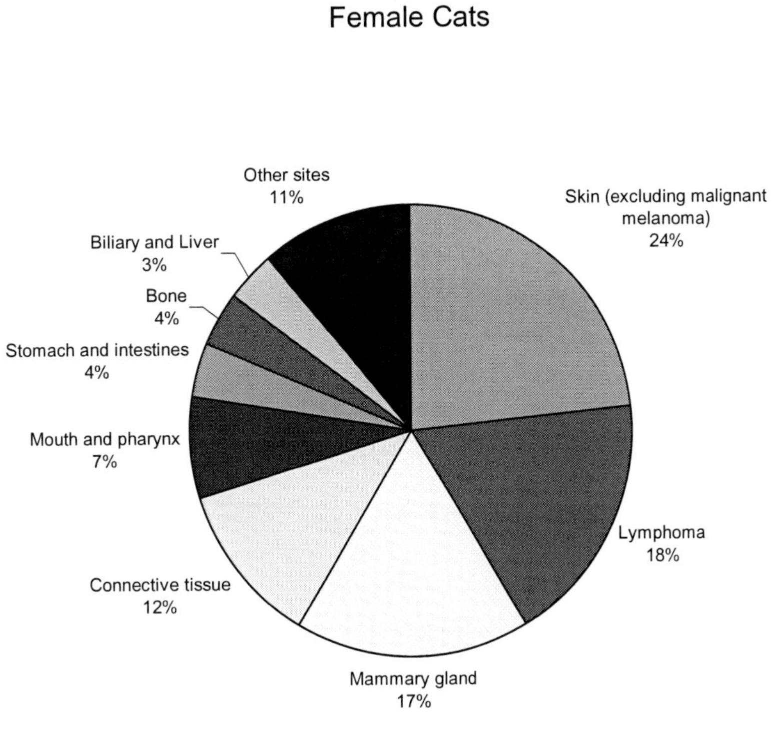

Figure 1. Most common cancer sites in male and female dogs and cats, Alameda and Contra Costa Counties, California, July 1963 – June 1966. Adapted from Dorn et al. [18].

Epidemiologic studies of cancer risk in companion animals are a valuable complement to human studies for several reasons. Dogs, and to some extent cats, have been well established as appropriate models for the study of human cancer because of similarities in cancer etiology between species [2,16]. In particular, canine cancers of the breast, testes, bladder, lung, nasal and sinus cavities, bone and lymphatic system all share clinical, pathologic, histologic and prognostic characteristics with their human counterparts [8,9]. These cancers occur commonly in dogs, and several studies suggest that incidence rates for many tumors are similar to those of humans. For certain malignancies, such as canine osteosarcoma and malignant lymphoma, incidence may be even greater than rates observed in humans.

Few studies in dogs and cats have systematically estimated the incidence of cancer on a population level. Dorn and colleagues conducted the first study to measure cancer incidence in a free-living canine population and estimated the annual incidence of all biopsy-confirmed cancers in two California counties between 1963 and 1966 [17,18]. The population at risk for the study was determined through a survey of a sample of households in Alameda County conducted in 1965. The population at risk only included those households that reported seeking veterinary care, in order to restrict the population to those animals that would be diagnosed with cancer and reported to the regional cancer registry by a veterinarian; this prevented underestimation of the cancer incidence rates because animals developing tumors that would not be diagnosed and reported to the registry were not included in the study population. For each dog and cat, owners reported sex, reproductive status (i.e., neutered or reproductively intact), and breed type. Results from the population sample were then used to estimate the total population of dogs and cats in the two counties in 1965. Malignant cancer cases were identified through a survey of the central animal neoplasm registry for Alameda and Contra Counties. Cases were classified by site according to the Manual of the International Statistical Classification of Diseases, Injuries, and Causes of Death, and benign cancers were excluded. The estimated annual incidence rates for all cancers were 381.2 per 100,000 dogs and 155.8 per 100,000 cats [18]. The distribution of cancers observed by Dorn and colleagues in male and female dogs and cats by tumor site (1963-1966) is presented in Figure 1. In comparison, the incidence of all human cancers except non-melanoma skin cancers in Alameda County during the same time period was estimated to be 272.1 per 100,000 [18]. Other studies have suggested that cancer incidence rates in dogs may be as much as twice those in humans [8], in large part because many dogs and cats with suspected cancer may be euthanized by a veterinarian without first having a biopsy-confirmed diagnosis. Thus, the rates estimated by Dorn and colleagues may underestimate the actual incidence rates in these species [2]. Rates for specific cancer types in cats and dogs may also vary between populations depending on the frequency of spaying and neutering. When spaying/neutering is common, rates of cancers of the mammary gland and testis in particular are considerably lower than those observed by Dorn et al [2].

Dogs and cats have considerably shorter life spans than humans. For humans, the average life span currently ranges from approximately 69 to 80 years [19]. In comparison, dogs live on average 7 to 14 years, depending on breed size [20], while the average life span in cats ranges from approximately 10 to 14 years [21]. Because of this shorter life span, the latency period between exposure to an environmental chemical such as ETS and the development of disease is shorter and the growth of a tumor may progress more quickly [8,9]. As a result, the effect of environmental factors on disease development can be assessed in a relatively short period of time, making epidemiologic studies in animals highly efficient to conduct. For example, Reif and colleagues investigated the relationship between cryptorchidy (i.e., undescended testicles) and incident testicular cancer in a prospective study of 938 dogs [15]. In this investigation, one half of all the incident tumors observed developed during the first year of follow-up. In comparison, prospective studies of human cancers may require long periods of follow-up, sometimes 10 to 20 years, to obtain enough cases to study the effects of environmental factors with statistical precision. Because of the shorter follow-up period required for studying incident cancers, prospective studies of cancers in animals are often less time-consuming and expensive than studies in humans.

Companion animals serve as useful sentinels for risks associated with environmental exposures they share with humans. Pets living in households are undoubtedly exposed to the same environmental contaminants as their human owners, including ETS [22]. Both the routes of exposure to ETS for companion animals and exposure dose may be physiologically relevant to humans. For example, dogs and cats may be exposed to ETS through multiple routes: 1) inhalation of airborne smoke; 2) trans-dermal absorption of particulates and residues that may be concentrated on fur and skin after contact with carpets, furniture and bedding; and 3) oral ingestion during oral grooming of particulates deposited on their fur. In cats in particular, oral grooming may provide a substantial source of exposure [22]. Because exposure may be through these multiple routes, pets may serve as appropriate models for exposure patterns of young children in a household, who may have closer contact with contaminated carpeting and bedding than adults, and who may frequently mouth household objects [23].

Preliminary research by our group indicates that domestic cats living in households with active smokers both absorb a substantial dose of ETS and metabolize nicotine in levels similar to those in humans. In 2002, we assessed the relationship between ETS exposure and urinary cotinine level in a cross-sectional study of cats presenting to Foster Hospital for Small Animals at Cummings School of Veterinary Medicine at Tufts University [24,25]. Owners of 184 cats completed a questionnaire measuring household smoking level in the previous 24 hours, as well as other demographic and lifestyle factors. Urine samples were also collected from 70 of these cats during the same clinic visit. We found that cats' urinary cotinine increased significantly with the total number of cigarettes smoked per day in the household. Mean urinary cotinine levels (ng/ml) in cats exposed to 0, 1 – 19, and 20 or more cigarettes per day were 7.0 (SD 4.1), 12.6 (10.2), and 40.0 (20.8), respectively ($P < 0.001$) (Figure 2) [24]. These levels are comparable to those observed in humans exposed to similar smoking levels; the standard cut-off values for the assay used in urine are 3 – 10 for no substantial ETS exposure, 11 – 30 for passive exposure or light smoking, and 30 – 500+ ng/ml for active smoking [26]. Our results suggest that cats living with smokers do receive a dose of ETS similar to that of humans exposed to household passive smoke. In dogs, Reif and colleagues observed a similarly strong association between the mean urinary cotinine level of dogs and the number of cigarettes smoked per day in the household [2]. In a laboratory study on cigarette smoke-exposed ferrets, urinary cotinine equivalents were similar to that of humans who smoke two packs of cigarettes per day [27].

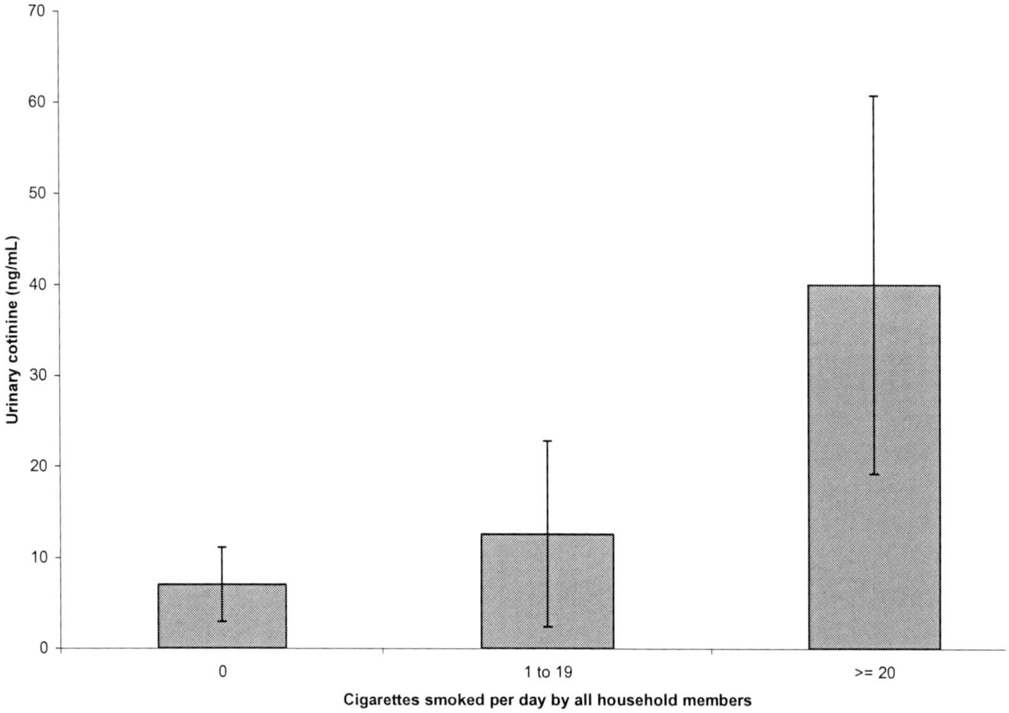

Figure 2. Mean urinary cotinine levels (ng/mL) of 70 cats by household smoking level. Adapted from Bertone-Johnson [24].

A companion animal's level of exposure to environmental chemicals such as ETS is often more consistent than that of humans, thereby offering another advantage to conducting epidemiologic studies in these populations. In contrast to humans who may travel and/or occupy many different households throughout their lives, cats and dogs generally spend a large proportion of their lives in one location or household. For example, Reif and colleagues evaluated the relationship between risk of canine lymphoma and residential exposure to electromagnetic fields (EMF) in a case-control study in Colorado [28]. While each dog's exposure to EMF was only assessed once, based on levels at a single residence, this level represented approximately 65% of the dog's lifetime exposure because the subjects spent such a high proportion of their lives in a single home. Whereas humans leave the house for work or school on a daily basis, companion animals spend considerable time indoors in a single location, suggesting their daily exposure to indoor contaminants is highly consistent over time.

While laboratory animal studies offer valuable insights into the carcinogenicity of tobacco smoke and its effect on susceptible tissues, there are several limitations to such studies. First, it is difficult and sometimes unfeasible to expose laboratory animals to levels of smoke similar to exposure patterns of humans [22]. Experimental short-term and high-level inhalation studies often result in increased mortality among laboratory dogs, limiting the statistical power of these studies [29,30]. High levels of illness and suffering of study subjects are common in laboratory inhalation studies. Alternatives to traditional experimental animal studies on smoke exposure are thus warranted. Epidemiologic observational studies on ETS and spontaneously occurring tumors, as compared to induced tumors in laboratory animals, offer a method to studying smoke-related tumors that more closely resemble cancer development in humans.

Epidemiologic studies of risk factors for disease in cats and dogs may also be less subject to many types of bias that are common in studies of humans, and have a lower likelihood of confounding by other factors related to both the exposure and disease. Confounding factors may cause an under- or overestimate of the true exposure-disease relationship depending on the relationship between the third factor and both the exposure and the disease. In humans, associations between cancer and factors such as passive smoking may be confounded by inadequate control for other strong risk factors including active smoking and occupational chemical exposures [2]. For example, occupational exposures to harmful chemicals such as asbestos or radiation may bias relative risk estimates of the relationship between ETS and cancer if these factors are not well controlled for in human studies [2]. However, these factors generally do not apply to pets and are therefore not likely to lead to confounding [2]. Similarly, in human studies the presence of factors such as active smoking and alcohol use, which are often strongly associated with increased risks of many cancers [31], often make evaluation of the contribution of other factors more difficult [32]. While some factors that are potential confounders in human studies are not relevant to studies on pets, other factors may exist that can bias the relationship between passive smoking and cancer, such as age or breed type. As in all epidemiologic studies, these factors should be assessed and adjusted for in statistical analyses.

In any case-control study, recall bias may lead to an inaccurate estimation of the association between exposure and disease when participants provide incorrect assessments of their exposure histories. This may occur if participants are aware of the study's hypothesis and answer questions about environmental exposures differently based on their disease status. For example, if subjects with cancer overestimate their previous exposure to passive smoke and the control subjects tend to provide accurate or slightly underestimates of their previous exposure, the RR would be spuriously overestimated. The likelihood of this occurring is somewhat reduced in studies of companion animals because few studies of this kind have been conducted to date; because few risk factors for disease in pets have been identified and most veterinarians generally do not discuss with clients the potential health hazards of exposing pets to household environmental exposures, owners are less likely to make connections between ETS and cancer in their pets than they are in themselves [22]. Consequently, reporting is likely to be more accurate and relative risk estimates are less likely to be biased.

In summary, epidemiologic studies of companion animals offer a complementary means by which to identify and evaluate risk factors for cancer of relevance to both animals and humans. Similarities in cancer incidence and biology between humans, cats and dogs make these species appropriate models for human cancer etiology. Shorter life spans, higher exposure doses, fewer confounding factors, and reduced likelihood of recall bias make pets ideal subjects for assessment of the health effects of passive smoke exposures of relevance to humans.

Studies of ETS Exposure and Cancer in Companion Animals

Malignant Lymphoma

Feline malignant lymphoma (FML) and canine malignant lymphoma (CML) have been proposed as appropriate models for human non-Hodgkin's lymphoma (NHL), as the three diseases share common clinical, pathologic and histologic features and respond similarly to treatment [8,9,33-38]. Malignant lymphoma is the most common cancer in cats [33] and the third most prevalent cancer in dogs [8], with reported incidence rates of approximately 125 per 100,000 [33] and 13-110 per 100,000 [8,18,35,38-40], respectively. In contrast, the annual US incidence rates of human NHL are considerable lower, at 22.6 per 100,000 in males and 16.0 cases per 100,000 in females [41].

Several biologic and clinical similarities have been identified between NHL in humans and malignant lymphomas in cats and dogs. Several studies suggest that as many as 84% of canine and feline lymphomas are multicentric [36,42]. The clinical presentation of CML is similar to that of human NHL, and generally involves the enlargement of peripheral lymph nodes, while FML often has visceral involvement. Histologic and morphologic similarities between CML, FML and human NHL allow for the classification of tumors using criteria developed for NHL [9,36,38,42-44]. As in humans, dogs and cats with high grade tumors tend to respond better to treatment and experience longer remission times than those with low grade lymphomas [8,44].

CML and NHL tumors are all largely B-lymphocytic in origin [2,36,45,46]. In dogs, Vail et al. estimates that 70-80% of canine tumors are B-cell derived [9]. This proportion is similar to that of human NHL in Western populations, in which only approximately 5-20% of tumors are classified as T-cell [38,39,47]. In cats, alimentary, mediastinal and multicentric tumors tend to be more commonly of T-cell origin than tumors occurring at other anatomic sites [48]. In humans, cats and dogs, T-cell lymphomas are associated with shorter survival time and poorer prognosis [9,36,38]. In addition, structurally similar proto-oncogenes located in the pathway of NHL development, such as the MYC gene, have been identified in humans, cats and dogs [2,9,49].

Previously, FML was believed to be largely the result of infection by feline leukemia virus (FeLV), as the majority of cats diagnosed with lymphoma also tested positive for FeLV [50]. However, in recent years increased frequency of vaccination against FeLV has greatly reduced the prevalence of this infection in domestic cats, and the proportion of lymphoma cases with concurrent FeLV infection has substantially decreased [33,51]. The reduced role of FeLV in the etiology of FML raises questions about whether lifestyle and environmental factors may influence disease risk in cats as they do in humans.

The potential roles of exposure to household ETS in the development of NHL, FML and CML have not been thoroughly evaluated. While no clear mechanism has been proposed to explain an association between active or passive smoking and the development of NHL in humans, several components of tobacco smoke may be carcinogenic to lymphoid tissue and may cause mutation in lymphocyte precursors [52-54]. Several recent studies in humans have suggested that active smoking may increase the risk of NHL, although results have been inconsistent. Of the four cohort studies [52-55] to evaluate this association, three [52,53,55] observed a significant increase in risk of incident NHL in current smokers, with relative risks ranging from 1.4 [55] to 3.8 [52]. A positive association between smoking and NHL has also been suggested by the results of several [56-61] but not all [62-66] case-control studies. In addition, while few studies have evaluated the role of exposure to ETS in the development of NHL, several studies have suggested a relationship between parental smoking prior to a child's birth and risk of childhood lymphoma [67-69].

A recent study by our research group investigated the association between ETS and risk of FML [3]. Recruitment for both cases and controls took place through the Foster Small Animal Hospital at Tufts University School of Veterinary Medicine (TUSVM) (now Cummings School of Veterinary Medicine) in central Massachusetts in June 2000 via mailed invitations to participate. Eligible cases were all cats diagnosed with biopsy-confirmed FML between January 1993 and June 2000, while eligible controls were cats diagnosed with renal failure between January 1993 and June 2000 at the same hospital. Cats with renal disease were chosen as appropriate controls because renal disease is a serious condition but is not known to be associated with ETS in cats or humans. Completed questionnaires were received from owners of 80 cases (64.5%) and 114 controls (67.9%) and comprised the final study population.

The questionnaire asked owners of eligible cases and controls about the characteristics, care, and home environment of their pet two years before the diagnosis date of lymphoma for cases and renal disease for controls. Several questions pertaining to household smoking level were included to quantify the level of ETS exposure. Owners were asked to report if the cat ever lived with a smoker, the types of tobacco products smoked, the number of years the cat lived with the smoker, the total number of smokers in the household, and the average number of cigarettes smoked per day by all household members. An ETS exposure index was created to simultaneously evaluate exposure duration and intensity by multiplying the number of years of exposure by the average number of cigarettes smoked in the house per day. Additional questions on age, sex, breed, hair length, reproductive status, use of flea and tick control products, diet, general medical history, and characteristics of the home environment were included in the questionnaire.

Results suggested a significant positive association between ETS exposure and risk of FML. After adjusting for age at diagnosis, location of residence, and hair length, cats with any exposure to ETS had a statistically significant two-fold increased risk of lymphoma (RR = 2.4; 95% Confidence Interval (CI) = 1.2-4.5) (Table 1). Risk increased with both the duration and quantity of exposure with evidence of a linear trend. Compared to those with no ETS exposure, cats living with smokers for 5 or more years had a three-fold increased risk (RR = 3.2; 95% CI = 1.5-6.9; P for trend = 0.003). Cats living with 2 or more smokers had a RR of 4.1 compared to those in non-smoking households (95% CI = 1.4 – 12.1; P for trend = 0.005), while cats exposed to a pack of cigarettes or more per day had a significant three-fold increase in risk (RR = 3.3; 95% CI = 1.3 – 8.1; P for trend = 0.006).

This study was the first to investigate the association between household ETS exposure and lymphoma in cats or other domestic animals. In our population, the majority of lymphomas were of gastrointestinal and nasal origin. Given this anatomical distribution, it seems biologically plausible that lymphoid tissues at these sites would be susceptible to the potentially harmful effects of inhaled and/or orally ingested ETS. This hypothesis is supported by the observation that tumor location varied slightly by ETS exposure status, with gastrointestinal tumors accounting for 56% of the lymphomas in ETS exposed cats compared to 39% in unexposed animals, though this difference was not statistically significant. Given the similarities between FML and NHL in humans, results from this study suggest that further research into ETS exposure as a risk factor for NHL in humans and other species is warranted.

Table 1. Multivariable relative risk (RR)* of feline malignant lymphoma by level of exposure to household cigarette smoking. Adapted from Bertone et al [3]

Exposure level	**Cases**	**Controls**	**RR (95% CI)**	***p* for trend†**
Household smoking				
None	47	82	1.0	
Any	33	32	2.4 (1.2 - 4.5)	
Number of years of ETS exposure				
0	47	82	1.0	
> 0 - < 5	9	16	1.3 (0.5 - 3.2)	
≥ 5	24	16	3.2 (1.5 - 6.9)	0.003
Number of smokers in household				
0	47	82	1.0	
1	22	24	1.9 (0.9 - 3.9)	
≥ 2	11	7	4.1 (1.4 - 12.1)	0.005
Number of cigarettes/day in household				
0	47	82	1.0	
1 - 19	16	17	1.9 (0.9 – 4.3)	
≥ 20	16	10	3.3 (1.3 – 8.1)	0.006
ETS exposure index‡				
0	47	82	1.0	
1 – 99	17	18	1.8 (0.8 – 4.0)	
≥ 100	15	9	3.8 (1.4 – 9.8)	0.008

* Multivariable relative risks adjusted for age at diagnosis, location of residence and hair length; CI = confidence interval;

† Test for trend calculated using the median value of each category as a continuous variable in the regression model;

‡ Years of exposure to ETS x number of cigarettes smoked per day by all household members.

A potential limitation of this study is inaccurate recall of smoking history by both case and control owners. Many owners were required to recall household smoking that occurred several years earlier, which may be difficult to report accurately and may therefore lead to bias in the assessment of the ETS-cancer relationship. The degree to which misclassification and bias may exist in studies of companion animals is unknown. However, research in humans suggests that misclassification of smoking status tends to be low [70] and that the effect of misclassification on risk estimates in studies of ETS and cancer is small [71,72]. If such a misclassification occurred at the same rate in both cases and controls, the results would most likely underestimate the relationship between ETS and risk of FML.

The association between ETS and canine malignant lymphoma has not been directly investigated to date, though a large case-control study of herbicide use and CML risk conducted by Hayes et al reported that household smoking was slightly more common in CML cases (47.5%) than in a group of control dogs without tumors (46.4%), and slightly less common than in control dogs with other types of malignant and benign tumors (48.2%) [73]. Our research group is currently conducting a case-control study of this relationship in dogs diagnosed with CML at the Foster Hospital at Tufts between 2000 and 2005.

Lung Cancer

In contrast to humans, lung cancer is a rare tumor in dogs and cats. Lung cancer accounts for only 1% of all canine cancers diagnosed [8] and an even lower proportion of feline tumors [42], whereas it is the second most common malignancy in humans, accounting for approximately 13% of new cancers diagnosed annually [41]. Secondary lung cancer resulting from metastatic disease is much more common in the dog and cat [8]. In the only study to survey the prevalence of cancer in a free-living population of canines, Dorn et al. reported a prevalence of 4.2 primary lung cancer cases per 100,000 among dogs living in two California counties [18]. As part of a controlled study to document spontaneous lung neoplasms in two colonies of beagle dogs followed for life, Hahn et al. observed a crude incidence rate for lung carcinomas of 8.8% (35 cases in 398 dogs); this high incidence rate was influenced by the high frequency of lung cancer in aged dogs, specifically in those over 13.6 years [74]. However, this observed rate in colonized beagle dogs may not represent the true incidence of lung cancer in free-living populations of domestic dogs of different geographies and breeds.

Primary lung cancer in dogs has several similarities to human lung cancer, making dogs an appropriate sentinel species in which to study environmental causes of human lung cancer. In canines, most primary tumors of the lung are carcinomas arising from bronchial or alveolar epithelium and adenocarcinomas, while squamous cell carcinomas appear less frequently [42,75]. The most common histologic types of lung tumor observed in humans are squamous cell carcinoma, adenocarcinoma, and small cell (oat) carcinoma [76]. Squamous cell carcinomas are more often related to smoking than are adenocarcinomas [76]. In humans, dogs and cats, tumor histologic type does not appear to influence survival times and disease-free intervals [42,76]. In addition, laboratory studies have noted similarities in the expression of epidermal growth factor receptor (EGF-R) between canine and human lung carcinomas. In a study by Gillett et al., 17 of 36 (47%) canine lung tumors exhibited expression of EGF-R, indicating a striking similarity to human lung tumors [77].

Research on the association between passive smoking and risk of lung cancer in humans was first investigated in 1981, when two studies reported an increased risk of lung cancer among nonsmoking women married to smokers [78,79]. Since that time, more than thirty epidemiologic studies have examined ETS exposure as a risk factor for lung cancer, which taken together suggest an approximate 30% increased risk associated with passive smoke exposure [80,81]. Risks generally increased with dose of ETS exposure, with an approximately 70% higher risk among those most heavily exposed [76]. However, it remains unclear whether passive smoking is entirely the cause of this excess risk. Exposure to occupational and other airborne pollutants such as arsenic, asbestos, chloromethyl ethers, chromium, nickel refining, mustard gas, polycyclic hydrocarbons, and radon may also explain part of the excess risk of lung cancer observed in nonsmokers [76]. Because companion animals are generally not exposed to industrial factors and air pollution to the same extent as humans and generally spend most of their time indoors, epidemiologic studies on risk of lung cancer in animal populations may allow researchers to better identify an excess risk caused by ETS exposure.

The effect of tobacco exposures on canine lung tissue has been explored in several laboratory studies. In experimental studies on beagle dogs exposed to mainstream smoke, exposed dogs developed both neoplastic lesions and basal and epithelial cell metaplasia, which often precede malignant tumor development [82]. Other laboratory studies in dogs showed that direct inhalation of tobacco smoke induced pulmonary tumors in beagle dogs [29,30]. The histopathologic changes in lungs of dogs exposed to ETS suggest that canine lung tissue responds to tobacco smoke similarly to human tissue. Because of these similarities, the dog has been deemed the best model for smoke inhalation studies of relevance to humans [83].

In the first study to examine the association between environmental tobacco smoke in the home and the risk of canine lung cancer, Reif and colleagues conducted a case-control study using oncology records of two university veterinary hospitals, the University of Illinois and Colorado State University [13]. All histologically confirmed lung cancer cases diagnosed between 1985 and 1987 were identified, (n = 70) along with randomly selected controls (n = 106) with other forms of cancer not suspected to be related to cigarette smoking that were diagnosed during the same period. Letters of solicitation were mailed to owners along with questionnaires examining smoke exposures and other lifestyle and environmental characteristics. The questionnaire queried owners on demographics and several aspects of the home environment. The number of smokers in the household, number of cigarette packs smoked daily by the heaviest smoker, and the proportion of time spent indoors by the dog were assessed. An exposure index was created by multiplying the number of smokers, the number of packs smoked by the heaviest smoker, and the proportion of time spent indoors by the dog. Age, sex, hospital, proportion of day spent indoors, body size, and skull shape were also evaluated. Completed responses were received from 73% of cases and 78% of controls, yielding 51 cases and 83 controls.

After adjustment for age, sex, time spent indoors and other factors, dogs exposed to any household ETS had a non-significant 60% higher risk of lung cancer (OR = 1.6; 95% CI = 0.7 – 3.7) compared to those in non-smoking households. Among dogs aged 10 years or less, the risk of lung cancer increased to almost three-fold as compared to unexposed dogs (OR = 2.7, 95% CI = 1.0-7.2), while risk among older dogs was 0.8 (95% C.I. 0.3-2.2). Risk did not appear to increase linearly with either number of packs smoked per day or the calculated exposure index.

Results from secondary analyses suggested that dog's skull shape may significantly modify the relationship between ETS and lung cancer risk. Reif et al divided the study population into two groups: 1) brachycephalic (i.e., short-length skull) breeds, such as pugs, boxers and bulldogs, combined with mesocephalic (i.e., medium-length skull) breeds, such as beagles, golden retrievers, Labrador retrievers, and German Shepherds; and 2) dolichocephalic (i.e., long-length skull) breeds, such as collies, greyhounds, Afghan hounds and Dobermans. In short/medium nosed dogs, exposure to >= 2 packs/day was associated with a non-significant 2-fold increase in risk (OR= 2.4; 95% CI = 0.7-7.8) (Table 2). In contrast, no increase in risk with ETS was observed for long-nosed dogs.

Table 2. Multivariable relative risk (RR)* of canine lung cancer by level of exposure to household cigarette smoking: results for Brachycephalic/mesocephalic vs. Dolichocephalic dogs. Adapted from Reif et al. [13]

	Brachy/mesocephalic dogs				Dolichocephalic dogs			
Risk factor	**Cases**	**Controls**	**RR***	**95% CI**	**Cases**	**Controls**	**RR***	**95% CI**
Smoker in household								
None	12	29	1.0		15	23	1.0	
Smoker	15	17	2.4	0.7 – 7.8	9	14	0.9	0.3 – 2.9
Number of smokers in household								
0	12	29	1.0		15	23	1.0	
1	9	9	3.4	0.8 – 15.0	7	8	0.8	0.2 – 3.2
>= 2	6	8	1.9	0.4 – 9.3	2	6	0.6	0.1 – 6.2
Packs per day†								
0	12	29	1.0		15	23	1.0	
< 2	10	11	2.5	0.6 – 10.0	5	11	0.7	0.2 – 2.5
>= 2	5	6	2.4	0.4 – 13.1	4	3	2.1	0.2 – 25.3
*Exposure index***								
one	12	29	1.0		15	23	1.0	
0.25 – 2.0	11	6	7.6	1.6 – 35.8	5	8	0.7	0.2 – 2.4
> 2.0	4	11	1.2	0.2 – 5.4	4	6	0.6	0.1 – 4.0

*Relative risk estimated by odds ratio, adjusted for age, sex, hospital and time spent outdoors;

CI = confidence interval;

† Number of packs of cigarettes smoked per day by heaviest smoker;

** Number of smokers x packs per day smoked by heaviest smoker x percentage of time dog spent; indoors; results from this analysis not adjusted for time spent indoors.

While not statistically significant, the results of this study suggest an association between passive smoking and canine lung cancer among short and medium-length nosed dogs. The finding of modification of the relationship between ETS exposure and lung cancer risk by skull length supports the hypothesis that long-nosed dogs may have more efficient filtration systems to rid the lower respiratory system of carcinogens in tobacco smoke [13]. An enhanced air filtration system may also explain the overall low incidence of lung cancer among dogs, as compared to a higher incidence in humans. In any case, the results are suggestive of an increased risk of lung cancer, especially among younger dogs, in which a borderline significant 2.5-fold increased risk for those exposed to the highest level of smoking was observed.

The study by Reif and colleagues raises important questions for further analysis. It would be interesting to evaluate the effect of duration of ETS exposure and the timing of exposure in relation to tumor development. In addition, while the authors assessed the number of smokers in the household, only the number of cigarettes smoked per day by the heaviest smoker was queried, which may underestimate the dogs' total level of smoke exposure. Finally, in this study all of the controls were patients diagnosed with other forms of cancer, including mammary cancer, soft tissue sarcoma, skin and connective tissue cancers. While ETS has not been associated with these tumors in dogs, many have been positively related to active and/or passive smoking in humans [31]. Their inclusion in the control group may potentially lead to an underestimation of the effect of ETS exposure on lung cancer risk. Given the provocative nature of these findings, additional studies of ETS exposure and canine lung cancer are clearly warranted.

To our knowledge, no studies have evaluated whether ETS may be associated with risk of lung cancer in cats.

Oral Cancer

Cancer of the oral cavity is the 4th most common malignancy of both domestic cats and dogs [42,84], while in humans it ranks 7th among blacks and 12th among whites in cancer incidence in the United States [85]. An estimated 30,990 new cases of human oral and pharyngeal cancer and 7,430 related deaths are reported each year in the United States, as estimated by the National Cancer Institute's Surveillance, Epidemiology, and End Results (SEER) Program [41]. There is no apparent breed predilection for oral cancers in the cat or dog [84]. Older dogs and cats are most often affected by this disease [84] and in humans, incidence rates rise progressively with advancing age [85]. The median age at diagnosis in humans is 63 years and the median age at death is 65 years [85]. The average age at diagnosis is 9 years in the dog and 11-12 years in the cat [84].

Numerous similarities in the histology of oral tumors in dogs, cats, and humans have been identified that suggest that findings from studies in animals may be applicable to humans. The three most common oral tumors in the dog are malignant melanoma, squamous cell carcinoma (SCC), and fibrosarcoma [84], whereas in cats and in humans, SCC is the predominant tumor type [84,85]. Among dogs and cats, most tumors of the oral cavity are malignant, highly locally invasive, and have a variable degree of metastasis [84]. Similarly, oral cancers in humans are likely to metastasize into second primary cancers of the oral cavity and adjacent sites [85]. Oral SCC in dogs is usually found in the gingival tissue of the rostral area and in cats most often occurs at the base of the tongue [42]. The most common sites of human oral SCC are the floor of the mouth and the tongue, followed by the soft palate and tonsillar region [86,87]. In dogs, cats, and humans, small tumors with only localized involvement at the time of diagnosis have better prognosis than tumors that have spread regionally or distantly [42,85].

The most important risk factor for human oral cancer is tobacco smoking, which may affect cancers of the tongue, mouth, and pharynx [88]. Cohort studies of male cigarette smokers have been conducted in various populations around the world and typically report large relative risks of oral cancer for smokers compared to nonsmokers, ranging from 3 to 13 [85]. Results from a large multi-site case-control study in the United States observed that relative risks of oral cancer increase according to the amount of tobacco smoked for both males and females [89]. Compared to non-smokers, risk of oral cancer was four times greater in the heaviest smoking men and 10 times greater in women, after adjusting for alcohol intake, another known risk factor for oral cancer [89]. In the same study, pipe or cigar smokers experienced a statistically significant 2-fold increased risk of oral cancer, compared to nonsmokers [89]. Smokeless tobacco has also been associated with oral cancer in numerous studies [80]. Case-control studies have reported 4 to 5-fold increases in risk of oral cancer among nonsmoking tobacco chewers, and relative risks as high as 50 have been reported for long-term users of chewing tobacco [85]. To date, studies examining the relationship between passive smoking and risk of oral cancer have not been conducted in humans. However, given the strength of evidence of the relationship between active smoking and oral cancer, studies on the role of ETS in the etiology of oral cancer are clearly warranted.

Our research group recently conducted a hospital-based case-control study of domestic cats presenting to the Foster Small Animal Hospital at Tufts University School of Veterinary Medicine (now Cummings School of Veterinary Medicine) between January 1994 and June 2000 [12]. Eligible cases were all cats receiving biopsy-confirmed diagnoses of oral SCC made by board-certified pathologists between January 1994 and June 2000, and eligible controls were cats diagnosed with renal failure at TUSVM during the same time period; cats with renal failure were chosen as controls because this disease is a serious condition but is nonmalignant and not known to be related to passive smoking in either cats or humans. In June 2000, all owners of eligible cases and controls were mailed a questionnaire about general characteristics of their pet's care and home environment. Thirty-six owners of cases (59%) and 112 owners of controls (67%) returned completed questionnaires.

ETS exposure and other characteristics of the study population were determined from the questionnaire completed by owners. The questions pertained to the 2-year period prior to the diagnosis of oral SCC or renal failure. Questions pertaining to ETS exposure included whether the cat ever lived with a smoker, the types of tobacco products smoked, number of years living with a smoker, total number of smokers in the household, and average number of cigarettes smoked per day by all household members combined. Other characteristics of the subjects queried included age, birth year, sex, breed, hair length, intact vs. neutered/spayed, medical history, year's owned, grooming type and frequency, flea product usage, aspects of diet, amount of time spent outdoors, and home size, location, and heating source.

Multivariate relative risks suggested an overall increase in risk of SCC for cats exposed to ETS compared to unexposed cats. After controlling for age, intake of canned food, intake of tuna fish, use of flea collars, and use of flea shampoo, cats that had ever lived with a smoker had a 2-fold increased risk of oral SCC, with marginal statistical significance (RR=2.3, 95% C.I. 0.8-6.5) (Table 3). Risk was also increased for those cats that had lived with a smoker for 5 or more years and in those that lived with 2 or more smokers compared to those living in nonsmoking households, although results were not statistically significant. A statistically significant 4-fold increased risk (RR = 4.0, 95% C.I. 1.1-14.8) was observed for cats living in households where 1-19 cigarettes were smoked per day compared to those unexposed, whereas cats living in homes where greater than 20 cigarettes were smoked per day were not at an increased risk (RR = 1.3, 95% C.I. 0.3-5.5).

Table 3. Multivariable relative risk (RR) of feline oral squamous cell carcinoma by level of exposure to household cigarette smoking. Adapted from Bertone et al. [12]

	Cases	Controls	RR	95% CI	P value**
Any household ETS					
No	22	81	1.0		
Yes	13	31	2.3	0.8 – 6.5	0.11
Years of ETS exposure					
0	22	81	1.0		
> 0 – 4	2	16	0.9	0.2 – 4.8	0.86
>= 5	9	16	2.7	0.8 – 9.0	0.12
Number of household smokers					
0	22	81	1.0		
1	7	24	2.0	0.6 – 7.1	0.26
2	5	7	2.8	0.6 – 12.6	0.20
Number of cigarettes smoked/day in household					
0	22	81	1.0		
1 – 19	8	17	4.0	1.1 – 14.8	0.04
>= 20	4	10	1.3	0.3 – 5.5	0.77

* Multivariable relative risks adjusted for age, intake of canned cat food, intake of tuna fish, use of flea collars and use of flea shampoo; CI = confidence interval;
** P value from Wald test in multivariable logistic regression modeling.

To our knowledge, this is among the first studies to examine the association between ETS and oral cancer in any species. Although no clear dose-response relationship was observed, cats with prolonged exposure to tobacco smoke experienced an increased risk of oral SCC. These results suggest that the relationship between ETS and oral cancer should be explored in human populations.

In the second study to examine the relationship between ETS exposure among domestic cats and oral SCC, our research group conducted a case-only study to determine the prevalence of overexpression of the tumor suppressor gene p53 in feline oral SCC and to determine the association between p53 and environmental exposures, including ETS [90]. Because the p53 gene is the most commonly mutated gene in human cancer and overexpression of this gene, particularly in oral SCC, has been associated with exposure to carcinogens found in tobacco products, it was of interest to determine if overexpression may occur as a result of passive smoking exposure [90]. Eligible cases for this study included all cats presenting to the Harrington Oncology Program at Tufts between January 1991 and June 2000 with a biopsy-confirmed diagnosis of oral SCC and a paraffin-embedded biopsy sample available (n = 32). Characteristics of the cats' home environment, care, medical history, diet, use of flea control products, demographics and ETS exposure were assessed via questionnaire mailed to the case owners. Questions pertaining to ETS exposure queried whether the cat had ever lived with a smoker, the types of tobacco products smoked, the number of years the cat had lived with a smoker, the total number of smokers in the household, and the average number of cigarettes smoked in total per day. To assess p53 overexpression, immunohistochemical analysis of the biopsy sample was performed on all samples that had not been decalcified. The final study population included 23 subjects with both completed survey information and available tumor biopsy sample.

The results of the p53 staining in tumor biopsy samples were assessed for correlation with the survey results of ETS exposure. Of the 23 biopsy samples examined, 15 (65%) demonstrated nuclear staining of the p53 protein. Tumor samples from cats exposed to ETS were 4.5 times more likely to overexpress p53 than tumors from unexposed cats, although results were not statistically significant ($p = 0.19$). Compared to cats with less than 5 years of ETS exposure, cats with ≥ 5 years of ETS exposure were 7 times more likely to overexpress p53 ($p = 0.38$).

Results of this study suggest that tumor tissue from cats with oral SCC often expresses a mutated form of the p53 tumor suppressor gene and that resultant disruption of cell signaling may play a role in the development of this malignancy. Although not statistically significant, the results on the relationship between ETS exposure and p53 overexpression suggest that ETS exposure may be associated with p53 mutation. Because of the small sample size and lack of other studies of ETS and feline oral SCC, additional studies are needed to further investigate this relationship.

To date, similar studies on ETS and oral SCC have not been conducted in dogs.

Bladder Cancer

Bladder cancer is a relatively uncommon malignancy in dogs and cats. The estimated incidence of urinary system cancers in dogs and cats is 4.2 per 100,000 and 2.4 per 100,000, respectively [18]. In comparison, the age-adjusted annual incidence of bladder cancer in the US (1998-2002) is 38.9 per 100,000 in males and 10 per 100,000 in females [41], although incidence rates vary almost 10-fold internationally [91]. Canine studies suggest that older dogs and female dogs are more often affected, whereas in humans the disease is more common in males [2]. Two studies [92-94] reported that female dogs had a 1.5 to 3-fold increased risk of bladder cancer compared to males, while neutered dogs of either sex seem to experience a higher risk compared to those that were intact [95]. The excess risk among female dogs may result from less frequent urination compared to males (1:3 ratio), thus the female bladder epithelium may have more prolonged contact with urine-borne carcinogens [96]. Furthermore, experimental studies of induced bladder cancer in dogs have shown the latency period to be less than 10 years compared with an estimated 25 years in humans [97], demonstrating the expediency of studying dogs as sentinels for human bladder cancer.

The histology and structure of the bladder is similar in both canines and humans, thus the etiology of bladder cancer is suspected to be comparable in both populations. In dogs as well as in humans, transitional cell carcinoma (TCC) is the most common form of bladder cancer [92-94]. The sensitivity of the human and canine bladder to environmental carcinogens, particularly aromatic amines, and studies linking human bladder cancer to occupational chemicals has led to hypotheses of bladder cancer's environmental origin [92,93]. Experimental bladder tumors in dogs have been produced by aromatic hydrocarbons including para-aminobiphenyl and paranitroliphenyl [98], suggesting the role of exogenous carcinogens in the development of these tumors. In addition, in both dogs and humans, tumors with similar histology were produced after exposure to beta-naphthylamine and benzidine, both of which are found in tobacco smoke [93], further suggesting similarities in bladder cancer etiology between species. Because domestic canines largely share their environment with their owners, studies on the relationship between environmental chemicals, including tobacco smoke, and the risk of bladder cancer may further understanding of bladder cancer etiology in both populations.

Cigarette smoking has been extensively studied in relation to bladder cancer in humans and is well established as a risk factor. An association between cigarette smoking and bladder cancer has been observed in more than 30 case-control studies and in 10 cohort studies [91]. Overall, smokers appear to have two to three times the risk of nonsmokers [91]. Risk increases with increasing intensity of smoking (packs per day), with relative risk estimates for moderate to heavy smokers ranging from 2 to 5, compared to nonsmokers [91].

Studies of the relation between ETS and risk of bladder cancer are few in number and results are inconsistent [99]. Studies of ETS and risk of bladder cancer in nonsmoking humans may be confounded by occupational and dietary exposures. For example, increased risks of bladder have been observed among industrial workers including painters, farmers, rubber workers, electrical workers, pesticide applicators, truck drivers, and workers in the petroleum and chemical industries [100,101], who may also have substantial exposure to active smoking and occupational ETS. Studies of ETS and bladder cancer may also be confounded by factors such as alcohol, artificial sweeteners, and analgesic use, although a consistent association between these exposures and bladder cancer has not been reported [91]. Studies of ETS and risk of bladder cancer in companion animals may help to disentangle the association between ETS and bladder cancer with less confounding by occupational and dietary factors.

To date, only one study has investigated the relation between ETS exposure and the risk of canine bladder cancer [94]. Glickman et al. conducted a case-control study of canine TCC at the University of Pennsylvania School of Veterinary Medicine between January 1982 and June 1985. All dogs with histologically confirmed TCC in the specified time frame were eligible for inclusion. Eighty-nine dogs with TCC were identified as cases, while eligible controls were 110 dogs selected from among all non-TCC biopsy reports. Control dogs with diseases of the urinary tract were excluded. Trained interviewers contacted the identified cases and controls to collect information regarding the dogs' residential and drug history, home environment, diet and body conformation one year prior to diagnosis, along with smoking patterns in the home during the dog's lifetime.

Owners of 59 of 89 (66.3%) cases and 71 of 110 (64.5%) controls were successfully interviewed. The number of pack-years smoked in the home during the dog's lifetime was calculated and risk of bladder cancer in dogs living in households with 1-3000 and >3000 pack-years were compared to risk in dogs living in non-smoking households. After controlling for age and breed size, an increased risk of bladder cancer was not observed for either category of smoking exposure. The odds ratios for dogs exposed to 1-3000 and >3000 lifetime pack-years of passive cigarette smoke compared to unexposed dogs were 1.3 (95% C.I. = 0.5-3.1) and 0.8 (95% C.I. = 0.3-2.0), respectively.

Results of this study do not suggest an increased risk of canine bladder cancer associated with household ETS exposure. However, the small sample size and relatively small number of exposed subjects may have prohibited the authors from observing a modest effect, if one exists. Given the strong relationship between active smoking and bladder cancer in humans, additional studies of ETS exposure and the disease in dogs may yield important new information.

Cancers of the Nasal Cavity and Paranasal Sinuses

Sinonasal cancer (SNC) accounts for 1% of all canine neoplasms [8] with an estimated incidence rate of approximately 40 per 100,000 hospitalizations, or approximately 5% of all hospitalized canine cancer patients [102]. In comparison, SNC is a rare disease in humans with an estimated yearly incidence in the US of less than 1 per 100,000 persons [6,103]. The incidence rate of canine SNC increases with age and the average age of affected dogs is 10 years [8]. Similarly, population-based incidence rates increase with age in humans with a median age of diagnosis of 63 in men and 65 in women [103].

Canine and feline nasal cancers are similar in clinical presentation and pathology to human nasal and paranasal sinus tumors, making companion animals a useful sentinel for studying environmental causes of human SNC [6]. Carcinomas, mainly adenocarcinoma and squamous cell carcinoma, make up two-thirds of SNC in dogs and cats, while squamous cell and undifferentiated carcinomas are the most common tumor types in human SNC [8,103,104]. Nasal tumors in both dogs and cats remain locally invasive and rarely metastasize to distant sites until late in the course of the disease [42,104], whereas in humans, approximately 31% of SNC cancers remain localized, 40% metastasize regionally, and 22% metastasize remotely [103].

The relationship between active and passive smoking and risk of human SNC has not been studied as extensively as other tumors in the respiratory tract, such as those of the pharynx, larynx, and lung. Information on the role of tobacco in the etiology of SNC has been generated mainly from descriptive epidemiology and case-control studies. Case-control studies of active smoking and risk of SNC tend to show either no association or only a modest elevation in risk, and tend to be limited to squamous cell carcinoma or undifferentiated carcinomas [103]. Furthermore, there are very few data available on the relationship between passive smoking and SNC in humans. Studies on ETS and canine SNC can fill this research gap and generate new information on the role of ETS in the development of this disease.

An environmental etiology for canine SNC has been suggested by several authors [102,105]. Numerous associations between industrial activity and location of residence with SNC in humans have been documented [106,107], but only speculated in canines. Hayes et al. noted similar risks of canine SNC among mixed breed and purebred dogs, suggesting an environmental rather than genetic etiology [102]. However, some "high-risk" breeds, such as the collie, have been identified in some studies [102], but it is still unclear whether this excess risk is due to nasal length or due to genetics. While both human and canine nasal cavities function as environmental filters, the canine nasal cavity is believed to be more complex and efficient in filtering pollutants; the extensive filtering experience by dogs may contribute to SNC by prolonging contact of nasal epithelium with carcinogens such as ETS [102].

Two case-control studies in dogs have evaluated the relationship between ETS exposure and SNC [6,14]. Reif and colleagues identified participants from oncology records systems from the veterinary teaching hospital at the Colorado State University [14]. All histologically-confirmed cases of cancer of the nasal cavity and paranasal sinuses from the years 1986-1990 were identified. Controls with other forms of cancer diagnosed during the same time period were randomly selected, and included dogs with lymphoma (n = 126 dogs), bone cancer (95), oral cancer (33), melanoma (19), hemangiosarcoma (15), and breast cancer (12). Telephone interviews were used to collect information on demographics, chemical exposures to pesticides, herbicides, flea and tick products, wood dust and household ETS exposure. Skull shape was ascertained by medical record based on specified breed or a description of the dog. An exposure index to represent lifetime exposure to ETS was created by multiplying the number of packs smoked per day by each smoker during the dog's lifetime and the time spent indoors by the dog. Subjects that lived in homes with no smokers were considered to receive no exposure to ETS. The final analysis was based on 103 cases and 378 controls.

Table 4. Multivariable relative risk (RR)* of canine nasal/sinus cancer by level of exposure to household cigarette smoking: results for Brachycephalic/mesocephalic vs. Dolichocephalic dogs. Adapted from Reif et al. [14]

	Brachy/mesocephalic dogs				Dolichocephalic dogs			
Risk factor	**Cases**	**Controls**	**RR***	**95% CI**	**Cases**	**Controls**	**RR***	**95% CI**
Smoker in household								
None	33	68	1.0		21	138	1.0	
Smoker	17	75	0.5	0.3 - 0.9	32	97	2.0	1.0 - 4.1
Packs smoked								
None	33	68	1.0		21	138	1.0	
1 to < 12	9	40	0.5	0.2 - 1.0	17	54	1.7	0.7 - 4.1
>= 12	8	35	0.4	0.2 - 0.9	15	43	2.4	1.0 - 5.9
Exposure index†								
None	34	73	1.0		22	141	1.0	
0 to <= 4.5	7	24	0.5	0.2 - 1.0	11	32	1.5	0.6 - 4.1
> 4.5	9	46	0.5	0.3 - 1.1	20	62	2.5	1.1 - 5.7

*Relative risk estimated by odds ratio, adjusted for age, gender and use of flea control products;
CI = confidence interval;
† Number of packs smoked by all household smokers during dog's lifetime x proportion of time dog spent indoors.

Among all dogs, those living with a smoker were not found to be at increased risk of SNC (OR = 0.9; 95% C.I. = 0.6-1.5), after adjusting for age, breed, gender, and use of flea control products. Evidence of a dose-response relationship did not exist for either pack-years smoked or the exposure index and risk of SNC. However, while an increased risk of SNC with ETS exposure was not observed among all dogs, skull shape was an important modifying factor of the ETS-cancer relationship. Among dolichocephalic dogs (i.e., long-nosed), dogs living with a smoker had twice the risk of SNC as unexposed dogs (OR = 2.0; 95% C.I. 1.0-4.1), and those with the highest level of exposure had a significant 2.5-fold increase in risk (OR = 2.5; 95% C.I. 1.1-5.7) (Table 4). In contrast, brachycephalic (i.e., short-nosed) and mesocephalic (i.e., medium-nosed) dogs living with a smoker had a decreased risk of SNC (OR=0.5; 95% C.I. 0.3-0.9), compared to unexposed dogs. While a significant dose-response relationship with ETS exposure ($p<0.05$) was observed for long-nosed dogs, there was no evidence of a dose-response among short and medium-nosed dogs.

The elevated risk among long-nosed dogs living in smoking households suggests that ETS may be etiologically related to SNC risk in canines. These results, together with those from the previously discussed study of ETS and lung cancer by Reif et al. [13], suggest that exposure to ETS may increase risk of cancers in those respiratory tissues with the most prolonged contact with chemical carcinogens in tobacco smoke. In long-nosed dogs with extensive nasal filtration, the tissues at greatest risk are those of the nasal and sinus cavities. In contrast, in short-nosed dogs and humans, both of whom filter smoke less efficiently in the nasal passages, lung tissue has greater exposure to carcinogens in ETS.

The relationship between ETS and canine SNC was also assessed by Bukowski and colleagues in a case-control study conducted at the University of Pennsylvania School of Veterinary Medicine [6]. Cases included those diagnosed with canine intranasal and sinus cancer between 1989 and 1993, while controls were dogs diagnosed with stomach, bowel, omental (i.e., peritoneum lining the abdominal cavity), or liver cancers during the same years. Owners of case and control subjects were asked to participate by completing a mailed questionnaire that elicited information on canine factors, owner demographics, and household exposures including ETS and local pollution. High risk status was assigned to Airedale terriers, basset hounds, old English sheepdogs, Scottish terriers, collies, Shetland sheepdogs, and German shorthair pointers. Nasal length was ascertained by owner classification on a graphical scale 1-5, with 1 being the shortest and 5 the longest. To quantify exposure to ETS, information was collected on the number of household smokers, type of tobacco product smoked (cigar, cigarette, or pipe), percentage smoked at home, and duration of smoking in years while residing with the animal. If quantitative information on smoking was not provided, it was assumed that smokers smoked 1 pack of cigarettes daily for the life of the animal, with 50% of the smoking occurring at home. A total of 129 cases and 176 controls responded with completed questionnaires to make up the final study population. The overall response rate was 72% and characteristics of respondents were similar to that of non-respondents.

After adjusting for nose length, purebred status, heating source and other factors, the authors did not observe an increased risk of SNC in dogs exposed to household ETS (OR = 0.7; 95% C.I. 0.41-1.19). However, results were not stratified by skull length, though this factor was included in multivariate analysis. Had the authors calculated the association between ETS and SNC stratified by skull length, they may potentially have observed an increased risk among long-nosed dogs similar to that found by Reif et al. [13].

In both studies, the inclusion of controls with other types of cancers may have contributed to an underestimation of the relationship between ETS exposure and SNC. For example, in the study by Reif et al. a large proportion of controls had malignant lymphoma.

While it is as yet unknown whether CML risk is positively associated with ETS, studies in humans [52,53,55] and cats [3] suggest that lymphoma may indeed be related to ETS. In this case, the risk of SNC associated with ETS may actually be greater than estimated in both of these studies. Future studies of this relationship may benefit from the inclusion of controls with benign tumors or other chronic diseases instead of other malignancies potentially associated with ETS exposure.

Given the provocative findings of Reif and colleagues suggesting a complex relationship between ETS exposure, nasal filtration and risk of SNC, additional studies of this relationship in long and short/medium-nosed dogs are clearly warranted. Results from these studies may provide interesting new information about the role of ETS exposure on respiratory cancers in humans.

Conclusion

In summary, epidemiologic studies of companion animals suggest that exposure to environmental tobacco smoke may be associated with the development of a variety of cancers, including lymphoma, oral cancer, lung cancer and perhaps those of the nasal/sinus cavities. These studies can make a unique and valuable contribution to knowledge of the relationship between passive smoking and cancer in humans, for which many relationships remain unclear. Though the field of companion animal epidemiology is still in its adolescence, provocative results from early investigations suggest that additional studies of the health effects of exposure to environmental tobacco smoke in animal populations, and in humans, are clearly warranted.

References

[1] National Research Council. Animals as Sentinels of Environmental Health Hazards. Washington, D.C.: National Academy Press; 1991.

[2] Kelsey JL, Moore AS, Glickman LT. Epidemiologic studies of risk factors for cancer in pet dogs. *Epidemiol.Rev.* 1998;20(2):204-17.

[3] Bertone ER, Snyder LA, Moore AS. Environmental tobacco smoke and risk of malignant lymphoma in pet cats. *Am. J. Epidemiol.* 2002; Aug 1;156(3):268-73.

[4] Gavazza A, Presciuttini S, Barale R, Lubas G, Gugliucci B. Association between canine malignant lymphoma, living in industrial areas, and use of chemicals by dog owners. *J. Vet. Intern. Med.* 2001; May-Jun;15(3):190-5.

[5] Cooley DM, Beranek BC, Schlittler DL, Glickman NW, Glickman LT, Waters DJ. Endogenous gonadal hormone exposure and bone sarcoma risk. *Cancer Epidemiol. Biomarkers Prev.* 2002; Nov;11(11):1434-40.

[6] Bukowski JA, Wartenberg D, Goldschmidt M. Environmental causes for sinonasal cancers in pet dogs, and their usefulness as sentinels of indoor cancer risk. *J. Toxicol. Environ. Health A* 1998; Aug 7;54(7):579-91.

[7] Garbe PL. The companion animal as a sentinel for environmentally related human diseases. *Acta Vet. Scand. Suppl.* 1988;84:290-2.

[8] MacEwen EG. Spontaneous tumors in dogs and cats: models for the study of cancer biology and treatment. *Cancer Metastasis Rev.* 1990; Sep;9(2):125-36.

[9] Vail DM, MacEwen EG. Spontaneously occurring tumors of companion animals as models for human cancer. *Cancer Invest.* 2000;18(8):781-92.

[10] American Pet Products Manufacturers Assoc. 2003-2004 Natl Pet Owners Survey 2004.

[11] Bertone-Johnson ER, Bundga M. Establishment of a prospective cohort of domestic dogs in western Massachusetts. *Am. J. Epidemiol.* 2005;161(Suppl):S126.

[12] Bertone ER, Snyder LA, Moore AS. Environmental and lifestyle risk factors for oral squamous cell carcinoma in domestic cats. *J. Vet. Intern. Med.* 2003; Jul-Aug;17(4):557-62.

[13] Reif JS, Dunn K, Ogilvie GK, Harris CK. Passive smoking and canine lung cancer risk. *Am. J. Epidemiol.* 1992; Feb 1;135(3):234-9.

[14] Reif JS, Bruns C, Lower KS. Cancer of the nasal cavity and paranasal sinuses and exposure to environmental tobacco smoke in pet dogs. *Am. J. Epidemiol.* 1998; Mar 1;147(5):488-92.

[15] Reif JS, Maguire TG, Kenney RM, Brodey RS. A cohort study of canine testicular neoplasia. *J. Am. Vet. Med. Assoc.* 1979;175:719-23.

[16] Misdorp W. Veterinary cancer epidemiology. *Vet. Q.* 1996; Mar;18(1):32-6.

[17] Dorn CR, Taylor DO, Frye FL, Hibbard HH. Survey of animal neoplasms in Alameda and Contra Costa Counties, California. I. Methodology and description of cases. *J. Natl. Cancer Inst.* 1968; Feb;40(2):295-305.

[18] Dorn CR, Taylor DO, Schneider R, Hibbard HH, Klauber MR. Survey of animal neoplasms in Alameda and Contra Costa Counties, California. II. Cancer morbidity in dogs and cats from Alameda County. *J. Natl. Cancer Inst.* 1968; Feb;40(2):307-18.

[19] Arias E. The United States Life Tables, 2002. Natl Vital Stat Rep 2004;53(6):1-38.

[20] Aldrich J. Geriatrics. In: Siegal M, editor. UC Davis School of Veterinary Medicine Book of the Dogs. Harper Collins; 1995.

[21] Thornton KC, Hamil J. Your Aging Cat. NY, NY: Macmillan USA/Howell Book House; 1997.

[22] Bukowski JA, Wartenberg D. An alternative approach for investigating the carcinogenicity of indoor air pollution: pets as sentinels of environmental cancer risk. *Environ. Health Perspect.* 1997; Dec;105(12):1312-9.

[23] Stanek EJ III, Calabrese EJ. Daily estimates of soil ingestion in children. *Environ. Health Perspect.* 1995; Mar;103(3):276-85.

[24] Bertone-Johnson ER. Re: Environmental tobacco smoke and risk of malignant lymphoma in pet cats. *Am. J. Epidemiol.* 2003; Dec 15;158(12):1227.

[25] Clancy EA, Moore AS, Bertone ER. Evaluation of cat and owner characteristics and their relationships to outdoor access of owned cats. *J. Am. Vet. Med. Assoc.* 2003; Jun 1;222(11):1541-5.

[26] Chilmonczyk BA, Knight GJ, Palomaki GE, Pulkkinen AJ, Williams J, Haddow JE. Environmental tobacco smoke exposure during infancy. *Am. J. Public Health.* 1990; Oct;80(10):1205-8.

[27] Liu C, Lian F, Smith DE, Russell RM, Wang XD. Lycopene supplementation inhibits lung squamous metaplasia and induces apoptosis via up-regulating insulin-like growth factor-binding protein 3 in cigarette smoke-exposed ferrets. *Cancer Res.* 2003; Jun 15;63(12):3138-44.

[28] Reif JS, Lower KS, Ogilvie GK. Residential exposure to magnetic fields and risk of canine lymphoma. *Am. J. Epidemiol.* 1995;141:352-9.

[29] Auerbach O, Hammond EC, Kirman D, Garfinkel L, Stout AP. The effect of direct cigarette smoke inhalation on the respiratory tree of dogs. *Natl. Cancer Inst. Monogr.* 1968; Jun;28:65-77.

[30] Auerbach O, Hammond EC, Kirman D, Garfinkel L. Effects of cigarette smoking on dogs. II. Pulmonary neoplasms. *Arch. Environ. Health* 1970; Dec;21(6):754-68.

[31] Baron JA, Rohan TE. Tobacco. In: Schottenfeld D, Fraumeni JF, editors. Cancer Epidemiology and Prevention. Second ed. New York: Oxford University; 1996. p. 269-89.

[32] Rothman KJ, Greenland S. Modern Epidemiology, 2nd Edition. Philadelphia: Lippincott-Raven. 1998.

[33] Vail DM, Moore AS, Ogilvie GK, Volk LM. Feline lymphoma (145 cases): proliferation indices, cluster of differentiation 3 immunoreactivity, and their association with prognosis in 90 cats. *J.Vet. Intern. Med.* 1998; Sep-Oct;12(5):349-54.

[34] Valli VE, Jacobs RM, Norris A, Couto CG, Morrison WB, McCaw D, et al. The histologic classification of 602 cases of feline lymphoproliferative disease using the National Cancer Institute working formulation. *J. Vet. Diagn. Invest.* 2000; Jul;12(4):295-306.

[35] Hahn KA, Bravo L, Adams WH, Frazier DL. Naturally occurring tumors in dogs as comparative models for cancer therapy research. *In Vivo.* 1994; Jan-Feb;8(1):133-43.

[36] Greenlee PG, Filippa DA, Quimby FW, Patnaik AK, Calvano SE, Matus RE, et al. Lymphomas in dogs. A morphologic, immunologic, and clinical study. *Cancer* 1990; Aug 1;66(3):480-90.

[37] Pierrepoint CG. Possible benefits to veterinary medicine of considering the dog as a model for human cancer. *J. Small Anim. Pract.* 1985;26:43-7.

[38] Teske E. Canine malignant lymphoma: a review and comparison with human non-Hodgkin's lymphoma. *Vet. Q.* 1994; Dec;16(4):209-19.

[39] Teske E, Wisman P, Moore PF, van Heerde P. Histologic classification and immunophenotyping of canine non-Hodgkin's lymphomas: unexpected high frequency of T cell lymphomas with B cell morphology. *Exp. Hematol.* 1994; Nov;22(12):1179-87.

[40] Clancy E, McConnell W, Patronek G, Moore A. Epidemiological study of canine lymphoma in New England. Veterinary Cancer Society Annual Conference Proceedings, 1999.

[41] Jemal A, Siegel R, Ward E, Murray T, Xu J, Smigal C, et al. Cancer statistics, 2006. *CA Cancer J. Clin.* 2006; Mar-Apr;56(2):106-30.

[42] Ogilvie GK, Moore AS. Managing the Veterinary Cancer Patient: A Practice Manual. Trenton, *NJ: Veterinary Learning Systems,* 1996.

[43] Fournel-Fleury C, Magnol JP, Chabanne L, Ghernati I, Marchal T, Bonnefond C, et al. Growth fractions in canine non-Hodgkin's lymphomas as determined in situ by the expression of the Ki-67 antigen. *J. Comp. Pathol.* 1997; Jul;117(1):61-72.

[44] Mooney SC, Hayes AA, MacEwen EG, Matus RE, Geary A, Shurgot BA. Treatment and prognostic factors in lymphoma in cats: 103 cases (1977-1981). *J. Am. Vet. Med. Assoc.* 1989; Mar 1;194(5):696-702.

[45] Teske E, Rutteman GR, Kuipers-Dijkshoorn NJ, van Dierendonck JH, van Heerde P, Cornelisse CJ. DNA ploidy and cell kinetic characteristics in canine non-Hodgkin's lymphoma. *Exp. Hematol.* 1993; Apr;21(4):579-84.

[46] Scherr P, Mueller NE. Non-Hodgkin’s Lymphomas. In: Schottenfeld D, Fraumeni JF, editors. Cancer Epidemiology and Prevention. Second ed. New York: Oxford University Press; 1996. p. 920-45.

[47] Groves FD, Linet MS, Travis LB, Devesa SS. Cancer surveillance series: non-Hodgkin's lymphoma incidence by histologic subtype in the United States from 1978 through 1995. *J. Natl. Cancer Inst.* 2000; Aug 2;92(15):1240-51.

[48] Vail DM, Thamm DH. Hematopoietic Tumors. In: Ettinger SJ, Feldman EC, editors. Textbook of Veterinary Internal Medicine. 6th Edition. ed. St. Louis: Elsevier Saunders; 2005. p. 732-47.

[49] Chaganti RS, Nanjangud G, Schmidt H, Teruya-Feldstein J. Recurring chromosomal abnormalities in non-Hodgkin's lymphoma: biologic and clinical significance. *Semin. Hematol.* 2000; Oct;37(4):396-411.

[50] Cotter SM, Hardy WD,Jr, Essex M. Association of feline leukemia virus with lymphosarcoma and other disorders in the cat. *J. Am. Vet. Med. Assoc.* 1975; Mar 1;166(5):449-54.

[51] Moore AS. Treatment of feline lymphoma. *Feline Pract.* 1996;24:17-20.

[52] Linet MS, McLaughlin JK, Hsing AW, Wacholder S, Co Chien HT, Schuman LM, et al. Is cigarette smoking a risk factor for non-Hodgkin's lymphoma or multiple myeloma? Results from the Lutheran Brotherhood Cohort Study. *Leuk. Res.* 1992; Jun-Jul;16(6-7):621-4.

[53] Parker AS, Cerhan JR, Dick F, Kemp J, Habermann TM, Wallace RB, et al. Smoking and risk of non-Hodgkin lymphoma subtypes in a cohort of older women. *Leuk. Lymphoma* 2000; Apr;37(3-4):341-9.

[54] Adami J, Nyren O, Bergstrom R, Ekbom A, Engholm G, Englund A, et al. Smoking and the risk of leukemia, lymphoma, and multiple myeloma (Sweden). *Cancer Causes Control* 1998; Jan;9(1):49-56.

[55] Herrinton LJ, Friedman GD. Cigarette smoking and risk of non-Hodgkin's lymphoma subtypes. *Cancer Epidemiol. Biomarkers Prev.* 1998; Jan;7(1):25-8.

[56] De Stefani E, Fierro L, Barrios E, Ronco A. Tobacco, alcohol, diet and risk of non-Hodgkin's lymphoma: a case-control study in Uruguay. *Leuk. Res.* 1998; May;22(5):445-52.

[57] Freedman DS, Tolbert PE, Coates R, Brann EA, Kjeldsberg CR. Relation of cigarette smoking to non-Hodgkin's lymphoma among middle-aged men. *Am. J. Epidemiol.* 1998; Nov 1;148(9):833-41.

[58] Brown LM, Everett GD, Gibson R, Burmeister LF, Schuman LM, Blair A. Smoking and risk of non-Hodgkin's lymphoma and multiple myeloma. *Cancer Causes Control* 1992; Jan;3(1):49-55.

[59] Franceschi S, Serraino D, Bidoli E, Talamini R, Tirelli U, Carbone A, et al. The epidemiology of non-Hodgkin's lymphoma in the north-east of Italy: a hospital-based case-control study. *Leuk. Res.* 1989;13(6):465-72.

[60] Miligi L, Seniori Costantini A, Crosignani P, Fontana A, Masala G, Nanni O, et al. Occupational, environmental, and life-style factors associated with the risk of hematolymphopoietic malignancies in women. *Am. J. Ind. Med.* 1999; Jul;36(1):60-9.

[61] Stagnaro E, Ramazzotti V, Crosignani P, Fontana A, Masala G, Miligi L, et al. Smoking and hematolymphopoietic malignancies. *Cancer Causes Control* 2001; May;12(4):325-34.

[62] Zahm SH, Weisenburger DD, Holmes FF, Cantor KP, Blair A. Tobacco and non-Hodgkin's lymphoma: combined analysis of three case-control studies (United States). *Cancer Causes Control* 1997; Mar;8(2):159-66.

[63] Siemiatycki J, Krewski D, Franco E, Kaiserman M. Associations between cigarette smoking and each of 21 types of cancer: a multi-site case-control study. *Int. J. Epidemiol.* 1995; Jun;24(3):504-14.

[64] Tavani A, Negri E, Franceschi S, Serraino D, La Vecchia C. Smoking habits and non-Hodgkin's lymphoma: a case-control study in northern Italy. *Prev. Med.* 1994; Jul;23(4):447-52.

[65] Matsuo K, Hamajima N, Hirose K, Inoue M, Takezaki T, Kuroishi T, et al. Alcohol, smoking, and dietary status and susceptibility to malignant lymphoma in Japan: results of a hospital-based case-control study at Aichi Cancer Center. *Jpn. J. Cancer Res.* 2001; Oct;92(10):1011-7.

[66] Nelson RA, Levine AM, Marks G, Bernstein L. Alcohol, tobacco and recreational drug use and the risk of non-Hodgkin's lymphoma. *Br. J. Cancer.* 1997;76(11):1532-7.

[67] Ji BT, Shu XO, Linet MS, Zheng W, Wacholder S, Gao YT, et al. Paternal cigarette smoking and the risk of childhood cancer among offspring of nonsmoking mothers. *J. Natl. Cancer Inst.* 1997; Feb 5;89(3):238-44.

[68] John EM, Savitz DA, Sandler DP. Prenatal exposure to parents' smoking and childhood cancer. *Am. J. Epidemiol.* 1991; Jan 15;133(2):123-32.

[69] Sorahan T, McKinney PA, Mann JR, Lancashire RJ, Stiller CA, Birch JM, et al. Childhood cancer and parental use of tobacco: findings from the inter-regional epidemiological study of childhood cancer (IRESCC). *Br. J. Cancer.* 2001; Jan 5;84(1):141-6.

[70] Wells AJ, English PB, Posner SF, Wagenknecht LE, Perez-Stable EJ. Misclassification rates for current smokers misclassified as nonsmokers. *Am. J. Public Health* 1998; Oct;88(10):1503-9.

[71] Nyberg F, Isaksoon I, Harris JRea. Misclassification of smoking status and lung cancer risk from environmental tobacco smoke in never-smokers. Epidemiology 1997;8:304-9.

[72] Wu AH. Exposure misclassification bias in studies of environmental tobacco smoke and lung cancer. *Environ. Health Perspect* 1999;107(suppl):873-7.

[73] Hayes HM, Tarone RE, Cantor KP, Jessen CR, McCurnin DM, Richardson RC. Case-control study of canine malignant lymphoma: positive association with dog owner's use of 2,4-dichlorophenoxyacetic acid herbicides. *J. Natl Cancer Inst.* 1991; Sep 4;83(17):1226-31.

[74] Hahn FF, Muggenburg BA, Griffith WC. Primary lung neoplasia in a beagle colony. *Vet. Pathol.* 1996; Nov;33(6):633-8.

[75] Nelson OL, Sellon RK. Pulmonary Parenchymal Disease. In: Ettinger SJ, Feldman EC, editors. Textbook of Veterinary Internal Medicine. 6th ed. St. Louis: Elsevier Saunders; 2005. p. 1241-2.

[76] Blot WJ, Fraumeni JF. Cancers of the lung and pleura. In: Schottenfeld D, Fraumeni JF, editors. Cancer Epidemiology and Prevention. Second ed. New York: Oxford University Press; 1996. p. 637-65.

[77] Gillett NA, Stegelmeier BL, Kelly G, Haley PJ, Hahn FF. Expression of epidermal growth factor receptor in plutonium-239-induced lung neoplasms in dogs. *Vet. Pathol.* 1992; Jan;29(1):46-52.

[78] Hirayama T. Non-smoking wives of heavy smokers have a higher risk of lung cancer: a study from Japan. 1981. *Bull. World Health Organ* 2000;78(7):940-2.

[79] Trichopoulos D, Kalandidi A, Sparros L, MacMahon B. Lung cancer and passive smoking. *Int. J. Cancer* 1981; Jan 15;27(1):1-4.

[80] Surgeon General. The health consequences of involuntary smoking. Washington, D.C.: U.S. Government Printing Office; 1986.

[81] National Research Council. Environmental Tobacco Smoke. Washington, D.C.: National Academy Press; 1986.

[82] Zwicker GM, Filipy RE, Park JF, Loscutoff SM, Ragan HA, Stevens DL. Clinical and pathological effects of cigarette smoke exposure in beagle dogs. *Arch. Pathol. Lab. Med.*1978; Dec;102(12):623-8.

[83] Reznik-Schuller H, Reznik G. Experimental pulmonary carcinogenesis. *Int. Rev. Exp. Pathol.* 1979;20:211-81.

[84] Parnell NK. Diseases of the Throat. In: Ettinger SJ, Feldman EC, editors. Textbook of Veterinary Internal Medicine. 6th ed. St. Louis: Elsevier Saunders; 2005. p. 1200-1.

[85] Blot WJ, McLaughlin JK, Devesa SS, Fraumeni JF, Jr. Cancers of the oral cavity and pharynx. In: Schottenfeld D, Fraumeni JF, editors. Cancer Epidemiology and Prevention. Second ed. New York: Oxford University Press; 1996. p. 666-80.

[86] Chen JK, Katz RV, Krutchkoff DJ. Intraoral squamous cell carcinoma. Epidemiologic patterns in Connecticut from 1935 to 1985. *Cancer* 1990; Sep 15;66(6):1288-96.

[87] Gervasio OL, Dutra RA, Tartaglia SM, Vasconcellos WA, Barbosa AA, Aguiar MC. Oral squamous cell carcinoma: a retrospective study of 740 cases in a Brazilian population. *Braz. Dent. J.* 2001;12(1):57-61.

[88] International Agency for Research on Cancer. Tobacco smoking. *IARC Monogr.* 1986;38:1-421.

[89] Blot WJ, McLaughlin JK, Winn DM, Austin DF, Greenberg RS, Preston-Martin S, et al. Smoking and drinking in relation to oral and pharyngeal cancer. *Cancer Res.* 1988; Jun 1;48(11):3282-7.

[90] Snyder LA, Bertone ER, Jakowski RM, Dooner MS, Jennings-Ritchie J, Moore AS. p53 expression and environmental tobacco smoke exposure in feline oral squamous cell carcinoma. *Vet. Pathol.* 2004; May;41(3):209-14.

[91] Silverman DT, Morrison AS, Devesa SS. Bladder cancer. In: Schottenfeld D, Fraumeni JF, editors. Cancer Epidemiology and Prevention. Second ed. New York: Oxford University Press; 1996. p. 1156-79.

[92] Hayes HM,Jr, Hoover R, Tarone RE. Bladder cancer in pet dogs: a sentinel for environmental cancer?. *Am. J. Epidemiol.* 1981; Aug;114(2):229-33.

[93] Hayes HM,Jr. Canine bladder cancer: epidemiologic features. *Am. J. Epidemiol.* 1976; Dec;104(6):673-7.

[94] Glickman LT, Schofer FS, McKee LJ, Reif JS, Goldschmidt MH. Epidemiologic study of insecticide exposures, obesity, and risk of bladder cancer in household dogs. *J. Toxicol. Environ. Health* 1989;28(4):407-14.

[95] Norris AM, Laing EJ, Valli VE, Withrow SJ, Macy DW, Ogilvie GK, et al. Canine bladder and urethral tumors: a retrospective study of 115 cases (1980-1985). *J. Vet. Intern. Med* 1992; May-Jun;6(3):145-53.

[96] Sprague RH, Anisko JJ. Elimination patterns in the laboratory beagle. *Behaviour* 1973; Nov;47(3):257-67.

[97] Poupko JM, Hearn WL, Radomski JL. N-Glucuronidation of N-hydroxy aromatic amines: a mechanism for their transport and bladder-specific carcinogenicity. *Toxicol. Appl. Pharmacol.* 1979; Sep 30;50(3):479-84.

[98] Coplan MM. Report on carcinogenic action of certain agents on urinary bladder of dogs. *JAMA* 1960; Apr 9;172:1611-8.

[99] Zeegers MP, Kellen E, Buntinx F, van den Brandt PA. The association between smoking, beverage consumption, diet and bladder cancer: a systematic literature review. *World J. Urol.* 2004; Feb;21(6):392-401.

[100] Claude J, Kunze E, Frentzel-Beyme R, Paczkowski K, Schneider J, Schubert H. Life-style and occupational risk factors in cancer of the lower urinary tract. *Am. J. Epidemiol.* 1986; Oct;124(4):578-89.

[101] Claude JC, Frentzel-Beyme RR, Kunze E. Occupation and risk of cancer of the lower urinary tract among men. A case-control study. Int J Cancer 1988; Mar 15;41(3):371-9.

[102] Hayes HM,Jr, Wilson GP, Fraumeni HF,Jr. Carcinoma of the nasal cavity and paranasal sinuses in dogs: descriptive epidemiology. *Cornell. Vet.* 1982; Apr;72(2):168-79.

[103] Roush GC. Cancers of the nasal cavity and paranasal sinuses. In: Schottenfeld D, Fraumeni JFJ, editors. Cancer Epidemiology and Prevention. 2nd ed. New York: Oxford University Press; 1996. p. 587-602.

[104] Venker-van Haagen AJ. Disease of the Nose and Nasal Sinuses. In: Ettinger SJ, Feldman EC, editors. Textbook of Veterinary Internal Medicine. 6th ed. St. Louis: Elsevier Saunders; 2005. p. 1194-5.

[105] Reif JS, Cohen D. The environmental distribution of canine respiratory tract neoplasms. *Arch. Environ. Health* 1971; Jan;22(1):136-40.

[106] Luce D, Leclerc A, Morcet JF, Casal-Lareo A, Gerin M, Brugere J, et al. Occupational risk factors for sinonasal cancer: a case-control study in France. *Am. J. Ind. Med.* 1992;21(2):163-75.

[107] Zheng W, Blot WJ, Shu XO, Diamond EL, Gao YT, Ji BT, et al. A population based case-control study of cancers of the nasal cavity and paranasal sinuses in Shanghai. *In. J. Cancer.* 1992;52(4):557-61.

In: Cancer Research Perspectives
Editor: Larissa S. Pereira, pp. 105-134
ISBN 978-1-60021-980-1

Chapter III

Circulating Endothelial Progenitor Cells: Relevant in Physiopathology, a Promise for Clinical Applications, and yet so Difficult to be Characterized

***Margherita Massa*[1,*], *Rita Campanelli*[2] *and Vittorio Rosti*[2]**
[1]Biotechnology Laboratory, [2]Organ Transplantation Laboratory, Fondazione Istituto di Ricovero e Cura a Carattere Scientifico (IRCCS) Policlinico San Matteo, Pavia, Italy.

Abstract

The recent identification of endothelial progenitor cells (EPCs) in the peripheral blood of adult individuals has highlighted the possibility that vasculogenesis can take place in the postnatal life. It has been reported that circulating EPCs can be recruited and incorporated into sites of active neovascularization but they can also play a role in replacing lost endothelial cells on the vessel wall mediating a mechanism of maintenance of the normal vascular homeostasis. An accurate and unique phenotypical and functional characterization of circulating EPC subsets is still matter of debate; infact, neither a precise and unique panel of cell surface markers nor universally accepted protocols are available up to now for their in vitro growth.

Methods for the identification and characterization of circulating endothelial cells able to participate to postnatal vasculogenesis and endothelial repair will be part of our review, that will be focused mainly on physiological and pathological conditions characterized by a spontaneous increase of the number of circulating EPCs. The possible role of a number of soluble factors able to induce the mobilization of EPCs from the bone marrow into the peripheral blood will be also discussed.

Keywords: endothelial progenitor cells, mobilization, vascular repair

---

* Correspondence concerning this article should be addressed to Dr. Margherita Massa, Fondazione IRCCS Policlinico San Matteo, Laboratorio Clinica Pediatrica, 19, P.le Golgi; 27100 Pavia, Italy. Fax: +39 0382 527976; telephone: +39 0382 502703; e-mail: m.massa@smatteo.pv.it.

INTRODUCTION

The first evidence that human adult circulating cells contain elements able to give rise to colonies of cells with an endothelial-like phenotype *in vitro*, and to incorporate into new vessels *in vivo* was reported in 1997 by Asahara and coll. in a seminal paper published in Science [1]. As a matter of fact, the presence of cells circulating in the peripheral blood with an endothelial-like phenotype was already known; however, these cells were shown to be mature, terminally differentiated endothelial cells, which are shed off from the vessel wall possibly because of senescence and/or following vessel wall injuries [2,3,4,5]. On the contrary, the cell population identified by Asahara and coll showed features that are typical of progenitor cells, namely the capability to proliferate, to form colonies of differentiated endothelial cells *in vitro*, and to migrate to sites of active vasculogenesis *in vivo*. These cells were referred to as circulating endothelial progenitor cells (EPCs) in order to distinguish them from their mature counterpart (circulating mature endothelial cells, ECs) and their importance was soon highlighted by several experiments which confirmed their involvement in neoangiogenetic processes associated with limb ischemia, myocardial infarction, atherosclerosis, wound healing, retinal neovascularization, and a possible use for therapeutic strategies [6,7].

This review will focus on some aspects of EPCs, by summarizing how they can be identified and enumerated in the peripheral blood (PB) of adult individuals and by discussing their involvement in human adult vessel wall homeostasis and in different pathological conditions. Finally, attention will be paid to the possible therapeutic role of these EPCs.

The existence of cells with the potential of proliferation and differentiation into mature endothelial cells was believed to pertain only to the embryonic development where the differentiation of mesodermal cells to angioblasts and subsequently to maturing endothelial cells is well known [8]. This principle was challenged by the experiments of Asahara and coll which showed that human adult circulating $CD34^+$ cells can differentiate into cells expressing some endothelial markers in vitro and have the functional capability to partecipate to neovessel formation at sites of ischemia in a murine model [1]. Following this report many efforts have been made in order to better identify and enumerate these cells, to understand their origin and to define "standard" conditions for their *in vitro* growth and differentiation (in an attempt similar to what has been done in the last 30 years with hematopoietic progenitor cells). This task quickly revealed to be quite hard because it emerged soon that an unique phenotypic marker for the EPCs able to differentiate them from mature endothelial cells and from other type of hematopoietic progenitor cells (HPCs) did not exist [6]. In addition, also from a functional point of view, it became evident that different culture conditions were able to allow the *in vitro* growth of different types of EPCs. Last but not least, things were further complicated by the low frequency of these cells in the human adult PB and bone marrow (BM).

PHENOTYPIC CHARACTERIZATION OF EPCs

Often, EPCs have been phenotipically characterized by the presence on their membrane of the CD34 antigen and of the type 2 receptor of the vascular endothelial growth factor (VEGFR-2) [1]. However, this couple of markers does not identify exclusively EPCs because they are also expressed by at least some mature ECs [9] and HPCs [10]. In 2000 Peichev and coll convincingly showed that EPCs, but not mature ECs, did express the early hematopoietic antigen CD133, thus suggesting that EPC should be regarded as a cell co-expressing the CD34 and the CD133 antigens, and the VEGFR-2, and that such kind of cell can be identified by flow cytometry at very low frequency in the adult PB, and at a higher frequency in the adult BM, adult mobilized PB, and umbilical cord blood [11]. In the same year, Gehling and coll confirmed at the functional level the importance of CD133 as a marker of EPCs by showing that purified CD133$^+$ cells were able to differentiate into endothelial cells in vitro [12]. Things however, turned out to be more complex because it was suggested [11,12] that this CD34$^+$CD133$^+$VEGFR-2$^+$ EPC could rather represent a multipotent progenitor cell capable of differentiating towards both the hematopoietic and the endothelial lineage, called hemangioblast [13,14,15,16]. The existence in the adult PB of a progenitor cell with a bi-potential hematopoietic and endothelial capability of differentiation such as the hemangioblast was regarded as a surprise but did not appear completely incomprehensible. In fact, an intimate association between endothelial and hematopoietic lineages is well described in the yolk sack of the developing embryo [17,18] and by experiments of gene knocking out in the animal model [19].

To further increase the list of surface antigens associated to the endothelial lineage, it has been reported that the CD117 antigen, the receptor of the hematopoietic cytokine stem cell factor (SCF), can identify cells able to participate to neovascularization of the injured myocardium of the mouse [20,21]. Indeed, in that experimental setting, only cells expressing at a high level the CD117 antigen could have part in this process. Subsequent experiments, again in the mouse model, confirmed the functional endothelial capacity of CD117$^+$ cells [22]. Unfortunately, as for CD133, also CD117 is expressed both on hematopoietic [23] and EPCs [24] and can not be regarderd as an unique marker of the endothelial lineage, neither when associated to other antigens such as CD34 and VEGFR-2. Besides these antigens, a number of other markers have been and are currently used to identify EPCs [6]. However, none of these is *per se* useful to identify EPCs because either they are also expressed on mature endothelial cells or they also belong to the hematopoietic lineage or both. For example Tie-2, VE-cadherin, CD146 and E-selectin are mainly or only expressed on mature or maturing endothelial cells, whereas CD31 (PECAM), von Willebrand factor (vWf), VEGFR-1 and Tie-2 (in addition to CD34, VEGFR-2, CD133 and CD117) are expressed on both endothelial and hematopoietic cells. Also the ability to incorporate 1,1'-dioctadecyl-3,3,3',3'-tetramethylindocarbocyanine-labeledacetylated low density lipoprotein (Di-LDL) and to bind lectins such as Ulex europeus or Bandeira semplicifolia, a combination of markers frequently used in the last years to identify EPCs, falls among these aspecific lineage markers [6]. Therefore, as it appears from the aforementioned considerations, the precise phenotype of the EPCs remains substantially indefinable. The assessment of the co-expression of multiple antigens seems to be an absolute requirement for the detection and consequently for the enumeration of circulating EPCs, and in keeping with this assumption, the assessment of the co-expression of CD34, VEGFR-2, and CD133 seems to be the more precise way for the identification, at the phenotype level, of at least a subset of "true" EPCs [25,26].

In Vitro Growth of EPCs

If the immuno-phenotypic characterization of the EPCs is still far from being exactly defined, the *in vitro* growth of EPCs is actually a matter of debate and controversy. In fact, *in vitro* attempts of growing EPCs made in these years have given different results suggesting that, at a functional level, different types of circulating cells can assume an endothelial phenotype. Moreover, *in vivo* studies have confirmed that these different type of putative EPCs can actively participate in effective neovascularization.

Asahara and coll [1] cultivated PB-derived $CD34^+$ cells on collagen or fibronectin coated dishes in the presence of Fetal Calf Serum and VEGF and after 7 days of culture obtained colonies of spindle shaped cells which were positive for a number of endothelial antigens, including CD31, Tie-2, E selectin, CD34 and Flk-1, and expressed endothelial nitric oxide synthase (eNOS) and VEGFR-2. Although this experiment remains a milestone in the history of circulating EPCs it was soon evident that this type of *in vitro* EPC derived colonies did not explained completely the proliferating and differentiating potential of the circulating EPCs. In fact, the purified $CD34^+$ cell population used was partially contaminated by mononuclear cells, thus leaving open the question of the precise identification and origin of the circulating EPCs, and the short term culture conditions suggested that other possible long term culture progenitors, endowed with a higher proliferative potential, could exist. These questions could be addressed by using different culture conditions including a more defined starting cell population, different culture medium favouring endothelial differentiation, and longer time of incubation. This turned out into a number of newly designed experiments for the *in vitro* growth of EPCs. A first evidence that more than one kind of EPC could exist came from the experiments of Lin and coll who showed that morphological and functional distinct type of EPCs can be grown *in vitro* starting from PB mononuclear cells [27]. They found that besides the small colonies of spindle-like cells obtained after 7 days of culture and endowed with a low proliferative potential, it was possible to obtain "late outgrowing cells" which appeared in culture after 3-4 weeks, had high proliferative potential, were able to form typical cobblestone areas, were positive for VE-cadherin, Flk-1, vWF, and CD36 and negative for some hematopoietic antigens such as CD45 and CD14. The Authors regarded these cells as true EPCs or angioblasts [27], probably derived directly from the putative hemangioblast. This experimental approach found a great success and was the starting point on which other experimental settings for the *in vitro* growth of EPCs were designed. In particular, Ingram and coll recently developed a culture system which basically stems from the work of Lin in which the Authors precisely identify both in the PB of adult individuals (at a very low frequency) and in the umbilical cord blood (at a 10 fold higher frequency than in PB) diverse sorts of EPCs able to form at different times of culture different types of colonies in a hierarchical model very similar to the well known hierarchical model of hematopoiesis

[28,29]. It should be noted that in all these types of protocols for the *in vitro* growth of EPCs, PB mononuclear cells were plated as a whole population and non-adherent cells were discarded after the first days of culture. In this way, however, contaminating adherent cells such as monocytes and mature ECs remain in the culture dish and cause a certain degree of heterogeneity of the cultivated cells, although it is likely that monocytes and mature ECs do not survive after the 4 weeks when the late outgrowing ECs emerge from the cultures. In this respect, some researchers have used the pre-plating of the mononuclear cells as a way for getting rid of adherent cells of monocytic origin [30,31]. However, yet again this method can eliminate some contaminating cells of myeloid origin, mainly monocytes, but not other not adherent cells of hematopoietic and non-hematopoietic origin which may participate to the *in vitro* growth and differentiation of cells with an endothelial phenotype and function. In fact, there is increasing evidence that also cells expressing mature hematopoietic antigens such as CD14 (a typical monocytic marker) can give rise to endothelial-like cells *in vitro*. In particular $CD14^+CD34^-$ PB derived cells can co-express endothelial markers, secrete angiogenic factors, and form tubular structures in matrigel [32, 33, 34] and when properly expanded *ex-vivo*, they can be incorporated in new vessels in an animal model [35]. Interestingly and in line with these observations, a subset of human PB monocytes has been reported to act as a pluripotent stem cell, *in vitro* [36, 37]. In addition to all these points, few studies suggest that other cells which are not of hematopoietic origin (neither immature, i.e. the hemangioblast, nor mature such as the aforementioned $CD14^+CD34$ cell population) can give rise to endothelial cells *in vitro* and *in vivo*. For instance, Hillebrands and coll reported that cells other than BM derived were responsible of the endothelial cell replacement in a mouse model of transplant arteriosclerosis [38]. In another *in vivo* experimental setting Verfaille's group showed that the so called MAPC (multipotent adult progenitor cell) which are circulating BM-derived cells different from hematopoietic stem cells (being $CD34^-$, $CD117^-$) can differentiate into distinct lineages, including endothelium [39]. Finally, cells belonging to the "side population" (a small circulating subset of $CD34^-$ stem cells, selected on the basis of Hoechst dye staining), are able to differentiate into various lineages including hematopoiesis, skeletal muscle, and endothelium [40].

These data suggest that a search for an unique definition of the real EPC is very difficult, at least at the functional level. It rather seems that a sort of heterogeneity of circulating EPCs exists and more in general, different subsets of circulating cells which are capable of assuming an endothelial phenotype and function are responsible for the different behaviour observed *in vitro*.

Mechanisms of Mobilization from Bone Marrow to Peripheral Blood

As reported in the previous paragraphs, EPCs have been mainly detected in the adult PB and in the umbilical cord blood. However, there are evidences that circulating EPCs derive from the BM [1,30,41], even when cells of non-hematopoietic origin are considered (see previous paragraph). How do EPCs leave the BM and mobilize to the PB? And how is possible to increase their otherwise very low frequency in the PB?

The spontaneous (not pharmacologically induced) mobilization of EPCs from the BM to the PB is a complex process regulated by a variety of factors, including growth factors and chemokines, receptors of adhesion molecules and enzymes [42].

A crucial step in the mobilization process is the loosening of the interactions between stromal cells (which are the main constituent of the bone marrow niche, the microenvironment where stem/progenitor cells are located) and EPCs which determines the recruitment of the progenitor cells from the BM to the PB. Activation of matrix metalloproteinase-9 (MMP-9) and of other proteinases (MMP-2, cathepsin G, elastases) mediates the cleavage of adhesion molecules and of the membrane bound form of Kit ligand (CD117) to its soluble form (s-Kit) [43]. These events are followed by the release of early $CD117^+$ progenitor cells (among which both hematopoietic and EPCs are included) from the niche to the vascular zone of the BM. In addition, also the BM derived e-NOS can play a role in EPCs mobilization since mice deficient in e-NOS showed reduced MMP-9 activity and impaired mobilization [44]. The most effective factor in inducing mobilization of EPCs from the BM to the PB is ischemia [45] which, by means of the Hypoxia Inducible Factor-1α-mediated up-regulation of VEGF and/or Stromal Derived Factor-1α (SDF-1α) [46] activates the cascade of events which causes proteinase activation and in turn EPC release from the marrow niches. A number of physiological and pathological conditions can affect the number of circulating EPCs, and these will be discussed below. Here, we will consider the effect of some pharmacological substances that can influence the EPC number in humans, namely Granulocyte-Colony Stimulating Factor (G-CSF), erythropoietin, VEGF, and statins. G-CSF is a cytokine commonly used for mobilization of $CD34^+$ cells in patients for HPC transplantation. It was shown that after G-CSF administration the proportion of circulating $CD34^+$ cells co-expressing VEGFR-2 and CD133 increased from a median of 0.4% to a median of 2.0% [11]. Another hematopoietic growth factor, erythropoietin, which is a well known modulator of erythroid progenitor and precursors proliferation and differentiation is also a potent mobilizer of EPCs from BM into PB [47, 48]. VEGF, administered via gene therapy in patients with critical limb ischemia, determined an increase in circulating EPCs up to 30 folds [49]. Last but not least, statins (the inhibitors of 3-hydroxy-3-methylglutaryl coenzyme A –HMG-CoA reductase) were shown to increase the number and functional activity of EPCs *in vitro* [50,51] and in patients with coronary artery disease [52]. This latter effect on EPC mobilization might further shed light onto the well known beneficial effects of statins as a medication against atherosclerotic vascular disease in addition to the already known effectiveness in lowering cholesterol levels.

Human EPCs in Healthy Subjects

The number of circulating EPCs in healthy subjects is rather low (0.01%) [6]. However, this number is not constant but it can change consistently. In fact, a variation in the number of circulating EPCs have been described in a number of physiological conditions, where pharmacologic interventions were absent. This phenomenon could have important consequences because circulating EPCs have been shown to participate in maintaining the vessel wall homeostasis, providing a circulating pool of cells that can take part in replacing dysfunctional endothelium or in repairing sites where a denuding injury occurred. This is quite relevant considering that endothelial injury leads to the loss of the anti-thrombotic properties of the vessel wall, and acts as a critical initial step in the development of atherosclerotic plaques [53]. The complete regeneration of injured endothelium may also occur by migration and proliferation of surrounding mature ECs as in adult angiogenesis; however, mature ECs are terminally differentiated cells with a low proliferative potential and their capacity to substitute damaged ECs and to create new vessels is relatively limited [54]. On the contrary, a role in vessel integrity could be played, rather than by mature ECs, by a functionally active population of EPCs, that has been recently described by Ingram and coll [55]. These EPCs are resident in the vessel wall and are able to proliferate and to differentiate *in vitro*.

Pregnancy

Evidences have been presented that circulating EPCs able to form late-outgrowth colonies are present in women during pregnancy, while in non pregnant women and in men the circulating ECs observed have the characteristic morphology of mature cells, uniform staining for vWF, and are unable to form this type of colonies [56]. The number of EPCs increases with gestation in normal pregnancies, and is directly correlated with both the gestational age and the plasma estradiol levels, suggesting that EPCs may play an important role in the regulation and maintenance of placental development and vascular integrity during pregnancy [57]. Previous reports have shown that in animal models of experimentally induced tissue injury estrogens increase the mobilization and influence the kinetics of EPCs that, leaving the bone marrow, incorporate into the neoendothelium contributing to the reendothelization process. This effect has been shown to be mainly dependent on eNOS expression, since both EPC mobilization and acceleration of reendothelization are absent in estradiol-treated eNOS null mice; in addition, both a mitogenic activity and an anti-apoptotic effect of estradiol on EPCs has been documented [58, 59].

Vascular Trauma

The normal menstrual cycle in women represents a physiological condition in which the endometrium undergoes shedding of the upper zone; this in turn induces a mechanism of cyclical repair, regeneration, and tissue remodelling that involves the growth of the vasculature [60]. Angiogenesis in the human uterus is required to support the reconstruction of endometrium and to provide a vascularized, receptive tissue for implantation and placentation three weeks later. By using the chick embryo chorioallantoic membrane *in vivo* assay for angiogenesis [61], it has been reported that human endometrial fragments, obtained at different phases of the menstrual cycle, have angiogenic potential, with a nadir in the late proliferative phase and significantly higher potential in the early proliferative, early secretory and late secretory phases [62]. VEGF and VEGFR-2 seem to play a role in the menstrual cycle, although data on their actual function are confusing both in animal models [63] and in humans [62, 64, 65]. Indeed, it has been suggested that during the premenstrual phase of the cycle there is an up-regulation of both the production of VEGF, and of the expression of its receptor VEGFR-2 on the stromal cells of the endometrium; however, at this stage of the cycle the physiologic role of this cytokine would be non angiogenic due to the fact that stromal cells expressing VEGFR-2 up-regulate the production of MMPs and induce the tissue expressing these factors to be eventually sloughed. Alternatively, the increase in VEGF levels in the early proliferative endometrium may be responsible for the elongation of the existing vessels, essential for tissue reconstruction [61].

There are no data regarding the possible recruitment of EPCs from the BM to the endometrium in order to support a vasculogenesis rather than an angiogenesis during the different phases of the physiological menstrual cycle. By both cytofluorimetric analysis and *in vitro* functional assay, we studied the percentage of circulating EPCs in a number of fertile women 24-48 hours before the beginning of the menstrual cycle, and 12, 24 hours, 15, and 23 days after the beginning of the menstrual cycle. Preliminary data suggest that fertile women, 24-48 hours before and 12 hours after the menstrual cycle, had a number of circulating EPCs, evaluated as $CD34^{+}VEGR\text{-}2^{+}$ cells, significantly higher than that found in a control group of age matched males; similarly, the percentage of circulating $CD34^{+}CD133^{+}VEGFR\text{-}2^{+}$ cells at 24-48 hours before and 15 days after the beginning of the menstrual cycle was significantly higher than that found in the control group (personal observations). No difference was found in the number of endothelial colonies obtained after 7 day culture assay of PB mononuclear cells, drawn from subjects of the control group or from fertile women tested at the defined different time points. In addition, no correlation was found between the number of circulating EPCs and plasma VEGF levels (personal observation). The possibility exists that the lack of correspondence between the increased number of circulating EPCs and the number of in vitro colonies during the different phases of the physiological menstrual cycle is due to the fact that we performed a culture assay which favours the growth of EPCs with a low proliferative potential and not the late-outgrowing EPCs. This, however, do not exclude their ability to participate in vascular repair processes or new vessel formation at the site of vascular injury (i.e. the endometrium). In a previous study, the number of circulating $34^{+}VEGFR\text{-}2^{+}$ EPCs was found increased in women with increased estrogen plasma levels due to ovarian hyperstimulation in the context of planned *in vitro* fertilization, and these cells also appeared to be resistant to *in vitro* induced apoptosis [58]. We did not find correlations between the increased number of circulating EPCs and plasma hormone levels (i.e. estrogens); this phenomenon may be less evident in physiological conditions, where both the variability between subjects that do not undergo any defined pharmacological treatment may be relevant, and the plasma levels are lower than those reached during hyperstimulation protocols. However, although further investigations are needed to understand the mechanisms underlying this finding, a physiological monthly amplification of EPC population may have a role in explaining the low rate of cardiovascular adverse events documented in fertile women with respect to men and to women that reached the menopause. In this regard, we found that the number of circulating $CD34^{+}CD133^{+}VEGFR\text{-}2^{+}$ EPCs was significantly higher in fertile women 24-48 hours before the beginning of the menstrual cycle than in women who met the criteria defining the menopause (personal observations).

Other less physiological vascular trauma induced by burn or by mechanical disruption, such as during surgical procedures, has been shown to lead to a cascade of events that results in an early increase of VEGF plasma levels promoting an increase in the number of circulating EPCs (VEGFR-2^+CD133^+) within 6-12 hours; these data further support the hypothesis that EPCs may enhance the re-endothelization of denuded prothrombotic injured vasculature [66].

PHYSICAL ACTIVITY

Physical activity is associated with an improvement of blood pressure, insulin sensitivity, and hemostatic and inflammatory parameters [67, 68]. However, despite the wealth of evidence derived from epidemiological and interventional trials, there is limited understanding of the underlying molecular mechanisms. Notably, physical training reduces vascular oxidative stress at least in part via increased activity of eNOS and extracellular superoxide dismutase, which in turn may exert beneficial vascular effects [69, 70]. Exercise is a non pharmacologic intervention that can acutely mobilize specific mononuclear cell subsets into circulation (i.e T suppressor/cytotoxic cells) [71, 72], and it has been recently observed that in voluntarily running mice there was an increase in the EPC number in BM, PB and spleen, which was mediated by a NO-dependent increase of VEGF plasma levels. Moreover, a decreased rate of EPC apoptosis, diminished neointima formation after vascular injury, and enhanced neoangiogenesis were also reported [73]. The effect of exercise (bicycle exercise test) on circulating EPCs in humans has been recently investigated [74]. In this study, an acute (within 5 to 10 minutes after the exercise was completed) increase of circulating CD133^+VE-Cadherin$^+$ cells (known to be involved in angiogenesis) was observed. In addition, after a 4 day culture period of PB-derived mononuclear cells, the Authors found that "angiogenic cells" able to bind Ulex lectin, and showing the typical uptake of Di-LDL, were increased compared with those grown in culture performed with blood obtained before the bicycle test. While the increase of EPCs, within 5 to 10 minutes after completion of exercise may indicate a mobilization either from BM or from the marginal pool, via beta adrenergic mechanisms similar to those of lymphocytes [71], the increase of EPCs after 4 days of culture seems to reflect a slower but more effective mobilization of functionally active progenitor cells. Interestingly, supernatants from these cultured cells were richer of endothelial growth factors such as VEGF, hepatocyte growth factors, G-CSF, and GM-CSF than those from cultured cells obtained from PB before the exercise was performed. According to these data, circulating EPCs may therefore be mobilized by exercise, possibly contributing to endothelial repair by homing to areas of dysfunctional endothelium and differentiate in new ECs or secreting vasculoprotective growth factors [74]. Alternatively but not exclusively, the beneficial effects of exercise can be at least in part attributed to an increase in blood flow. In fact, an increased flow enhances endothelium dependent vasodilatation by increasing the vascular expression of NO synthase and increases the release of NO inhibiting multiple processes involved in atherogenesis [75]. Another interesting finding of this study [74] was that exercise was also associated to an increase of CD133^+VE-cadherin$^-$ cells, which is likely to represent hematopoietic stem/progenitor cells. The increase of HPCs after exercise is reminiscent of a previous finding [76] obtained evaluating the number of circulating $CD34^+$ HPCs in healthy subjects trained to perform a marathon, half marathon, or sedentary controls. The runners had increased number of $CD34^+CD38^-$, $CD34^+CD33^-$ cell subsets with respect to the sedentary controls; however, no significant variation was noted, between the values obtained before and after they run the marathon or half marathon. Interestingly, there was a decrease of the number of circulating $CD34^+$ cells the morning after the race with respect to the values found before and immediately after the race. The physiological role of increased circulating HPCs is quite difficult to explain. It is possible that an increased turn over of polymorfonuclear (PMN) cells associated with exercise and the consequent inflammatory state may stimulate the HPC mobilization; in this case, the decrease of the HPCs after the race might reflect simply a maturation and replenishment of the peripheral PMN compartment. Alternatively, the HPC population may include cells with angioblastic potential having phenotypic markers in common with HPCs. Further supporting the role of exercise in EPC mobilization, it has been reported that a 44-year old healthy subject tested before, 1 day, and 45 days after a trek in the Himalayas, showed a significant increase of the number of both circulating EPCs ($CD45^-$ $CD146^+CD144^+$) and of endothelial colonies ($CD31^+CD105^+CD144^+CD146^{low}CD133^-$ vWf^{low}) 1 day after the exercise with respect to that found before and 45 days after the trek, and that found in a group of healthy controls [77]. According to these data, it is likely that the association of the effects of a higher oxygen demand induced by exercise, and of the hypoxia occurring at high altitude and determining a low oxygen saturation are strong stimuli for a rapid EPC mobilization. On the other hand, it has been shown that there was no significant change in the number of circulating $CD34^+VEGFR\text{-}2^+$ EPCs, in a group of healthy subjects undergoing a maximal exercise test on a calibrated electronically braked bicycle evaluated before and 2, 4, 6, 8, 24, and 48 hours after the test [78]. According with this finding, we also have unpublished data obtained in a group of healthy subjects and in a group of athletes who trained since at least 3 months, 3 times per week for a minimum of one hour. They all underwent the maximal test on a calibrated electronically braked bicycle, and the circulating EPCs were evaluated before the exercise and within 1 hour from the end of the exercise. No difference was found in the percentage of EPCs evaluated either as $CD34^+VEGFR\text{-}2^+$ or $CD34^+CD133^+VEGFR\text{-}2^+$ cells in healthy subjects or in athletes tested before and after the exercise; however, in athletes, the number of endothelial colonies obtained from 7 day culture of PB drawn before the exercise was higher than that found with PB from healthy sedentary controls. Similarly, the number of HPCs, tested by ISHAGE [79], were higher in athletes than in healthy sedentary controls evaluated before the test was performed. Taken together, these results suggest an influence of physical exercise in mobilization of progenitor cells (EPCs and/or HPCs) although they can not be considered conclusive. Further experiments are needed to define the relation between exercise and EPC mobilization. In fact, it has been suggested that EPC mobilization may in part explain the significant cardiovascular benefits of exercise; however, it is still a matter of debate whether healthy subjects and specific subsets of patients (i.e. patients with coronary artery disease) would demonstrate similar pattern of cell mobilization after acute/long lasting exercise.

AGING

Whereas pregnancy, menstrual cycle, and physical exercise seem to be able to increase the number of circulating EPCs, other factors have been described to negatively influence the number and function of these cells in healthy subjects. The most physiological of them, with no doubt, is the aging, that has been suggested to be associated with a decrease in the number and function of vascular stem and progenitor cells. Preliminary results from animal models indicated that transplantation of BM from old mice into young mice led to minimal neo-vascularization when compared to transplantation of young BM [80]. It was also demonstrated that EPCs from older patients with clinical ischemia had a significantly less therapeutic effect in rescuing ischemic hind limb of a nude mouse compared with those obtained from younger ischemic patients [80,81], providing evidence that an age dependent impairment in neo-vascularization may be heavenly influenced by the EPC phenotype. The mechanisms for this age-dependent impairment are largely unknown, and may be in part explained by the presence of a number of risk factors that are often associated to the older age and may constitute additional elements to be considered in studying the mechanisms that induce EPC impairment. Indeed, Hill et al [72] evaluated, by the Framingham risk factor score, the total burden of risk factors for cardiovascular disease, in a population of relatively healthy subjects, with a mean age of 50 years, who never had symptomatic cardiovascular diseases, or any condition in which angiogenesis may be present. Women were excluded from the study because of the possible confounding effects of the angiogenetic processes occurring during the menstrual cycle. The results showed that the EPCs, evaluated as number of colony forming units, in high-risk subjects were both fewer in number and become senescent more rapidly than those in low-risk subjects.

In addition, a decrease in VEGF plasma levels and the number of circulating EPCs has been found in subjects of advanced age (>62 years) compared with those with a younger age (<62 years) [83]. Recently, a comprehensive analysis of the association between age-related endothelial dysfunction and the number and function of EPCs, defined by the expression of $CD34^{+}VEGFR\text{-}2^{+}$ and $CD133^{+}VEGFR\text{-}2^{+}$, has been published [84]. No quantitative differences in EPCs were observed; however, culture-enriched EPCs from old but healthy subjects resulted impaired in terms of functional features like proliferation, migration, and survival. Changes in stem and progenitor cells may be of great importance for the aging process, potentially leading to progressive deterioration of functional and proliferative homeostasis in organs [85].

Recent studies support the notion that one possible mechanism for the vascular changes in advancing aging is the exhaustion of progenitor cells, in particular BM cells that are capable of vascular repair. Exhaustion of this component of BM in number, function, or both, could produce disequilibrium between vascular injury and vascular repair [82].

SMOKING

Smoking is another factor, although not a physiological one, that have been described to negatively influence the number of circulating EPCs in healthy subjects. Almost ten years ago, it was reported that long-term cigarette smoking might be involved in inducing an impairment in basal nitric oxide mediated vasodilation [86]. More recently, the number of circulating EPCs has been evaluated in chronic smokers and in non smoking subjects by both culture assay and cytofluorimetric analysis [87]. Interestingly, while the viability of mononuclear cells, assessed in an *in vitro* culture, from heavy smokers was similar to that of mononuclear cells derived from non smokers, the number of circulating EPCs (assessed by cytofluorimetric analysis as $CD45^{low}CD34^{+}CD133^{+}VEGFR\text{-}2^{+}$) from smokers was significantly lower than that of non smoking subjects. To be noted, the effect of smoking cessation was appreciable after two weeks, induced significant increase of circulating EPCs in chronic smokers in four weeks, and the phenomenon was more evident in light than in heavy smokers. The quick recovery of EPCs after quitting smoking rapidly disappeared when smoking was resumed.

The possibility exists that the rapid change in circulating EPC number associated with smoking status is related to an actual endothelial dysfunction in smokers. Injured vessels in smokers may benefit from EPCs for maintaining endothelial function, and their number may increase quitting smoking due to a decreased number of injured vessels; on the other hand, smoking may affect BM environment and EPC mobilization could be decreased by smoking.

EPCS IN HUMAN PATHOLOGICAL CONDITIONS

Cardiovascular Diseases

Age, hyperlipidemia, hyperglycemia, hypertension, familiarity for cardiovascular diseases, and smoking impair the function of the vascular endothelium and are considered cardiovascular risk factors. The number of circulating EPCs, that are involved in endothelial repair, have been negatively associated to risk factors, and it has recently been shown that the evaluation of their number in the PB may be a surrogate marker of vascular function, but also of cumulative cardiovascular risk, evaluated in term of Framingham risk score [88,82]. More importantly in a 2 year follow up study it has been shown that patients suffering from one cardiovascular event during the time of observation had significantly lower EPC number at the time of admission in the study than that of subjects who had an event free course, strongly suggesting that these cells contribute to ongoing vascular repair and their number may predict a disease progression [89]. In this study the evaluation of EPCs was performed by cytofluorimetric analysis and their phenotype was characterized by antibodies recognizing the CD34 antigen and the VEGFR-2 on the membrane; however, this is still one of the many ways used to count circulating EPCs, it may include a number of mature ECs, and it does not allow any conclusion about the functionality of these cells. So far, these limitations may give only a potential clinical value to this finding.

The number of circulating EPCs has been widely studied in patients with coronary artery disease (CAD) with a particular attention to verify the possible effect of ischemic or non ischemic condition. In the most of the studies patients were divided according with the presence of an angiografically documented stenotic, non stenotic, or ricanalized coronary artery. Actually, the number of EPCs evaluated the most of the time by cytofluorimetric analysis as $CD34^{+}VEGFR\text{-}2^{+}$ cells was decreased, although not significantly, in patients with CAD with respect to healthy controls, irrespectively of the presence of a stenotic coronary [78,90,89]. Low levels of circulating EPCs in patients with coronary artery disease could be the consequence of a number of mechanisms. It is possible that risk factors, by modulating the levels of oxidative stress, nitric oxide activity, or other physiologic processes, directly influence the mobilization or half life of EPCs. An alternative explanation supported by the data from Schmidt-Licke and coll [89] is that continuous endothelial damage or dysfunction leads to an eventual depletion or exhaustion of a presumable finite supply of EPCs.

To evaluate whether a single reversible episode of ischemia is sufficient to induce any measurable change in the number of circulating EPCs, additional investigations were performed in patients with CAD who underwent single symptom-limited exercise stress test. In the most of the studies the maximal exercise test was performed on a calibrated electronically braked bicycle, and the workload was increased progressively. Myocardial ischemia, when present, was evidenced by typical angina pectoris or a significant exercise induced ST-segment depression. Exercise was terminated when patients experienced chest pain, exhaustion, or when 3mm horizontal ST segment depression was reached. The results of these studies demonstrate that after the single exercise test a detectable increase of circulating EPCs is evident at 24-48 hours only in those patients that experienced a myocardial ischemia during the test; this was associated also to increased VEGF plasma levels [78]. Similarly, patients with documented peripheral arterial occlusive disease that reported an ischemic leg pain during the exercise showed a significantly increased number of circulating EPCs, with respect to patients who were enrolled after revascularization, or those with stable CAD [90]. On the other hand, Schmidt-Lucke et al evaluated the number of circulating EPCs in patients with CAD without acute coronary syndrome, and in patients with acute coronary syndrome and troponin T levels indicative of myocardial necrosis. The results showed that the number of circulating EPCs was significantly lower than that found in healthy controls in all the groups of patients, irrespectively of the presence of the acute coronary syndrome; however, it has to be pointed out that this finding may be influenced by the enrolment of patients with acute coronary syndrome who had a higher incidence of risk factors (i.e. smoking, CRP serum levels, LDL serum cholesterol levels) than patients with stable CAD, and were less likely to be treated with statins. Although it is difficult to compare the results obtained in this last study to those previously mentioned, it appears that the association between ischemia and EPCs mobilization is an actual finding.

An important question with respect to potential therapeutic approaches is whether the EPC pool can be increased in vivo in patients with CAD. Exercise training has evolved as an accepted therapy to improve endothelial cell number and function. To this regard, a number of studies have been performed in animal models [73] and humans with respect to exercise training and its effects on endothelial function and EPC number in different clinical contexts, especially in the presence of cardiovascular risk factors. In patients with CAD the endothelial dysfunction, documented by abnormal acetylcholine induced coronary vasoconstriction, resulted significantly improved after 4 weeks of intensive physical training, showing a coronary-artery constriction in response to acetylcholine reduced by 54% [91]; in addition, in a recently published trial [92] patients with CAD were randomly assigned to 12 months of exercise training or to percutaneous coronary intervention. Patients trained had a significantly higher event-free survival than those undergoing the standard intervention procedure. Further supporting the beneficial effects of training, Laufs and coll [73] described a significant increase of circulating EPCs after a 4 week rehabilitation training program in patients with stable CAD.

Acute Myocardial Infarction (AMI)

Differently from angina pectoris, AMI is characterized by the presence of the necrosis of the cardiac tissue. The combination of ischemia and necrosis can exert sinergistic effect on EPC mobilization and in turn in inducing reparative processes. The first report in this field [93] described an increased concentration of $CD34^+$ cells and increased VEGF plasma levels after AMI with a peak on the seventh day after the acute event. Culture assays of PB mononuclear cells showed also an increased number of attaching cells expressing endothelial lineage markers on day 7. These data were partially confirmed and extended by us [94]. We found that the highest mobilization of $CD34^+$ cells was evident at time of admission of patients with AMI (within 6 hours from the first symptoms), together with the highest number of endothelial colonies, and highest VEGF plasma levels. On day 7, the number of circulating $CD34^+$ cells was already reduced, but still higher than that found in healthy controls. The increased $CD34^+$ cells in patients with AMI at admission included an increase both in hematopoietic $CD34^+$ cells (defined by the International Society of Hematotherapy and Graft Engineering – ISHAGE- guidelines) [79], and an increase in circulating $CD34^+VEGFR\text{-}2^+$ cells. This last subset was shown to include increased percentages of $CD34^+CD133^+VEGFR\text{-}2^+$ and $CD34^+CD117^+VEGFR\text{-}2^+$ "true" EPCs. It seems intriguing to think that in the early phase of AMI HPCs and EPCs could play different roles, if any, in tissue repair, with EPCs devoted to neoangiogenesis, and HPCs, due to their "plasticity", to new myocardium generation.

So far, data suggesting that spontaneous mobilization of $CD34^+$ cells might contribute to determine a more favourable post-AMI remodelling are lacking. Recently, Leone and coll [95], in a limited number of patients tested at time of AMI and after 1 year follow up, showed a significant and favourable correlation between the number of circulating $CD34^+$ cells and changes of the left ventricular ejection fraction, the wall motion score index, and the left ventricular end-systolic volume. Further supporting the hypothesis of a "regeneration role" of the increased number of circulating $CD34^+$ cells at the onset of AMI, Wojakowski and coll [96] found a simultaneous increase in expression of mRNA for specific early cardiac, muscle, and endothelial markers in the population of PB mononuclear cells in patients after AMI. Although this finding is still a matter of debate mainly because the evaluation of the mRNA expression should have been performed on purified $CD34^+$ cells [97], all these data may contribute to a better understanding of the repairing processes spontaneously occurring after

AMI, and in turn may help in identifying the best strategy for the use of a cell-based therapy in the regeneration of human myocardium.

Diabetes Mellitus

A decreased number and/or function of circulating EPCs have been described in diabetic patients [98, 99], where they could be involved in the pathogenesis of the typical vascular complications of the disease. These observations were confirmed in a recent report [100] that showed that the number of circulating EPCs, evaluated by cytofluorimetric analysis as $CD34^{+}VEGFR\text{-}2^{+}$ cells, was reduced in diabetic patients with respect to healthy controls. However, the reduction was larger when the number of circulating EPCs of healthy subjects was compared either with that of patients with diabetes associated with peripheral vascular disease or of patients suffering from ischemic foot lesions complicating end-stage obstructive vascular disease. More importantly, a significant inverse correlation was found between the values of glucose and the absolute number of EPCs. It was suggested that the lower number of EPCs in diabetic patients may reflect a shortened peripheral survival of these cells rather than a weak BM mobilization. Supporting this hypothesis, it has been reported that high glucose concentration is able to induce apoptosis of cultured ECs *in vitro* [101].

Hematological Diseases

Myelofibrosis with Myeloid Metaplasia (MMM)

Myelofibrosis with myeloid metaplasia (MMM) is a clonal Philadelphia-negative chronic myeloproliferative disorder (Ph^{-} CMPD) characterized by a variable degree of BM fibrosis, extramedullary haematopoiesis, and presence of immature myeloid cells in the PB. [102,103]. Recently, it has been reported that an increased number of circulating $CD34^{+}$ HPCs is a diagnostic marker of the disease and that it is related to the progression of the disease [104]. Neoangiogenesis has been documented in the BM of patients with MMM, where microvessel density has been reported to be higher than in other CMPDs [105]. This finding was successively extended also to the spleen [106]. Indeed, in patients with MMM, spleen sectional area occupied by capillary vascular structures was found to be up to three times larger than the upper value of normal subjects; in addition, patients with the highest extent of spleen localization of $CD34^{+}$ cells had the highest extent of capillary vascular density [106]. These results, together with data showing that the number of spleen $CD34^{+}$ HPCs paralleled that of PB $CD34^{+}$ HPCs, are in keeping with the concept that a tight equilibrium exists between blood and spleen haematopoietic cell compartments and that spleen myeloid metaplasia and capillary neoangiogenesis are correlated mechanisms. Supporting this finding, $CD34^{+}CD133^{+}VEGFR\text{-}2^{+}$ EPCs were found in the spleen of patients with MMM, constituting up to 13% of $CD34^{+}$ cells, and were associated with a sustained spleen neoangiogenesis [106]. The frequency of $CD34^{+}CD133^{+}VEGFR\text{-}2^{+}$ EPCs was also increased in the PB of patients with MMM compared with healthy subjects [107]. Interestingly, a higher number of these cells resulted significantly associated with a younger age, a diagnosis of prefibrotic MMM and a reduced number of immature myeloid cells and blasts in PB. These observations support the hypothesis that increased trafficking of EPCs characterizes those patients with a mild clinical phenotype. In addition, circulating $CD34^{+}$ cells from MMM patients were able to form colonies whose cells were $CD31^{+}$VE-cadherin^{+}vWF^{+}CD45^{-}, confirming the presence of increased number of EPCs in the PB. The fact that both HPCs and EPCs are increased in the PB of MMM patients opens new perspectives in the interpretation of the pathogenesis of this disease. In fact, by assuming the same BM origin for EPCs and HPCs, high levels of circulating EPCs and HPCs in MMM could be the result of a common aberration of BM stem and progenitor cells or of BM microenvironment that could directly influence their mobilization. The finding of decreasing levels of circulating EPCs observed in patients with greater numbers of circulating HPCs [107] may be due to a competitive relationship between EPCs and HPCs mobilization or to an eventual depletion of a presumably limited supply of EPCs, caused by the continuous stimulation of the marrow compartment, or may be due to the progressive trapping of EPCs in extramedullary organs.

Multiple Mieloma (MM)

Neoangiogenesis has also been thought to have a governing role in multiple myeloma (MM) pathogenesis and progression. This has been indicated by the presence of an increased BM microvascular density that was positively correlated with disease activity, and by increased expression of angiogenic factors such as VEGF [108,109,110,111,112]. More recently, Hong Zhang and coll were the first to evaluate the number of circulating endothelial cells (CEC) in MM [113]. By cytofluorimetric analysis and culture assays they found that both the number of CEC and that of EPCs is elevated in patients with MM. In addition, as already shown for EPCs derived from the BM of patients with MM [114], also circulating EPCs were able to grow on matrigel and display a capillary network formation *in vitro*. The clinical relevance of this finding was due to the direct relation of both CEC and EPCs with β2 globulin and the monoclonal component, markers that reflect tumor mass and prognosis; in addition, the demonstration of a suppressive effect of thalidomide on circulating EPCs may represent the key mechanism by which the drug affects angiogenesis in MM, indicating that patients in whom thalidomide is ineffective can be identified by high colony growth and high monoclonal protein levels.

Clinical Applications of Endothelial Progenitor Cells

Several small–scale feasibility and safety clinical trials have been recently performed in humans to evaluate the use of BM cell transplantation for the treatment of myocardial infarction and peripheral limb ischemia. With the exception of the study by Stamm and coll [115] where autologous purified $CD133^{+}$ BM cells were injected into the infarct border zone, in the most of the other published studies the transplantation procedure, either by intracoronary delivery or by injection into the myocardial tissue, was performed with unfractioned autologous BM mononuclear cells [116,117]. Alternatively, unfractioned BM and *ex vivo* expanded PB derived mononuclear cells were intracoronary infused into a randomized group of patients with riperfused AMI [118,119]. The recently published 1 year follow up of this study showed sustained improvement in left ventricular function, and smaller infarct sizes in the 2 groups of patients receiving cell therapy [120]. Wollert and coll [121] reported recently the results of BOOST randomized controlled trial in two groups of patients treated with standard medical therapy for AMI alone, or in association with intracoronary infusion of autologous BM cells [121]. Similarly, in a small number of patients Fernandez-Aviles and coll used intracoronary delivery of BM cells that were injected about 13 days after AMI [122]. All the results obtained in these studies indicate that such therapeutic approach is feasible and safe. Moreover, an improvement in ventricular function and enhancement of coronary perfusion was reported after cell therapy in the BOOST study [121]. Autologous BM mononuclear cells were delivered also into the gastrocnemius muscle of patients with unilateral or bilateral leg ischemia caused by severe peripheral artery disease [123]. In this protocol, the BM mononuclear cell transplantation resulted a safe and an effective strategy for treatment of peripheral ischemic diseases. All these trials have a number of limitations. They consisted of a limited number of patients, were single center, and almost all of them were uncontrolled. Moreover, in the most of these studies there was not a pre-selection of a single cell population to be injected. Therefore, the encouraging results reported should be considered preliminary although of potential clinical interest and, due to the use of unselected cells, can not be attributed only to EPCs.

Pharmacological Mobilization of EPCs

An important question for designing potential therapeutic approaches based on the use of EPCs is whether the BM EPC pool can be mobilized *in vivo* by treatment with pharmacologic agents or cytokines [124]. Several studies performed in animal models have shown that treatment with hematopoietic and endothelial growth factors (SCF, G-CSF, SDF-1α, VEGF) can induce the recruitment of progenitor cells from the BM to the infarcted myocardium [125,126,49]. However, the principal concern in applying this strategy in humans is represented by the possible recruitment of EPCs not only to sites of vessel injuries but also to sites of occult neoplasia, leading to vascularization of dormant tumors. In addition, in a recent clinical trail that used G-CSF for the mobilization of EPCs in patients with AMI, the potential beneficial effects of EPC mobilization on damaged myocardium was counteracted by an increased rate of in-stent restenosis that led to the cancellation of the trial [127]. Besides this discouraging result, a number of studies have shown a possible role for erythropoietin (EPO) as EPC mobilizer. It has been reported that EPO treated mice showed an increased number of both BM and PB EPCs. In addition, in *in vivo* models of post natal vascularization, EPO significantly increased ischemia induced neovascularization [47]. In keeping with these data, Parsa and coll [128] described that EPO treatment leads to significant improvement of cardiac function in animal models of myocardial infarction; this protection, however, was mainly associated with a decreased apoptosis of cardiomyocytes. Preliminary studies in humans described an increased endogenous production of EPO in patients with unstable CAD with respect to patients with stable CAD, suggesting that ischemia may induce a spontaneous release of this cytokine acting on cell subsets different from those involved in erythropoiesis; interestingly, in patients with unstable CAD, EPO serum levels were correlated with both the number of $CD34^{+}VEGFR\text{-}2^{+}$ cells and the number of endothelial colonies [47]. The hypothesis that EPO stimulates EPCs in humans was further investigated in patients with renal anemia who received therapeutic standard doses of recombinant human EPO. The treatment induced an increase in the number of functionally active EPCs assessed in cell culture and in tube formation assays in patients treated with respect to those not treated [48], suggesting that patients with renal failure, often dying for cardiovascular complication such as AMI and stroke possibly caused by impaired vascular repair mechanisms, may gain some additional benefits in addition to the amelioration of anemia when treated with EPO. Moreover, a safety and efficacy trial has been performed in patients who received high doses of recombinant EPO intravenously ($3.3x10^4$ IU/day) for the first 3 days after cerebral ischemic stroke [129]: the results obtained indicated that high doses of recombinant EPO were well tolerated, and no safety concerns were identified. The treatment was associated with an improvement during the 1 month follow up, mainly sustained by a strong reduction in infarct size observed by magnetic resonance imaging. Longer follow up and larger scale controlled studies are needed to confirm these preliminary findings. In fact, the use of Epo outside the usual indication of correcting anemia, could be limited by a number of adverse effects such as an excessive increase of hematocrit and the appearance of anti-Epo auto-antibodies leading to serious pure red cell aplasia [130]. It has to be considered that regarding the possibility of an increase in hematocrit values, it is well known that the efficacy of infused EPO is reduced if the supplementation of Fe is lacking [131]; in addition, Ehrenreich and coll [129], although testing high doses of EPO, did not report significant changing of either the hematocrit or the red blood cell count during a 30 day follow up of the patients enrolled in the study. According to the possible appearance of anti-EPO antibodies, this side effect has been previously described in patients with chronic renal failure undergoing a chronic clinical treatment with EPO. This appeared to be mainly due to the use of an EPO formulation that has now been withdrawn; this resulted in an actual documented frequency of this event of 1 out of 100.000 [132]. However, the possibility to completely avoid these complications may be EPO derivatives, that have been recently described [133]. EPO derivatives are carbamylated EPO (CEPO), or certain EPO mutants that do not bind to the classical EPO receptor and lack hematopoietic activity, yet retain full tissue protection (i.e. anti apoptotic function). It has been well documented that there is a physical association [134] and functional interaction of EPO receptor with the common β receptor (βcR) subunit, which provides increased ligand-binding affinity to the receptor complex and it is also the signal-transducing component common to the GM-CSF, IL-3, and IL-5 receptors [135]. The hematopoietic and tissue protective activities of EPO are distinct and separate, implicating the existence of different receptors. In fact, EPO receptor exhibits no affinity for CEPO, while the βcR subunit binds this EPO derivative; in addition, CEPO has no cytoprotective effects on tissues from βcR knockout mice, that exhibit normal hematopoiesis [136]. These data demonstrate that CEPO exherts a protective function through the βcR subunit, and shows no effects on erythropoiesis. Therefore, CEPO may represent a new therapeutic approach for patients who may have benefits from the use of EPO either as anti-apoptotic agent or as mobilizer of EPCs, avoiding the side effects that may derive from the hematopoietic function of the natural molecule.

CONCLUSION

At present, no exclusive surface antigen, or combination of antigens, that could characterize the endothelial progenitor cell subset has been defined. Therefore, EPCs should still be considered as a pool of cells that, although sharing surface markers with different cell subsets of the HPCs, or deriving from a unique hemoangioblast, or from monocytes, are able to form endothelial colonies or vascular structures once seeded on the appropriate substrate or infused in *in vivo* models of vascular injury. Despite the lack of a definitive characterization of EPCs, in the last years many studies have investigated their role both in physiological and pathological conditions. In this last setting, EPCs have acquired a great relevance since they have been shown to be part of mechanisms of vascular repair, including both angiogenesis and vasculogenesis processes.

These findings have highlighted the possible use of EPCs for therapeutic approaches. Looking from this point of view to the past, the first pilot studies in which un-separated BM derived cells were injected in the infarcted zone of patients with AMI, have possibly been a solution to the alternative, still lacking, of properly characterize the actual EPC subset and than inject it. It is possible that the, although modest, clinical improvements obtained following injection of "EPCs" in the heart of patients with AMI is due to additional effects of different bone marrow cell subsets secreting factors helping the repairing function EPC mediated. To this regard, the most promising approach in the clinical practice may be the evaluation of the administration of mobilizing factors (ie EPO) in order to induce an increase in the number of circulating EPCs and possible "accessory cells" that will home to the site of the vascular injury. On the other hand, further studies aimed to identify EPCs may allow to discover soluble factors exclusively produced by these cells, paving the way for new therapeutic approaches.

ACKNOWLEDGMENT

The contribution of Dott. Maurizio Ferrario, Cardiology Department, IRCCS Policlinico San Matteo, and of Dott. Giovanni Barosi, head of the Laboratory of Clinical Epidemiology, IRCCS Policlinico San Matteo, is warmly acknowledged. We also thank Dott. Valentina Meli for the excellent technical assistance.

This work was supported by grants from IRCCS Policlinico San Matteo (Ricerca Corrente #80520 and #80545).

REFERENCES

[1] Asahara T, Murohara T, Sullivan A, Silver M, van der Zee R, Li T, Witzenbichler B, Schatteman G, Isner JM. Isolation of putative progenitor endothelial cells for angiogenesis. *Science 275*:964-967, 1997.

[2] Stump MM, Jordan GL Jr, Debakey ME, Halpert B. Endothelium grown from circulating blood on isolated intravascular Dacron hub. *Am J Pathol 43*:361-367, 1963.

[3] Hladovec J, Prerovsky I, Stanek V, Fabian J. Circulating endothelial cells in acute myocardial infarction and angina pectoris. *Klin Wochenschr 56*:1033- 1036, 1978.

[4] George F, Poncelet P, Laurent JC, Massot O, Arnoux D, Lequeux N, Ambrosi P, Chicheportiche C, Sampol J. Cytofluorometric detection of human endothelial cells in whole blood using S-Endo 1 monoclonal antibody. *J Immunol Methods 139(1)*:65-75, 1991.

[5] George F, Brisson C, Poncelet P, Laurent JC, Massot O, Arnoux D, Ambrosi P, Klein-Soyer C, Cazenave JP, Sampol J . Rapid isolation of human endothelial cells from whole blood using S-Endo1 monoclonal antibody coupled to immuno-magnetic beads: demonstration of endothelial injury after angioplasty. *Thromb Haemost* 67(1):147-153,1992.

[6] Rafii S, Lyden D. Therapeutic stem and progenitor cell transplantation for organ vascularization and regeneration. *Nat Med* 9:702-712, 2003.

[7] Carmeliet P. Angiogenesis in health and disease. *Nat Med* 9(6):653-660, 2003.

[8] Coffin JD, Harrison J, Schwartz S, Heimark R. Angioblast differentiation and morphogenesis of the vascular endothelium in the mouse embryo. *Dev Biol* 148(1):51-62, 1991.

[9] Flamme I, Breier G, Risau W. Vascular endothelial growth factor (VEGF) and VEGF receptor 2 (flk-1) are expressed during vasculogenesis and vascular differentiation in the quail embryo. *Dev Biol* 169(2):699-712, 1995.

[10] Ziegler BL, Valtieri M, Porada GA, De Maria R, Muller R, Masella B, Gabbianelli M, Caszella I, Pelosi E, Bock T, Zanjani ED, Peschle C. KDR receptor: a key marker definig hematopoietic stem cells. *Science* 285:1553-1558, 1999.

[11] Peichev M, Nayer AJ, Pereira D, Zhu Z, Lane WJ, Williams M, Oz MC, Hicklin DJ, Witte L, Moore MA, Rafii S. Expression of VEGFR-2 and AC133 by circulating human CD34(+) cells identifies a population of functional endothelial precursors. *Blood* 95(3):952-958, 2000.

[12] Gehling UM, Ergun S, Schumacher U, Wagener C, Pantel K, Otte M, Schuch G, Schafhausen P, Mende T, Kilic N, Kluge K, Schafer B, Hossfeld DK, Fielder W. In vitro differentiation of endothelial cells from AC133-positive progenitor cells. *Blood* 95(10):3106-3112, 2000.

[13] Pelosi E, Valtieri M, Coppola S, Botta R, Gabbianelli M, Lulli V, Marziali G, Masella B, Muller R, Sgadari C, Testa U, Bonanno G, Peschle C. Identification of the hemangioblast in postnatal life. *Blood 100(9)*:3203-3208, 2002.

[14] Choi K, Kennedy M, Kazarov A, Papadimitriou JC, Keller G. A common precursor for hematopoietic and endothelial cells. *Development* 4:725-732, 1998.

[15] Cogle CR, Wainman DA, Jorgensen ML, Guthrie SM, Mames RN, Scott EW. Adult human hematopoietic cells provide functional hemangioblast activity. *Blood* 103(1):133-135, 2004.

[16] Mikkola HK, Orkin SH. The search for the hemangioblast. *J Hematother Stem Cell Res* 11(1):9-17, 2002.

[17] Auerbach R, Huang H, Lu L. Hematopoietic stem cells in the mouse embryonic yolk sac. *Stem Cells* 14(3):269-280, 1996.

[18] Eichmann A, Corbel C, Nataf V, Vaigot P, breant C, Le Douarin NM. Ligand-dependent development of the endothelial and hematopoietic lineages from embryonic mesodermal cells expressing vascular endothelail growth factor receptor 2. *Proc Natl Acad Sci USA* 94:5141-5146, 1997.

[19] Shalaby F, Rossant J, Yamaguchi TP, Gertsenstein M, Wu XF, Breitman ML, Schuh AC. Failure of blood-island formation and vasculogenesis in Flk-1-deficient mice. *Nature* 376:62-66, 1995.

[20] Orlic D, Kajstura J, Chimenti S, Jakoniuk I, Anderson SM, Li B, Pickel J, McKay R, Nadal-Ginard B, Bodine DM, Leri A, Anversa P. Bone marrow cells regenerate infarcted myocardium. *Nature* 410:701-705, 2001.

[21] Orlic D, Kajstura J, Chimenti S, Limana F, Jakoniuk I, Quaini F, Nadal-Ginard B, Bodine DM, Leri A, Anversa P. Mobilized bone marrow cells repair the infarcted heart, improving function and survival. *Proc Natl Acad Sci U S A* 410:701-705, 2001.

[22] Li TS, Hamano K, Nishida M, Hayashi M, Ito H, Mikamo A, Matsuzaki M. CD117+ stem cells play a key role in therapeutic angiogenesis induced by bone marrow cell implantation. *Am J Physiol Heart Circ Physiol* 285(3):H931-H937, 2003.

[23] Orlic D, Fischer R, Nishikawa S, Nienhuis AW, Bodine DM. Purification and characterization of heterogeneous pluripotent hematopoietic stem cell populations expressing high levels of c-kit receptor. *Blood* 82(3):762-770, 1993.

[24] Kocher AA, Schuster MD, Szabolcs MJ, Takuma S, Burkhoff D, Wang J, Homma S, Edwards NM, Itescu S. Neovascularization of ischemic myocardium by human bone-marrow-derived angioblasts prevents cardiomyocyte apoptosis, reduces remodeling and improves cardiac function. *Nat Med* 7(4):430-436, 2001.

[25] Urbich C, Dimmeler S. Endothelial progenitor cells: characterization and role in vascular biology. *Circ Res* 95(4):343-353, 2004.

[26] Hristov M, Weber C. Endothelial progenitor cells:characterization, pathophysiology, and possible clinical relevance. *J Cell Mol Med* 8;4:498-508, 2004.

[27] Lin Y, Weisdorf DJ, Solovey A, Hebbel RP. Origins of circulating endothelial cells and endothgelail outgrowth from blood. *J Clin Invest* 105:71-77, 2000.

[28] Ingram DA, Mead LE, Tanaka H, Meade V, Fenoglio A, Mortell K, Pollok K, Ferkowicz MJ, Gilley D, Yoder MC. Identification of a novel hierarchy of endothelial progenitor cells using human peripheral and umbilical cord blood. *Blood* 104(9):2752-2760, 2004.

[29] Bessler M. Endothelial progenitor cells: reporting for duty. *Blood* 104:2616-2617, 2004.

[30] Shi Q, Rafii S, Wu MH, Wijelath ES, Yu C, Ishida A, Fujita Y, Kothari S, Mohle R, Sauvage LR, Moore MA, Storb RF, Hammond WP. Evidence for circulating bone marrow-derived endothelial cells. *Blood* 92(2):362-367, 1998.

[31] Ito H, Rovira II, Bloom ML, Takeda K, Ferrans VJ, Quyyumi AA, Finkel T. Endothelial progenitor cells as putative targets for angiostatin. *Cancer Res* 59(23):5875-5877, 1999.

[32] Schmeisser A, Garlichs CD, Zhang H, Eskafi S, Graffy C, Ludwig J, Strasser RH, Daniel WG. Monocytes coexpress endothelial and macrophagocytic lineage markers and form cord-like structures in Matrigel under angiogenic conditions. *Cardiovasc Res* 49(3):671-680, 2001.

[33] Rehman J, Li J, Orschell CM, March KL. Peripheral blood "endothelial progenitor cells"are derived from monocyte/macrophages and secrete angiogenic growth factors. *Circulation* 107:1164-1169, 2003.

[34] Gulati R, Jevremovic D, Peterson TE, Chatterjee S, Shah V, Vile RG, Simari RD. Diverse origin and function of cells with endothelial phenotype obtained from adult human blood. *Circ Res* 93(11):1023-1025, 2003.

[35] Urbich C, Heeschen C, Aicher A, Dernbach E, Zeiher AM, Dimmeler S. Relevance of monocytic features for neovascularization capacity of circulating endothelial progenitor cells. *Circulation* 108(20):2511-2516, 2003.

[36] Zhao Y, Glesne D, Huberman E,. A human peripheral blood monocyte subset acts as pluripotent stem cell. *Proc Natl Acad Sci USA* 100:2426-2431, 2003.

[37] Romagnani P, Annunziato F, Liotta F, Lazzeri E, Mazzinghi B, Frosali F, Cosmi L, Maggi L, Lasagni L, Scheffold A, Kruger M, Dimmeler S, Marra F, Gensini G, Maggi E, Romagnani S. CD14+CD34low Cells With Stem Cell Phenotypic and Functional Features Are the Major Source of Circulating Endothelial Progenitors. *Circ Res* 97:314-322, 2005.

[38] Hillebrands JL, Klatter FA, van Dijk WD, Rozing J. Bone marrow does not contribute substantially to endothelial-cell replacement in transplant arteriosclerosis. *Nat Med* 8(3):194-195, 2002.

[39] Reyes M, Dudek A, Jahagirdar B, Koodie L, Marker PH, Verfaillie CM. Origin of endothelial progenitors in human postnatal bone marrow. *J Clin Invest* 109(3):337-346, 2002.

[40] Jackson KA, Majka SM, Wang H, Pocius J, Hartley CJ, Majesky MW, Entman ML, Michael LH, Hirschi KK, Goodell MA. Regeneration of ischemic cardiac muscle and vascular endothelium by adult stem cells. *J Clin Invest* 107(11):1395-1402, 2001.

[41] Quirici N, Soligo D, Caneva L, Servida F, Bossolasco P, Deliliers GL. Differentiation and expansion of endothelial cells from human bone marrow CD133(+) cells. *Br J Haematol* 115(1):186-194, 2001.

[42] Lapidot T, Petit I. Current understanding of stem cell mobilization: the roles of chemokines, proteolytic enzymes, adhesion molecules, cytokines, and stromal cells. *Exp Hematol* 30(9):973-981, 2002.

[43] Heissig B, Hattori K, Dias S, Friedrich M, Ferris B, Hackett NR, Crystal RG, Besmer P, Lyden D, Moore MA, Werb Z, Rafii S. Recruitment of stem and progenitor cells from the bone marrow niche requires MMP-9 mediated release of kit-ligand. *Cell* 109(5):625-637, 2002.

[44] Aicher A, Heeschen C, Mildner-Rihm C, Urbich C, Ihling C, Technau-Ihling K, Zeiher AM, Dimmeler S. Essential role of endothelial nitric oxide synthase for mobilization of stem and progenitor cells. *Nat Med* 9(11):1370-1376, 2003.

[45] Lee SH, Wolf PL, Escudero R, Deutsch R, Jamieson SW, Thistlethwaite PA. Early expression of angiogenesis factors in acute myocardial ischemia and infarction. *N Eng J Med* 342:626-633, 2000.

[46] Ceradini DJ, Kulkarni AR, Callaghan MJ, Tepper OM, Bastidas N, Kleinman ME, Capla JM, Galiano RD, Levine JP, Gurtner GC. Progenitor cell trafficking is regulated by hypoxic gradients through HIF-1 induction of SDF-1. *Nat Med* 10(8):858-864, 2004.

[47] Heeschen C, Aicher A, Lehmann R, Fichtlscherer S, Vasa M, Urbich C, Mildner-Rihm C, Martin H, Zeiher AM, Dimmeler S. Erythropoietin is a potent physiologic stimulus for endothelial progenitor cell mobilization. *Blood* 102(4):1340-1346, 2003.

[48] Bahlmann FH, De Groot K, Spandau JM, Landry AL, Hertel B, Duckert T, Boehm SM, Menne J, Haller H, Fliser D. Erythropoietin regulates endothelial progenitor cells. *Blood* 103(3):921-926, 2004.

[49] Kalka C, Masuda H, Takahashi T, Gordon R, Tepper O, Gravereaux E, Pieczek A, Iwaguro H, Hayashi SI, Isner JM, Asahara T. Vascular endothelial growth factor(165) gene transfer augments circulating endothelial progenitor cells in human subjects. *Circ Res* 86(12):1198-1202, 2000.

[50] Llevadot J, Murasawa S, Kureishi Y, Uchida S, Masuda H, Kawamoto A, Walsh K, Isner JM, Asahara T. HMG-CoA reductase inhibitor mobilizes bone marrow--derived endothelial progenitor cells. *J Clin Invest* 108(3):399-405, 2001.

[51] Dimmeler S, Aicher A, Vasa M, Mildner-Rihm C, Adler K, Tiemann M, Rutten H, Fichtlscherer S, Martin H, Zeiher AM. HMG-CoA reductase inhibitors (statins) increase endothelial progenitor cells via the PI 3-kinase/Akt pathway. *J Clin Invest* 108(3):391-397, 2001.

[52] Vasa M, Fichtlscherer S, Adler K, Aicher A, Martin H, Zeiher AM, Dimmeler S. Increase in circulating endothelial progenitor cells by statin therapy in patients with stable coronary artery disease. *Circulation* 103(24):2885-2890, 2001.

[53] Davignon J, Ganz P. Role of endothelial dysfunction in atherosclerosis. *Circulation* 109(23 Suppl 1):27-32, 2004.

[54] Hristov M, Weber C Endothelial progenitor cells:characterization, pathophysiology, and possible clinical relevance. *J Cell Mol Med 8;4*:498-508, 2004.

[55] Ingram DA, Caplice NM, Yoder MC. Unresolved questions, changing definitions, and novel paradigms for defining endothelial progenitor cells. *Blood* 106:1525-1531, 2005.

[56] Gussin HAE, Bischoff FZ, Hoffman R, Elias S. Endothelial precursor cells in the peripheral blood of pregnant women. *J Soc Gynecol Investig* 9:357-361, 2002.

[57] Sugawara J, Mitsui-Saito M, Hoshiai T, Hayashi C, Kimura Y, Okamura K. Circulating endotheial progenitor cells during human pregnancy. *J Clin Endocrinol Metab* 90:1845-1848, 2005.
[58] Strehlow K, Werner N, Berweiler J, Link A, Dirnagl U, Priller J, Laufs K, Ghaeni L, Milosevic M, Bohm M, Nickenig G. Estrogen increases bone marrow derived endothelial progenitor cell production and diminishes neointima formation. *Circulation* 107:3059-3065, 2003.
[59] Iwakura A, Luedemann C, Shastry S, Hanley A, Kearney M, Aikawa R, Isner JM, Asahara T, Losordo DW. Estrogen-mediated, endothelial nitric oxide synthase-dependent mobilization of bone marrow- derived endothelial progenitor cells contributes to reendothelization after arterial injury. *Circulation* 108:3115-3121, 2003.
[60] Gordon JD, Shifren JL, Foulk RA, Taylor RN, Jaffe RB. Angiogenesis in the human female reproductive tract. *Obset Gynecol Surv* 50:688-697, 1995.
[61] Maas JWM, Groothuis PG, Dunselman GAJ, de Goeij AFPM, Struyker Boudier HAJ, Evers JLH. Endometrial angiogenesis throughout the human menstrual cycle. *Hum Reprod* 16(8):1557-1561, 2001.
[62] Brenner RM, Nayak NR, Slayden OD, Critchley HO, Kelly RW. Premenstrual and menstrual changes in the macaque and human endometrium: relevance to endometriosis. *Ann N Y Acad Sci* 955:60-74, 2002.
[63] Nayak NR, Brenner RM. Vascular proliferation and vascular endothelial growth factor expression in the rhesus macaque endometrium. *J Clin Endocrinol Metab* 87(4):1845-1855, 2002.
[64] McIlhenny C, George WD, Doughty JC. A comparison of serum and plasma levels of vascular endothelial growth factor during the menstrual cycle in healthy female volunteers. *Br J Cancer* 86(11):1786-1789, 2002.
[65] Print C, Valtola R, Evans A, Lessan K, Malik S, Smith S. Soluble factors from human endometrium promote angiogenesis and regulate the endothelial cell transcriptome. *Hum Reprod* 19(10):2356-2366, 2004.
[66] Gill M, Dias S, Hattori K, Rivera ML, Hicklin D, Witte L, Girardi L, Yurt R, Himel H, Rafii S. Vascular trauma induces rapid but transient mobilization of VEGFR2(+)AC133(+) endothelial precursor cells. *Circ Res* 88:167-174, 2001.
[67] Stewart KJ. Exercise training and the cardiovascular consequence of type 2 diabetes and hypertension: plausible mechanisms for improving cardiovascular health. *JAMA* 288:1622-1631, 2002.
[68] Wannamethee SG, Lowe GD, Whincup PH, Rumley A, Walker M, Lennon L. Physical activity and hemostatic and inflammatory variables in elderly men. *Circulation* 105:1785-1790, 2002.
[69] Kojda G, Cheng YC, Burchfield J, Harrison DG. Dysfunctional regulation of endothelial nitric oxide synthase (eNOS) expression in response to exercise in mice lacking one eNOS gene. *Circulation* 103:2839-2844, 2001.
[70] Fukai T, Siegfried MR, Ushio-Fukai M, Cheng Y, Kojda G, Harrison DG. Regulation of the vascular extracellular superoxide dismutase by nitric oxide and exercise training. *J Clin Invest* 105:1631-1639, 2000.

[71] Maisel AS, Knowlton KU, Fowler P, Rearden A, Zieglel MG, Motulsky HJ, Insel PA, Michel MC. Adrenergic control of circulating lymphocyte subpopulations. Effects of congestive heart failure, dynamic exercise, and terbutaline treatment. *J Clin Invest* 85:462-467, 1990.

[72] Barret AJ, Longhurst P, Sneath P, Watson JG. Mobilization of CFU-C by exercise and ACTH induced stress in man. *Exp Hematol 6*:590-594, 1978.

[73] Laufs U, Werner N, Link A, Endres M, Wassmann S, Jurgens K, Miche E, Bohm M, Nickenig G. Physical training increases endothelial progenitor cells, inhibits neointima formation, and enhances angiogenesis. *Circulation* 109(2):220-226, 2004.

[74] Rehman J, Li J, Parvathaneni L, Karlsson G, Panchal VR, Temm CJ, Mahenthiran J, March KL. Exercise acutely increases circulating endothelial progenitor cells and monocyte-/macrophage-derived angiogenic cells. *J Am Coll Cardiol* 43(12):2314-2318, 2004.

[75] Niebauer J, Cooke JP. Cardiovascular effects of exercise: role of endothelial shear stress. *J Am coll Cardiol* 28:1652-1660, 1996.

[76] Bonsignore MR, Morici G, Santoro A, Pagano M, Cascio L, Bonanno A, Abate P, Mirabella F, Profita M, Insalaco G, Gioia M, Vignola AM, Majolino I, Testa U, Hogg JC. Circulating hematopoietic progenitor cells in runners. *J Appl Physiol* 93(5):1691-1697, 2002.

[77] Ciulla MM, Giorgetti A, Lazzari L, Cortiana M, Silvestris I, Annoni G, De Asmundis C, Fiore AV, Montelatici E, Paliotti R, Magrini F, Rebulla P, Cortelezzi A. High-altitude trekking in the Himalayas increases the activity of circulating endothelial cells. *Am J Hematol* 79(1):76-78, 2005.

[78] Adams V, Lenk K, Linke A, Lenz D, Erbs S, Sandri M, Tarnok A, Gielen S, Emmrich F, Schuler G, Hambrecht R. Increase of circulating endothelial progenitor cells in patients with coronary artery disease after exercise-induced ischemia. *Arterioscler Thromb Vasc Biol* 24(4):684-690, 2004.

[79] Sutherland DR, Anderson L, Keeney M, Nayar R, Chin-Yee I. The ISHAGE guidelines for CD34+ cell determination by flow cytometry. International Society of Hematotherapy and Graft Engineering. *J Hematother* 5(3):213-226, 1996.

[80] Edelberg JM, Tang L, Hattori K, Lyden D, Rafii S. Young adult bone marrow-derived endothelial precursor cells restore aging-impaired cardiac angiogenic function. *Circ Res* 90(10):E89-93, 2002.

[81] Murayama T, Kalka C, Silver M, Ma H, Asahara T. Aging impairs therapeutic contribution of human endothelial progenitor cells to postnatal neovascularization. *Circulation* 104 Suppl II:68, 2001.

[82] Hill JM, Zalos G, Halcox JPJ, Schenke WH, Waclawiw MA, Quyyumi AA, Finkel T. Circulating endothelial progenitor cells, vascular function, and cardiovascular risk. *NEJM* 7:593-600, 2003.

[83] Scheubel RJ, Zorn H, Silber RE, Kuss O, Morawietz H, Holtz J, Simm A. Age-dependent depression in circulating endothelial progenitor cells in patients undergoing coronary artery bypass grafting. *J Am Coll Cardiol* 42(12):2073-2080, 2003.

[84] Heiss C, Keymel S, Niesler U, Ziemann J, Kelm M, Kalka C. Impaired progenitor cell activity in age-related endothelial dysfunction. *J Am Coll Cardiol* 45(9):1441-1448, 2005.

[85] Van Zant G, Liang Y. The role of stem cells in aging. *Exp Hematol 31*:659-672, 2003.

[86] Mc Veigh GE, Lemay L, Morgan D, Cohn JN. Effects of long-term cigarette smoking on endothelium-dependent responses in humans. *Am J Cardiol* 78(6):668-72, 1996.

[87] Kondo T, Hayashi M, Takeshita K, Numaguchi Y, Kobayashi K, Iino S, Inden Y, Murohara T. Smoking cessation rapidly increases circulating progenitor cells in peripheral blood in chronic smokers. *Arterioscler Thromb Vasc Biol* 24(8):1442-1447, 2004.

[88] Vasa M, Fichtlscherer S, Aicher A, Adler K, Urbich C, Martin H, Zeiher AM, Dimmeler S. Number and migratory activity of circulating endothelial progenitor cells inversely correlate with risk factors for coronary artery disease. *Circ Res* 89(1):E1-E7, 2001.

[89] Schmidt-Lucke C, Rossig L, Fichtlscherer S, Vasa M, Britten M, Kamper U, Dimmeler S, Zeiher AM. Reduced number of circulating endothelial progenitor cells predicts future cardiovascular events: proof of concept for the clinical importance of endogenous vascular repair. *Circulation* 111(22):2981-2987, 2005.

[90] Sandri M, Adams V, Gielen S, Linke A, Lenk K, Krankel N, Lenz D, Erbs S, Scheinert D, Wilhelm Mohr F, Schuler G, Hambrecht R . Effects of exercise and ischemia on mobilization and functional activation of blood-derived progenitor cells in patients with ischemic syndromes: results of 3 randomized studies. *Circulation* 111(25):3391-3399, 2005.

[91] Hambrecht R, Wolf S, Gielen S, Linke A, Hofer J, Erbs S, Schoene N, Schuler G. Effect of exercise on coronary endothelial function in patients with coronary artery disease. *N Engl J Med* 342(7):454-460, 2000.

[92] Hambrecht R, Walther C, Mobius-Winkler S, Gielen S, Linke A, Conradi K, Erbs S, Kluge R, Kendziorra K, Sabri O, Sick P, Schuler G. Percutaneous coronary angioplasty compared with exercise training in patients with stable coronary artery disease: a randomized trial. *Circulation* 109(11):1371-1378, 2004.

[93] Shintani S, Murohara T, Ikeda H, Ueno T, Honma T, Katoh A, Sasaki K, Shimada T, Oike Y, Imaizumi T. Mobilization of endothelial progenitor cells in patients with acute myocardial infarction. *Circulation* 103(23):2776-2779, 2001.

[94] Massa M, Rosti V, Ferrario M, Campanelli R, Ramajoli I, Rosso R, De Ferrari GM, Ferlini M, Goffredo L, Bertoletti A, Klersy C, Pecci A, Moratti R, Tavazzi L. Increased circulating hematopoietic and endothelial progenitor cells in the early phase of acute myocardial infarction. *Blood* 105(1):199-206, 2005.

[95] Leone AM, Rutella S, Bonanno G, Abbate A, Rebuzzi AG, Giovannini S, Lombardi M, Galiuto L, Liuzzo G, Andreotti F, Lanza GA, Contemi AM, Leone G, Crea F. Mobilization of bone marrow-derived stem cells after myocardial infarction and left ventricular function. *Eur Heart J* 26(12):1196-1204, 2005.

[96] Wojakowski W, Tendera M, Michalowska A, Majka M, Kucia M, Maslankiewicz K, Wyderka R, Ochala A, Ratajczak MZ. Mobilization of CD34/CXCR4+, CD34/CD117+, c-met+ stem cells, and mononuclear cells expressing early cardiac, muscle, and endothelial markers into peripheral blood in patients with acute myocardial infarction. *Circulation* 110(20):3213-3220, 2004.

[97] Wolf D, Rumpold H, Gunsilius E. Correspondence. Circulation 111:e307-e308, 2005.

[98] Tepper OM, Galiano RD, Capla JM, Kalka C, Gagne PJ, Jacobowitz GR, Levine JP, Gurtner GC. Human endothelial progenitor cells from type II diabetics exhibit impaired proliferation, adhesion, and incorporation into vascular structures. *Circulation* 106(22):2781-2786, 2002.

[99] Loomans CJ, de Koning EJ, Staal FJ, Rookmaaker MB, Verseyden C, de Boer HC, Verhaar MC, Braam B, Rabelink TJ, van Zonneveld AJ. Endothelial progenitor cell dysfunction: a novel concept in the pathogenesis of vascular complications of type 1 diabetes. *Diabetes* 53(1):195-199, 2004.

[100] Fadini GP, Miorin M, Facco M, Bonamico S, Baesso I, Grego F, Menegolo M, de Kreutzenberg SV, Tiengo A, Agostini C, Avogaro A. Circulating endothelial progenitor cells are reduced in peripheral vascular complications of type 2 diabetes mellitus. *J Am Coll Cardiol* 45(9):1449-1457, 2005.

[101] Baumgartner-Parzer SM, Wagner L, Pettermann M, Grillari J, Gessl A, Waldhausl W. Hight glucose-triggered apoptosis in cultured endothelial cells. *Diabetes* 44:1323-1327, 1995.

[102] Barosi G. Myelofibrosis with myeloid metaplasia: diagnostic definition and prognostic classification for clinical studies and treatment guidelines. *J Clin Oncol* (7): 2954-2970, 1999.

[103] Tefferi A. Myelofibrosis with myeloid metaplasia. *N Engl J Med* 342(17):1255-1265, 2000.

[104] Barosi G, Viarengo G, Pecci A, Rosti V, Piaggio G, Marchetti M, Frassoni F. Diagnostic and clinical relevance of the number of circulating CD34(+) cells in myelofibrosis with myeloid metaplasia. *Blood* 98(12):3249-3255, 2001.

[105] Mesa RA, Hanson CA, Rajkumar SV, Schroeder G, Tefferi A. Evaluation and clinical correlations of bone marrow angiogenesis in myelofibrosis with myeloid metaplasia. *Blood* (96): 3374-3380, 2000.

[106] Barosi G, Rosti V, Massa M, Viarengo GL, Pecci A, Necchi V, Ramajoli I, Campanelli R, Marchetti M, Bazzan M, Magrini U. Spleen neoangiogenesis in patients with myelofibrosis with myeloid metaplasia. *Br J Haematol* (124): 618-625, 2004.

[107] Massa M, Rosti V, Ramajoli I, Campanelli R, Pecci A, Viarengo G, Meli V, Marchetti M, Hoffman R, Barosi G. Circulating CD34+,CD133+, and vascular endothelial growth factor receptor 2-positive endothelial progenitor cells in myelofibrosis with myeloid metaplasia. *J Clin Oncol* (24):5688-5695, 2005.

[108] Vacca A, Ribatti D, Roncali l, Ranieri G, Serio G, Silvestris F, Dammacco F. Bone marrow angiogenesis and progression in multiple myeloma. *Br J Haematol* 87(3):503-8, 1994.

[109] Rajkumar SV, Mesa RA, Fonseca R, Schroeder G, Plevak MF, Dispenzieri A, Lacy MQ, Lust JA, Witzig TE, Gertz MA, Kyle RA, Russell SJ, Greipp PR. Bone marrow angiogenesis in 400 patients with monoclonal gammopathy of undetermined significance, multiple myeloma, and primary amyloidosis. *Clin Cancer Res* 8(7):2210-2216, 2002.

[110] Pruneri G, Ponzoni M, Ferreri AJ, Decarli N, Tresoldi M, Raggi F, Baldessari C, Freschi M, Baldini L, Goldaniga M, Neri A, Carboni N, Bertolini F, Viale G. Microvessel density, a surrogate marker of angiogenesis, *is significantly related to survival in multiple myeloma patients. Br J Haematol 118(3)*:817-820, 2002.

[111] Sezer O, Niemoller K, Kaufmann O, Eucker J, Jakob C, Zavrski I, Possinger K. Decrease of bone marrow angiogenesis in myeloma patients achieving a remission after chemotherapy. *Eur J Haematol* 66(4):238-244, 2001.

[112] Rajkumar SV, Fonseca R, Witzig TE, Gertz MA, Greipp PR. Bone marrow angiogenesis in patients achieving complete response after stem cell transplantation for multiple myeloma. *Leukemia* 13(3):469-472, 1999.

[113] Zhang H, Vakil V, Braunstein M, Smith EL, Maroney J, Chen L, Dai K, Berenson JR, Hussain MM, Klueppelberg U, Norin AJ, Akman HO, Ozcelik T, Batuman OA. Circulating endothelial progenitor cells in multiple myeloma: implications and significance. *Blood* 105(8):3286-3294, 2005.

[114] Vacca A, Ria R, Semeraro F, Marchionne F, Coluccia M, Boccarelli A, Scavelli C, Nico B, Gernone A, Battelli F, Tabilio A, Guidolin D, Petrucci MT, Ribatti D Dammacco F. Endothelial cells in the bone marrow of patients with multiple myeloma. *Blood* 102(9):3340-3348, 2003.

[115] Stamm C, Westphal B, Kleine HD, Petzsch M, Kittner C, Klinge H, Schumichen C, Nienaber CA, Freund M, Steinhoff G. Autologous bone-marrow stem-cell transplantation for myocardial regeneration. *Lancet* 361(9351):45-46, 2003.

[116] Strauer BE, Brehm M, Zeus T, Kostering M, Hernandez A, Sorg RV, Kogler G, Wernet P. Repair of infarcted myocardium by autologous intracoronary mononuclear bone marrow cell transplantation in humans. *Circulation* 106(15):1913-1918, 2002.

[117] Tse HF, Kwong YL, Chan JK, Lo G, Ho CL, Lau CP. Angiogenesis in ischaemic myocardium by intramyocardial autologous bone marrow mononuclear cell implantation. *Lancet* 361(9351):47-49, 2003.

[118] Assmus B, Schachinger V, Teupe C, Britten M, Lehmann R, Dobert N, Grunwald F, Aicher A, Urbich C, Martin H, Hoelzer D, Dimmeler S, Zeiher AM. Transplantation of Progenitor Cells and Regeneration Enhancement in Acute Myocardial Infarction (TOPCARE-AMI). *Circulation* 106(24):3009-3017, 2002.

[119] Britten MB, Abolmaali ND, Assmus B, Lehmann R, Honold J, Schmitt J, Vogl TJ, Martin H, Schachinger V, Dimmeler S, Zeiher AM. Infarct remodeling after intracoronary progenitor cell treatment in patients with acute myocardial infarction (TOPCARE-AMI): mechanistic insights from serial contrast-enhanced magnetic resonance imaging. *Circulation* 108(18):2212-2218, 2003.

[120] Schachinger V, Assmus B, Britten MB, Honold J, Lehmann R, Teupe C, Abolmaali ND, Vogl TJ, Hofmann WK, Martin H, Dimmeler S, Zeiher AM. Transplantation of progenitor cells and regeneration enhancement in acute myocardial infarction: final one-year results of the TOPCARE-AMI Trial. *J Am Coll Cardiol* 44(8):1690-1699, 2004.

[121] Wollert KC, Meyer GP, Lotz J, Ringes-Lichtenberg S, Lippolt P, Breidenbach C, Fichtner S, Korte T, Horning B, Messinger D, Arseniev L, Hertenstein B, Ganser A, Drexler H. Intracoronary autologous bone-marrow cell transfer after myocardial infarction: the BOOST randomised controlled clinical trial. *Lancet* 364(9429):141-148, 2004.

[122] Fernandez-Aviles F, San Roman JA, Garcia-Frade J, Fernandez ME, Penarrubia MJ, de la Fuente L, Gomez-Bueno M, Cantalapiedra A, Fernandez J, Gutierrez O, Sanchez PL, Hernandez C, Sanz R, Garcia-Sancho J, Sanchez A. Experimental and clinical regenerative capability of human bone marrow cells after myocardial infarction. *Circ Res* 95(7):742-748, 2004.

[123] Tateishi-YuyamaE, Matsubara H, Murohara T, Ikeda U, Shintani S, Masaki H, Amano K, Kishimoto Y, Yoshimoto K, Akashi H, Shimada K, Iwasaka T, Imaizumi T. Therapeutic angiogenesis using cell transplantation (TACT) study investigators. Therapeutic angiogenesis for patients with limb ischaemia by autologous transplantation of bone-marrow cells: a pilot study and a randomised controlled trial. *Lancet* 360(9331):427-435, 2002.

[124] Dimmeler S, Vasa-Nicotera M. Aging of progenitor cells: limitation for regenerative capacity? *J Am Coll Cardiol* 42(12):2081-2082, 2003.

[125] Orlic D, Kajstura J, Chimenti S, Limana F, Jakoniuk I, Quaini F, Nadal-Ginard B, Bodine DM, Leri A, Anversa P. Mobilized bone marrow cells repair the infarcted heart, improving function and survival. *Proc Natl Acad Sci U S A* 410:701-705, 2001.

[126] De Falco E, Porcelli D, Torella AR, Straino S, Iachininoto MG, Orlandi A, Truffa S, Biglioli P, Napolitano M, Capogrossi MC, Pesce M. SDF-1 involvement in endothelial phenotype and ischemia-induced recruitment of bone marrow progenitor cells. *Blood* 104(12):3472-3482, 2004.

[127] Kang HJ, Kim HS, Zhang SY, Park KW, Cho HJ, Koo BK, Kim YJ, Soo Lee D, Sohn DW, Han KS, Oh BH, Lee MM, Park YB. Effects of intracoronary infusion of peripheral blood stem-cells mobilised with granulocyte-colony stimulating factor on left ventricular systolic function and restenosis after coronary stenting in myocardial infarction: the MAGIC cell randomised clinical trial. *Lancet* 363(9411):751-6, 2004.

[128] Parsa CJ, Matsumoto A, Kim J, Riel RU, Pascal LS, Walton GB, Thompson RB, Petrofski JA, Annex BH, Stamler JS, Koch WJ. A novel protective effect of erythropoietin in the infarcted heart. *J Clin Invest* 112(7):999-1007, 2003

[129] Ehrenreich H, Hasselblatt M, Dembowski C, Cepek L, Lewczuk P, Stiefel M, Rustenbeck HH, Breiter N, Jacob S, Knerlich F, Bohn M, Poser W, Ruther E, Kochen M, Geffeler O, Gleiter C, Wessel TC, De Ryck M, Itri L, Prange H, Cerami A, Brines M, Siren AL. Erythropoietin therapy for acute stroke is both safe and beneficial. *Mol Med* 8(8):495-505, 2002.

[130] Casadevall N, Nataf J, Viron B, Kolta A, Kiladjian JJ, Martin-Dupont P, Michaud P, Papo t, Ugo V, Teyssandier I, Varet B, Mayeux P. Pure red-cell aplasia and antierythropoietin antibodies in patients treated with recombinant erythropoietin. *N Engl J Med* 346(7):469-475, 2002.

[131] Macdougall IC, Hutton RD, Cavill I, Coles GA, Williams JD. Poor response to treatment of renal anaemia with erythropoietin corrected by iron given intravenously. *BMJ* 299(6692):157-158, 1989.

[132] Bennet CL, Luminari S, Nissenson AR, Tallman MS, Klinge SA, McWilliams N, McKoy JM, Kim B, Lyons EA, Trifilio SM, Raisch DW, Evens AM, Kuzel TM, Schumock GT, Belknap SM, Locatelli F, Rosset J, Casadevall N. Pure red-cell aplasia and epoetin therapy. *N Engl J Med* 351(14):1403-1408, 2004.

[133] Leist M, Ghezzi P, Grasso G, Bianchi R, Villa P, Fratelli M, Savino C, Bianchi M, Nielsen J, Gerwien J, Kallunki P, Larsen AK, Helboe L, Christensen S, Pedersen LO, Nielsen M, Torup L, Sager T, Sfacteria A, Erbayraktar S, Erbayraktar Z, Gokmen N, Yilmaz O, Cerami-Hand C, Xie QW, Coleman T, Cerami A, Brines M. Derivatives of erythropoietin that are tissue protective but not erythropoietic. *Science* 305(5681): 239-242, 2004.

[134] Jubinsky PT, Krijanovski OI, Nathan DG, Tavernier J, Sieff CA. The beta chain of the interleukin-3 receptor functionally associates with the erythropoietin receptor. *Blood* 90:1867-1873, 1997.

[135] D'Andrea RJ, Gonda TJ. A model for assembly and activation of the GM-CSF, IL-3 and IL-5 receptors: insights from activated mutants of the common beta subunit. *Exp Hematol* 28:231-243, 2000.

[136] Brines M, Grasso G, Fiordaliso F, Sfacteria A, Ghezzi P, Fratelli M, Latini R, Xie QW, Smart J, Su-Rick CJ, Pobre E, Diaz D, Gomez D, Hand C, Coleman T, Cerami A. Erythropoietin mediates tissue protection through an erythropoietin and common beta-subunit heteroreceptor. *Proc Natl Acad Sci U S A* 101(41):14907-1412, 2004.

In: Cancer Research Perspectives
Editor: Larissa S. Pereira, pp. 135-165
ISBN 978-1-60021-980-1

Chapter IV

ENVIRONMENTAL TOBACCO SMOKE AND CANCER

Jinfu Hu* and Marie DesMeules
Centre for Chronic Disease Prevention and Control; Public Health Agency of Canada; Ottawa, Ontario; Canada.

ABSTRACT

Environmental tobacco smoke (ETS) is a widespread contaminant of indoor air where smoking is not prohibited. It is a significant source of exposure to a large number of substances known to be hazardous to human health. Over the last several decades there has been a growing interest in examining the health consequences of ETS. The International Agency for Research on Cancer (IARC) has evaluated the evidence of a carcinogenic risk from exposure to ETS, and has classified it as an established human carcinogen. Except for lung cancer, the evidence of a causal association between ETS exposure and other cancers is inconclusive. In this review chapter, we reviewed recent publications on exposure to ETS and cancers to add more evidence of the risk of passive smoking in lung cancer, which has been established as a causal association, and in other types of cancer in adults and in children.

* Correspondence concerning this article should be addressed to: Jinfu Hu, MD; Evidence and Risk Assessment Division; Centre for Chronic Disease Prevention and Control; Public Health Agency of Canada; 120 Colonnade Road, AL: 6701 A; Ottawa, Ontario; Canada K1A 0K9; Phone: (613) 957-1070; Fax: (613) 941-2633; E-mail: Jinfu_hu@phac-aspc.gc.ca.

ABBREVIATIONS

ETS	environmental tobacco smoke;
OR	odds ratio;
RR	relative risk;
HR	hazard ratio;
CI	confidence interval;
IARC	International Agency for Research on Cancer;
PHA	polycyclic aromatic hydrocarbons;
NAT2	N-acetyltransferase 2;
NPC	nasopharyngeal cancer;
NNK	4-(methylnitrosamino)-1-(3-pyridyl)- 1 butanone;
NNAL	4-(methylnitrosamino)-1-(3-pyridyl)-1 butanol;
HSIL	high-grade squamous intraepithelial lesion;
CNS	central nervous system;
ALL	acute lymphocytic leukemia;
AML	acute mylogenous leukemia;
ANLL	acute non-lymphocytic leukemia;
NHL	non-Hodgkin's lymphoma;
GCT	germ cell tumours;
RCC	renal cell carcinoma;
EPIC	The European Prospective Investigation into Cancer Nutrition;
UKCCS	United Kingdom Childhood Cancer Study;
IRESCC	Inter-Regional Epidemiological Study of Childhood Cancer;
OSCC	Oxford Survey of Childhood Cancer.

INTRODUCTION

Tobacco smoke is the main known cause of cancer-related deaths worldwide. It has been estimated that tobacco causes approximately 25% of all cancers in men and 4% in women [1]. As a cause of human cancer, tobacco smoke is uniquely important. In the previous International Agency for Research on Cancer (IARC)(1986) monograph on tobacco smoking, it was concluded that there was sufficient evidence for establishing a causal association between tobacco use and cancer of the lung, the upper aeridigestive tract, pancreas and lower urinary tract [2]. Recently, IARC provided further evidence that cancer of the stomach, liver and cervix, renal-cell carcinoma and myeloid leukemia can be caused by smoking. According to the evaluation by IARC, there is sufficient evidence on the carcinogenicity of Environmental Tobacco Smoke (ETS) in humans, and thus ETS has been classified as a human carcinogen [3]. ETS can cause sudden infant death, cancer and other diseases [4-6]. Estimations in the USA reported that 88% of nonsmokers were exposed to ETS during 1988-1991 based on the detection in serum of the nicotine metabolite cotinine [7]. An estimated 50,000 people die from passive smoking each year in The USA [8]. At least 3000 non-smokers die from passive smoke each year in France [9].

ETS has received particular attention, being reportedly associated with increased morbidity and mortality in nonsmokers [10,11]. ETS (or secondhand smoke) is a mixture of exhaled mainstream smoke and sidestream smoke produced from the smoldering tobacco. [3]. Cigarette smoke is the main source for involuntary exposure. There are a number of studies that have addressed the composition of ETS beyond the 'common' constituents such as nicotine and carbon monoxide (CO) [3]. Tobacco smoke consists of more than 4000 chemical compounds, and more than 60 of these are known carcinogens [3,12]. ETS contains higher concentrations of some toxins than does mainstream smoke [13]. Carcinogens are present at higher concentrations by unit of volume in sidestream smoke than in mainstream smoke. People can be exposed to ETS from a spouse, in the work place, in public areas, and exposure during childhood. This review chapter focuses on currently available epidemiological publications related to ETS and cancer at sites in adult non-smokers and children.

Environmental Tobacco Smoke and Cancer in Adults

The first indication of ETS was in the 1980s, with the report of an increased risk for lung cancer among non-smoking women married to smokers [14,15]. Since then, more epidemiological studies on the association between passive smoking (or involuntary smoking) and lung cancer have been published. From the mid' 80s to the mid' 90s, studies concentrated on chronic long term effects of exposure to ETS in adults, in particular, evaluation of lung cancer risk for exposed women. Only a few studies have reported on ETS and cancer from sites other than the lung in adults [16]. Recently more epidemiologic research has reported that ETS also increases the risk of other cancers. Except for lung cancer, the evidence of a causal association between ETS exposure and other cancers is inconclusive [3].

Lung Cancer

For lung cancer, the effect of ETS exposure on non-smokers is recognised. Involuntary smoking causes lung cancer in never smokers with an excess risk in the order of 20% for women and 30% for men [3]. The evidence on exposure-response relationships provided a causal relationship between exposure to involuntary smoking and the development of lung cancer by IARC [3]. A review on carcinogen derived biomarkers of exposure to ETS by Hecht [17] showed that the elevated biomarkers in people exposed to ETS was 4-(methylnitrosamino)-1-(3-pyridyl)-1 butanol (NNAL) and its glucuronides (NNAL-Gluc) and urinary metabolites of the tobacco specific lung carcinogen 4-(methylnitrosamino)-1-(3-pyridyl)-1 butanone (NNK), which provides evidence that ETS causes lung cancer in non-smokers.

Cohort Study

The European Prospective Investigation into Cancer Nutrition (EPIC) study, including more than 500 000 healthy volunteers recruited in 10 European countries among men and women with over 7 years follow-up with 97 newly diagnosed cases, showed that exposure to ETS was associated with increased risk of lung cancer [18]. For the whole cohort, the hazard ratio (HR) was 1.34 (95% confidence interval (CI), 0.85-2.13), and odds ratio (OR) was 1.76 (95% CI, 0.96-3.23) in the nested case-control study. The EPIC study added further evidence on the carcinogenicity of ETS in human and exposure to ETS as a cause of lung cancer. The EPIC study included more adjustments for potential confounders such as diet, and laboratory analyses, for example, cotinine measurements and polymorphisms in genes involved in carcinogenesis.

Meta-Analyses

A meta-analysis, including 51 studies and 7369 non-smoking lung cancer cases, examined the association between exposure to secondhand smoke and the risk of lung cancer in lifelong non-smokers [19]. The relative risk (RR) was 1.25 (95% CI, 1.15-1.37) for exposure to the spouse; no evidence existed of RR difference between the two genders. A pooled analysis of data, using 2 previously reported large case-control studies from the USA and Europe, included 1263 never smoking lung cancer cases [20]. The odds ratios (ORs) were 1.18 (95%CI, 1.01-1.37) for exposure to spousal smoking and 1.23 (95%CI, 1.01-1.51) for long-term exposure. A dose-response relationship was presented with increasing duration of exposure to ETS from a spouse.

Exposure to ETS at Work

The IARC revealed a general increase in the relative risk for lung cancer associated with exposure to secondhand smoke at work. The associations are stronger with better assessment of exposure and other aspects of study design [3]. In the workplace, exposure to ETS is associated with an increase of 16%-19% risk of lung cancer among never smokers [3]. A meta-analysis study showed that the summary RR was 1.17 (95%CI, 1.04-1.32) for workplace exposure [19]. An excess risk for exposure to ETS in the work place was also observed in a pooled analysis of two large studies [20]. The ORs were 1.16 (95%CI, 0.99-1.57), and 1.27 (95%CI, 1.03-1.57) for long-term exposure. A dose-response effect was observed (p=0.01) with increased duration of exposure.

ETS is a significant occupational health hazard for food-service workers. A study in Hong Kong estimated that death from heart disease or lung cancer in the Hong Kong catering workforce of 200 000 occurred at the rate of 150 per year for a 40-year working-lifetime exposure to ETS [21]. The study modeled workers' mortality risks using average cotinine levels, estimates of workplace respirable particulates, risk data for cancer and heart disease from the cohort study, and national (US) and regional (Hong Kong) mortality from heart disease and lung cancer. Another study on ETS exposure in hospitality workers in Spain reported that excess lung cancer mortality risk associated with ETS exposure was higher than 145 deaths per 100 000 workers [22].

An increased risk was observed for those who reported ever exposure to ETS in social settings (OR, 1.17; 95% CI, 1.00-1.36) [20]. ETS exposure in the service workplace such as restaurants and bars presents a potential health hazard to employees and non-smoking patrons. Levels of ETS in restaurants were approximately 1.6 to 2.0 times higher than in office workplaces of other businesses, and 3.9 to 6.1 times higher in bars than in office workplaces [23]. A review estimated that excess lung cancer mortality risk from lifetime exposure to ETS in bars, bowling alleys, billiard halls, betting establishments and bingo parlours was between 1.0-4.1/1000, which greatly exceeded the typical de manifestis risk level of 0.3/1000 [24]. The study on biomarkers of a tobacco-specific lung carcinogen in non-smokers who work in restaurants, bars [25], casinos [26] and other service places [24] and exposure to ETS in the USA also demonstrated that exposure of non-smokers to ETS in commercial settings resulted in uptake metabolites of a tobacco-specific lung carcinogen (i.e., nicotine, total cotinine, total NNAL), and had important health effects on non-smoking employees.

ETS Exposure and Genetic Susceptibility to Lung Cancer

It is well recognized that 80%-90% of all lung cancer is attributable to cigarette smoking. Only 15% of all smokers develop this disease and approximately 10% of all diagnoses are among never smokers [27]. This suggests that there is great individual variation in susceptibility to lung carcinogens. Most never smokers with lung cancer have been exposed to ETS. A clinical investigation in the USA reported that 82% (170/207) female lung cancer patients in never smokers were exposed to ETS; the mean years of exposure were 27 from a smoking spouse, 19 from parents, and 15 from co-workers [28]. The etiology of lung cancer in non-smoking females has emphasized host factors and ETS exposure. A review of molecular epidemiology of lung cancer in female passive smokers concluded that proper exposure monitoring of ETS and consideration of susceptibility markers were recommended to obtain undistorted mechanisms of etiology in ETS exposure [29]. Interindividual variability in the susceptibility to carcinogens may be particularly important at low degrees of environmental exposure.

The common tumour suppressor p53 gene mutation is a sensitive marker of tobacco-related carcinogenesis [30,31]. The p53 gene mutation in lung tumours varies between women smokers and non-smokers, suggesting different origins or mechanisms of formation of this mutation in the two groups [32]. Biomarkers of tobacco smoke exposure in human lung cancer pointed to levels of p53 gene mutation in tumours increased from never smokers involuntarily exposed to tobacco smoke [33].

Studying gene-environment interactions in relation to risk of cancer may be valuable because positive findings would clearly implicate the substrates with which the gene interacts as disease causing exposure, clarify cancer etiology and point to environmental modifications for disease prevention. A population–based study in the USA evaluated the association between GSTM1, GSTT1 and GSTP1 polymorphisms and the risk of lung cancer in never smokers with low levels of ETS exposure. The results showed that the carrying GSTM1 null genotype was associated with 2.3-fold increase in risk (95% CI, 1.05-5.13) in never smoking individuals with 20 or more years of household ETS exposure, carrying the GSTM1 null/GSTP1 Val combination were associated with increased lung cancer risk at over 4-fold for developing lung cancer (OR, 4.56; 95% CI, 1.21-17.21). In the presence of ETS, the GSTM1 genotype both alone and in combination with the GSTP1 genotype alters the risk of developing lung cancer among never smokers [34]. The author also evaluated a possible role of CYP1A1 and CYP1B1 polymorphisms and risk of lung cancer among never smokers using the same study population mentioned above [35]. The results showed that CYP1B1 Leu^{432}

Val was significantly associated with lung cancer susceptibility among Caucasians. The combination of CYP1B1 Leu^{432} and $NQ01C^{609}$ T appeared to be associated with the highest risk of lung cancer. A study in France pointed to the role of O^6–alkylguanine DNA alkyltransferase (AGT) polymorphisms in lung cancer susceptibility among nonsmokers, in particular among subjects exposed to environmental carcinogens [36].

Breast Cancer

A number of epidemiologic studies have assessed the association between active and passive smoking and risk of breast cancer. The results are inconsistent [37-41]. A review by Lee [42] concluded that a relationship between ETS and breast cancer has not been established based on thirteen studies including four cohort studies. However, another review on the effect of environment on breast cancer risk concluded that environmental exposure in combination with genetic pre-disposition, age at exposure, and hormonal milieu had a cumulative effect on breast cancer risk [43]. Recently some studies of passive smoking and breast cancer implicate pre-menopausal women [44,45], but not in other studies [41,46,47].

Cohort Studies

Based on eight cohort studies, no association between exposure to ETS and breast cancer was reported in four prospective studies in the USA [46,48-50]. There was a small non-significantly increased risk of breast cancer associated with ETS exposure to a spouse (RR, 1.27; 95% CI, 0.91-1.77) in South Korea [51] and Japan (RR, 1.32; 95% CI, 0.83-2.09) [52]. The sources of ETS exposure most investigated in ETS exposure from the spouse, excluded one prospective study, which included both at home and at work [50]. Another prospective study in middle-aged Japanese women showed exposure to ETS increased the risk of female breast cancer in premenopausal women (RR,2.6; 95%CI, 1.3-5.2), but not in postmenopausal women (RR, 0.7; 95% CI, 0.4-1.0) [44]. This was consistent with a positive association between active smoking and breast cancer (RR, 3.9; 95%CI, 1.5-9.9 for premenopausal breast cancer and RR, 1.1; 95% CI, 0.5-2.5 for postmenopausal breast cancer). In this study, the passive exposure to ETS was collected from residential and occupational /or public settings. In contrast, an inverse association between passive smoking and breast cancer was found in one prospective study only in Japanese non-smoking women (RR,0.58; 95%CI, 0.32-1.10; $p=0.078$) [53].

Case-Control Studies

A number of case-control studies on ETS exposure and breast cancer was conducted in the USA [41,47,54-58], Canada [59], The United Kingdom [60], Germany [40], Switzerland [61], Poland [62], Japan [63] and China [64,65]. Three studies only were designed as hospital-based case-control studies [54,63,64]. Some studies reported a positive association between passive smoking and breast cancer [40,57,59-61,63,64]. A significant trend was observed with increased ETS exposure at home and at work ($p<0.05$) [61] and with increased ETS exposure in lifetime ($p=0.009$) [40]. A Canadian study reported a strong dose-response trend ($p=0.0007$) with an OR of 2.9 (95% CI, 1.3-6.6) for more than 35 years of passive residential and /or occupational exposure in premenopausal women [59]. Although there was no apparent association between any passive smoke exposure or exposure to a husband's smoke and breast cancer in the study; however, an elevated breast cancer risk was observed in ETS exposure of 5 hours or more per day at work (OR, 1.6; 95% CI, 1.0-2.4; p=0.02) in a Chinese study [65]. Also, another study in the USA reported that an increased risk of breast cancer for non-smokers who lived with a smoking spouse for over 27 years (OR, 2.1; 95% CI, 1.47-3.02) [55]. Some of those studies have provided neither evidence of an increase in the risk of breast cancer from ETS exposure [41,47,54,56,58,62], nor differences between ETS exposure and breast cancer in premenopausal and postmenopausal women [41,47,65].

Meta-Analysis

Breast cancer risks differed based on menopausal status [66]. Pooled relative risk estimates for breast cancer were conducted from nineteen published studies of passive smoking and breast cancer risk among non-smoking women [45]. Results showed that the risk of breast cancer was associated with exposure to ETS (RR, 1.27; 95% CI, 1.11-1.45). The RRs were 1.68 (95%CI,1.33-2.12) for premenopausal breast cancer, and 2.19 (95% CI, 1.68-2.84) for 5 studies with more completed assessment for ETS exposure, but not in postmenopausal breast cancer. This was consistent with the prospective study by Hanaoka [44].

Interaction Between N-Acetyltransferase 2 and ETS Exposure

Studies have demonstrated that tobacco related carcinogens have been detected in human breast tissues [67,68]. A number of case-control studies was conducted to evaluate the interaction between NAT2 acetylation status and active and passive exposure to tobacco smoke as related to breast cancer [58,62,69-71]. The results are inconsistent. A case-control study in Germany showed passive smoking was associated with higher risk in rapid than in slow acetylators, with ORs of 2.0 (95% CI, 1.0-4.1) and 1.2 (95% CI, 0.7-2.0), respectively [69]. However, a case-only study of 502 women with incident primary breast cancer in The USA did not suggest any substantial interaction between acetylation status and exposure to tobacco smoke in the etiology of breast cancer [70]. A study in The USA also did not support NAT2 as a risk factor for breast cancer or that it altered susceptibility to tobacco smoke [58]. A recent study by Lissowska [62] reported NAT2 slow vs. rapid/intermediate acetylation genotype was not related to breast cancer risk (OR, 0.99; 95% CI, 0.87-1.13), and did not significantly modify the relationship with smoking. Another population-based case-control study in Germany reported that no evidence was found in the interaction of SULT1A1genotype with smoking [71]; however, the SULT1A1*1/*1 genotype in combination with NAT2 fast acetylator status appeared to increase breast cancer risk.

Brain Cancer

An association between cigarette smoking and brain cancer has not been established. A number of case-control studies reported no association with cigarette smoke [72-75]. However, two recent prospective cohort studies supported a positive association between cigarette smoke and risk of glioma [76,77]. In addition, two case-control studies also reported a positive association between cigarette smoke and meningioma in men [78] and women [79].

A cohort study in non-smoking Japanese women whose husbands smoked, found significantly increased mortality from brain tumours among the wives (p=0.004) [80]. A population-based case-control study in Australia showed an increased risk of meningioma was associated with exposure to ETS from a spouse, especially amongst women (OR, 2.7; 95% CI, 1.2-6.1) based on 48 non-smoking cases and 206 non-smoking controls [72]. Another population-based case-control study in The USA, based on 95 non-smoking cases and 202 non-smoking controls, also reported an increased risk of meningioma in men and women combined with exposure to a smoking spouse (OR, 2.0; 95% CI, 1.1-3.5) [78]. Increased duration of passive smoking from a spouse was associated with increased risk of meningioma (p=0.02).

Cancer of the Nasosinus, Nasopharynx, Head and Neck

Nasopharyngeal and Nasal Sinus Cavity Cancer

Nasal Sinus Cavity Cancer

A review by Benninger [81] pointed out tobacco smoking and ETS were associated with nasal and sinus disease such as allergic rhinitis and nasosinus cancer. Cancer of the nasal cavity and sinuses is quite rare. A few studies investigated the association between ETS and nasosinus cancer.

In a Japanese prospective study by Hiryama based on 28 cases, women with ETS exposure had a significantly increased risk of nasosinus cancer by exposure to the husband's increased number of cigarettes per day. The RRs were 2.0 (95%CI, 0.6-6.3) for 15-19 cigarettes per day and 2.55 (95% CI, 1.0-6.3) for 20 or more cigarettes per day (p =0.02) [80].

A case-control study in Japan, including 44 cases and 88 controls, showed an increased risk of squamous cell neoplasm of the maxillary sinus in non-smoking women only with an increased number of smokers in the household (OR, 5.7 for two or more smokers), but not in men [82]. Another case-control study, using data from the 1986 US National Mortality Followback Survey based on 28 cases and 99 controls, showed that non-smoking men who had a wife who smoked had a three–fold increased risk of nasalsinus cancer (95% CI, 1.0-8.9) [83]. When the analysis of cases was restricted to those with cancer of the maxillary sinus, the risk was somewhat higher (OR, 4.8; 95% CI, 0.9-24.7). The study subjects were selected from a systematic sample of death certificates, and data were collected by next-of-kin.

Nasopharyngeal Cancer

Nasopharyngeal cancer (NPC) is rare in most countries; the highest incidence in the world is southeast China [84]. A case-control study in Taiwan provided no evidence of an increased in risk of NPC from exposure to ETS [85]. Another case-control study in China reported a non-significant negative association with NPC for cumulative exposure to ETS during adulthood by pack-person–years [86]. However, one case-control study in the USA reported a significant positive association between ETS exposure in childhood and NPC (OR, 2.28; 95% CI, 1.21-4.28), but not in adulthood [87]. Another case-control study in China also reported a strong statistically significant positive association between the risk of NPC and exposure to ETS in children or adults among non-smoking women, but not in men [88]. Among non-smoking women during childhood, a consistent increase in risk of NPC related to exposure to ETS (OR, 3.36; 95% CI, 1.41-8.05 for exposure to mother smoking and OR, 2.95; 95% CI, 1.41-6.19 for exposure to father smoking) [88]. During adulthood, the ORs were 3.09 (95% CI; 1.48-6.46) for exposure to a spouse smoking and 3.28 (95% CI, 1.48-7.27) for exposure to 3 or more hours per day from co-worker smokers [88].

Cancer of the Head and Neck

Few studies has been conducted on exposure to ETS and cancer of the head and neck. No significant association between exposure to ETS and head and neck cancer was reported in two studies [52,89]. However, another study reported significant association with ETS exposure at home and at work (OR, 8.0; 95% CI, 2.55-25.1 for women and OR, 3.78; 95% CI, 1.37-10.4 for men) [90]. The estimations seem implausibly high and may have resulted from the non-comparability of the way the data were collected for cases and controls [42].

Cancer of the Digestive System

Stomach Cancer

The major determinants of gastric cancer are environmental rather than host-related [91]. Among environmental factors, smoking is the most important risk factor for cancer overall. There is sufficient evidence that smoking causes stomach cancer [3]. A few studies reported exposure to ETS and the risk of stomach cancer.

A population based case-control study in Canada, based on 305 non-smoking cases and 726 non-smoking controls, examined the role of ETS exposure in the risk of stomach cancer [92]. The results showed that a significant trend ($p<0.05$) is related to exposure to ETS with combined residential years and occupational years exposed in male cardial cancer only (OR, 3.7; 95%CI, 1.0-13.7 for high vs. never exposure). It is notable that the study also reported correspondingly the association with active smoking. However, the sample size for cardial cases among never smokers was small, based on 31 cases only. Further research with a large sample size could clarify the role of passive smoking in stomach cancer by subsite. However, a large prospective study of Korean women, based on 197 incident stomach cases, reported that spousal smoking was not associated with an increased risk of stomach cancer in non-smoking women (RR, 1.0; 95%CI, 0.7-1.5 for ex-smokers and RR 0.9; 95%CI, 0.6-1.2 for current smoker spouse) [51].

Pancreatic Cancer

Tobacco smoke, with its complexity of constituents, damages the pancreas in multiple ways. Smoking not only affects pancreatic secretion patterns via its nicotine content but also induces inflammatory reactions and exerts carcinogenic effects by several other constituents. Smoking contributes to pancreatic carcinogenesis, and to a hypothetical opening to pancreatic cancer development [93]. An experimental study provided further evidence on mechanisms whereby inhalation of ETS that leads to focal chronic pancreatic inflammation in rats [94].

One population-based case–control study in Canada, based on 105 non-smoking cases and 1145 non-smoking controls, reported no significant association of pancreatic cancer with either as a child or as an adult exposure to ETS (OR, 1.21; 95% CI, 0.60-2.44) [95].

Other Cancers in the Digestive System

Colorectal Cancer

A prospective study was conducted in Washington County, USA with 12-year follow up to examine the incidence of colorectal cancer in women in relation to passive exposure to smoke (i.e., having lived with a person who smoked) [96]. A statistically significant reduction in risk for colorectal cancer was observed among non-smoking women who were exposed to ETS (RR, 0.74; 95% CI, 0.56-0.97), but an increased risk for this cancer was found for non-smoking men exposed to ETS in the household (RR, 2.99; 95%CI, 1.77-5.04). In contrast, a population-based case-control study in the USA reported that ETS was significantly associated with rectal cancer in men (ORs, 1.5; 95% CI, 1.1-2.0 for total exposure to ETS (h/wk) both 10 and 20 years respectively), but not in women [97]. A population-based case-control study in Germany reported that exposure to ETS was associated with an increased risk for colorectal cancer only among NAT2 fast acetylators (OR, 2.6; 95% CI, 1.1-5.9 for exposure in childhood and adulthood) [98].

Liver Cancer

A large prospective study of Korean women, based on 83 incident liver cancer cases, found no increased risk with exposure to a spouse who smoked (RR, 0.8; 95% CI, 0.5-1.5 and RR, 0.7; 95% CI, 0.4-1.1 for ex-smoker and current smoker spouse respectively) [51].

Cancer of the Urine System

Kidney Cancer

Exposure to ETS and the risk of kidney cancer is reported in only two Canadian studies.

One study included 119 non-smoking cases of kidney cancer and 524 non-smoking population controls based on whether or not subjects were exposed to ETS from cohabitants or co-workers (h/day) [99]. The highest exposure level (more than 8 hours per day) was associated with a risk of 1.6 (95%CI, 0.5-4.7; p=0.68) for men and 1.7 (95%CI, 0.8-3.4; p=0.03) for women. Another large population-based case-control study involved 260 non-smoking cases of renal cell carcinoma (RCC) and 803 non-smoking controls according to lifetime exposure to ETS for years of residential plus occupational exposure and total smoker-years of residential plus occupational exposure. Men and women with 43 or more years of passive residential and/or occupational exposure were associated with RCC (OR, 3.9; 95% CI, 1.4-10.6; p=0.001 for men and OR, 1.8; 95% CI, 1.0-3.3; p=0.09 for women). A statistically significant positive association with RCC was also shown in both genders for total smoker-years of exposure with a dose-response relationship (p=0.0004 for men and p=0.01 for women) [100].

Bladder Cancer

About one-half of bladder cancer incidences in the United States can be attributed to known causes, mainly cigarette smoking [101]. Cigarette smoking is a well-established risk factor for bladder cancer [2]. The relationship between ETS exposure and bladder cancer has been investigated in a few studies. Little evidence has suggested an association between ETS exposure and risk of bladder cancer.

A Japanese prospective study found no significant increased risk of cancer of urinary organs (mainly cancer of bladder and kidney) in women in relation to smoking by the husband [52]. Another prospective study from The Netherlands, based on 55 cases of never smokers exposed to ETS from spouses, parents, or co-workers, reported that ETS was not associated with an increased risk of bladder cancer [102]. A case-control study involving 86 non-smoking cases and 266 non-smoking hospital controls in the USA showed no significant association between any index of ETS exposure and risk of bladder cancer in both genders [103]. Another population-based case-control study involving 142 non-smoking cases and 217 non-smoking population controls in Canada also revealed that risk of bladder cancer was not related to ETS exposure at home and at work [104]. However, a hospital-based case control study on the interaction between ETS and arsenic methylation ability was conducted in Taiwan, based on 12 non-smoker cases and 81 non-smoker controls with known exposure to arsenic in drinking water [105]. The results showed that ETS significantly elevated the risk of bladder cancer among men (OR, 4.6; 95%CI, 1.87-27.4), but not in women. Arsenic methylation abilities played an important role in reducing the risk of bladder cancer for both non-smokers and smokers exposed to ETS.

Cigarette smoke is an important source of 4- and 3- minobiphenyl (ABP) exposure. Quantitative analysis of haemoglobin adducts of 4- and 3-ABP was used to assess aromatic amine exposure in tobacco smoke in a population-based case-control study in the USA, involving 761 case patients with bladder cancer and 770 individually matched controls. Findings suggested that environmental exposure to arylamines might account for a significant proportion of non-smoking-related bladder cancer in the general population [106].

Cancer of the Genital System in Women

Cervical Cancer

A number of studies on ETS and cervical cancer have been conducted. The results are inconsistent. A long-term two-cohort study established in 1963 and 1975 based on the private census of the residents of Washington County in The USA, involved 94 cases of never smokers in the 1963 cohort and 55 cases of never smokers in the 1975 cohort [107]. The results showed that passive smoking was associated with cervical cancer, and stronger in the 1963 cohort (RR, 2.1; 95% CI, 1.3-3.3) than in the 1975 cohort (RR, 1.4; 95% CI, 0.8-2.4). The increased risk of cervical cancer revealed an exposure to the spouse or solely from other persons in the household who smoked. In contrast, another prospective study of 9675 Japanese non-smoking women found no increased risks of cervical cancer in non-smoking women who had husbands who smoked (RR, 1.1; 95% CI, 0.3-4.5) [53]. The results were based on only 9 cases of cervical cancer. Also, a large prospective study of Korean women, based on 203 incident cervix cancer cases, found no association between spousal smoking and cervix cancer (RR, 0.9; 95% CI, 0.6-1.3, for ex-smokers and RR, 0.9; 95%CI, 0.6-1.2 for current spousal smoking) [51].

A community-based nested case-control study from cervical cancer screen program of Taiwanese women, including 89 non-smoker cases and 175 non-smoker controls, reported that lifetime ETS exposure was a major determinant for the risk of cervical neoplasms (OR, 2.99; 95% CI, 1.10-8.09 for more than 20 pack-years exposure) [108]. A population-based case-control study in The USA also reported that risk from passive smoking was greater in women who were not smokers (OR, 3.43; 95% CI, 1.23-9.54 exposed for 3 hours or more per day) than in women who smoked (OR, 2.59; 95% CI, 0.23-29.24) [109]. However, no statistically significant association was found between exposure to ETS, either at home or at work, and cervical intraepithelial neoplasma in another case-control study in The USA, including 36 non-smoking cases and 170 non-smoking controls [110].

A prospective cohort study of 623 Singapore women showed that the risk of detection of high-grade squamous intraepithelial lesion (HSIL) increased with the spouse's smoking habit [111]. A case-control study in the USA observed that increased risk of HSIL was increased with exposure to ETS with high-risk human papillomaviruses (HR-HPVs) [112].

In addition, a study of women in India, including 103 cases and 103 controls, reported that cervix cancer increased in passive smokers with GSTM1, GSTT1 and GSTP1 genotypes [113].

Ovarian Cancer

The results in the research on the role of smoking in ovarian cancer are inconsistent [3,114,115]. A few studies have reported results relating ETS exposure to ovarian cancer risk. A population-based case-control study in the USA, based on 351 non-smoking cases and 367 non-smoking controls, showed no association between gestation and childhood exposure to ETS and the risk of invasive or borderline ovarian cancer [115]. However, another hospital-based case-control study in the USA, involving 246 non-smoking cases and 470 non-smoking controls, reported a significant decreased risk of ovarian cancer among nonsmokers exposure to ETS (OR, 0.68; 95%CI, 0.47-0.99) [114].

Leukemias

A population based case-control study in Canada, involving 266 non-smoker cases and 1326 non-smoker controls, reported that the risk for chronic lymphocytic leukemia was associated with ETS exposure (OR, 2.3; 95% CI, 1.2-4.5 for more than 83 smoker-years of residential exposure, and OR, 2.4; 95% CI, 1.3-4.3 for more than 72 smoker-years of occupational exposure), but not in other types of leukemia [116]. As well, Kasim, et al [117] reported no association of active smoking with chronic lymphocytic leukemia. The two studies used the same data.

Environmental Tobacco Smoke and Cancer in Children

The evidence on the harmful effects of ETS on children starts with the effects on the foetus and carries on throughout childhood [118,119]. Both prenatal and postnatal exposure to chemicals in cigarette smoke has negative significant influences on infants' health in the early periods of life [120]. Smoking during pregnancy is associated with an increased frequency of perinatal complications, such as preterm delivery, low birth weight, intrauterine growth restriction, and sudden infant death syndrome [121]. Many constituents of cigarette smoke, including nicotine and polycyclic aromatic hydrocarbons (PHA), have been shown to pass through the placenta [122,123]. Higher levels of PAH-DNA adducts were found in fetal than in maternal tissue [124]. Activation of procarcinogens in human fetal and placental tissues has been demonstrated, as has smoke-induced damage to DNA in the human placenta [125]. Exposure to ETS can be both ways during gestation and childhood.

A review by Preston-Martin [126] concluded that findings on parental cigarette smoking and risk of cancer in childhood were not consistent. In another review, Tredaniel, et al [127] suggested no clear associations between maternal smoking during pregnancy and childhood cancer or specific sites. Later, a review by Sasco and Vainio [128] concluded no strong association between maternal smoking in pregnancy and/or exposure to ETS and childhood cancer. Tumours most often found associated with maternal smoking in pregnancy or ETS exposure are childhood brain tumours and leukemia-lymphoma, with risk up to two or greater in selected studies. The effect of gestational exposure to cigarette smoking on childhood cancer risk is still being debated [128].

Epidemiologic studies have indicated that offspring of mothers who smoke might be at greater risk for developing cancer in later life [129-133]. A mate-analysis revealed an almost seven-fold increased level of haemoglobin adducts in newborns exposed to ETS in utero than in non-exposed newborns [124]. Active maternal smoking and secondary maternal exposure to ETS produce quantitatively and qualitatively indistinguishable increases in fetal HPRT mutation [134].

A toxicology study demonstrated that exposure of pregnant mice to a relevant dose of mainstream cigarette smoke decreased offspring resistance to transplanted tumour cells and persistently reduced cytotoxic T-lymphocyte activity in prenatally exposed pups [135].

Exposure by Parental Smoking and Risk of Childhood Cancer

Exposure by Paternal Smoking

A review by Tredaniel, et al [127] showed that a significantly increased risk of specific types of childhood cancer have not been linked to smoking by a father. A national case-control study used records of the Oxford Survey of Childhood Cancer (OSCC) (deaths from 1971 to 1976), including the parents of 2587 children who died with cancer and the parents of 2587 healthy controls matched for sex and date of birth [136]. The results showed a statistically significant positive trend between paternal daily consumption of cigarettes and the risk of childhood cancer (RR, 1.63; 95% CI, 1.23-2.15 for 40 or more cigarettes per day; $p<0.001$). About 14% of all childhood cancer in this series could be attributable to paternal smoking. Another large case-control study in the UK from the Inter-Regional Epidemiological Study of Childhood Cancer (IRESCC), including the parents of 555 children diagnosed with cancer and two separate matched pairs controls, reported a statistically significant positive trend ($p<0.02$) between the risk of childhood cancer and paternal daily consumption of cigarettes before the pregnancy when cases were compared to General Practitioner, but not in cases compared to hospital controls [137].

A population-based case control study was conducted in China, including 642 childhood cancer patients (less than age 15) of non-smoking mothers and individual matched controls. Results showed that a father who had ever smoked cigarettes was 30% more likely (OR, 1.3; 95% CI, 1.0-1.7) to have an offspring who developed cancer than fathers who never smoked [138]. The risk increased with fathers' smoking pack-years before conception (OR, 1.7; 95% CI, 1.2-2.5 for 5 or more smoking pack-years; $p=0.006$).

Exposure by Maternal Smoking

The results from IRESCC in the UK showed a statistically significant negative trend ($p<0.001$) between the risks of childhood cancer and maternal smoking (cigarettes per day) before pregnancy when cases were compared with hospital controls [137]. But, when cases were compared with General Practitioner, a non-significant positive trend ($p=0.53$) was shown with a significantly elevated point estimate for the two lowest smoking categories (RR, 1.77; 95% CI, 1.07-2.92 for less 10 cigarettes per day and RR, 1.51; 95% CI, 1.08-2.13 for 10-19 cigarettes per day). The same pattern of risk of childhood cancer was also shown during the fifth month of pregnancy (cases vs. General Practitioner). The two results were different using two control groups. The approach on controls' selection might have influenced the results.

A nationwide population-based case-control study in the United Kingdom Childhood Cancer Study (UKCCS), including 3838 children with cancer and 7629 control children under the age of 15 years, reported a negative association between maternal preconception cigarette smoking and childhood cancer of all sites (OR, 0.86; 95% CI, 0.75-0.99 for 20 or more cigarettes per day; $p=0.07$) [139]. Under reporting of smoking mothers by case mothers resulted in a statistically significant negative association between mother cigarette smoking during pregnancy and childhood cancer.

Children Cancer

Brain and Central Nervous System

Brain Tumours

Epidemiological studies have examined maternal smoking prior to or during pregnancy in relation to brain tumours in childhood, and a number of case-control studies showed no significantly increased risk [138,140-148]. Recently, a large prospective study of 1.4 million live births in Sweden from 1983-1997 (under 15 years old) with 8 years follow-up found a modest increase in the risk of brain tumours in the offspring of women who smoked during pregnancy (HR, 1.24; 95% CI, 1.01-1.53) [133]. The effect of smoking on occurrence of brain tumours was most apparent for astrocytoma and most strong in 2-4 year-old children [133]. In this cohort, smoking explained about 5% of cases. However, adjustment for measured variables from birth records was limited. Information on other sources of exposure to tobacco such as parental smoking prior to pregnancy, maternal exposure to ETS during pregnancy and parental smoking during early childhood was lacking.

A case-control study in Italy observed an elevated risk of brain tumours among non-smoking mother; the relative risks for light and heavy exposure to ETS were 1.7 (95% CI, 0.8-3.6) and 2.2 (95% CI, 1.1-4.5; p=0.02) [129]. A meta-analysis reported that exposure to paternal cigarette smoke showed an association with brain tumours (RR, 1.22; 95% CI, 1.05-1.40; based on 10 studies) [149]. However, another meta-analysis from 12 studies did not support an association between maternal smoking during pregnancy and childhood brain tumours with a summary relative risk estimate of 1.05 (95% CI, 0.9-1.21) [150].

Central Nervous System Tumours

Tumours of the central nervous system (CNS) is the second most common malignancy of childhood, accounting for approximately 20% of all cases of childhood cancer in developed countries [151]. CNS tumours are the second most common cancers in under 15-year-olds in many areas of Europe [152].

A cohort study by Pershagen et al [153] found no association between maternal smoking in pregnancy and risk for tumours of the central nervous system. A population-based case-control study in Italy, including the mothers of 244 children aged 0-15 years with CNS tumours and 502 control mothers, reported that an increased risk of CNS tumours was found in the children of non-smoking mothers exposed regularly to tobacco smoke both in early pregnancy (OR, 1.8; 95% CI, 1.0-2.3) and in later pregnancy (OR, 1.7; 95% CI, 1.2-2.5) [130]. The results confirmed their previous findings [129]. However, A meta-analysis reported that no association between exposure to maternal tobacco smoke during pregnancy and CNS tumours was found in 12 studies (RR, 1.04; 95%CI, 0.92-1.18) [149]. A large population-based case-control study in Germany, including 466 cases of CNS and 2458 controls under the age of 15 years, also reported no association between maternal exposure to ETS and CNS tumours [131]; but an elevated risk of ependymoma with maternal smoking during pregnancy was observed (OR, 5.66; 95%CI, 2.01-15.9 for more than 10 cigarettes per day). No association between mother smoking during pregnancy or paternal smoking before pregnancy and CNS tumours was found in another German study [154]. The UKCCS based on 635 CNS cases showed no association between cigarette smoking by paternal or maternal preconception and the risk of CNS tumours in their children [139]; however, a statistically significant negative association (p=0.01) was found among maternal cigarette smoking during pregnancy.

Leukemias and Lymphomas

Leukemias

The effects of parent smoking during pregnancy and the risk of leukemia have been addressed in some epidemiological studies. The results are inconsistent. A large cohort study of Swedish children, including 750 hemopoietic cancer occurring between 1983 and 1997, using the same data source on brain tumours, indicated maternal smoking during pregnancy affected the risk of childhood leukemia in the offspring [155]. Results revealed a higher risk of acute mylogenous leukemia (AML) (HR, 1.41; 95% CI, 0.74-2.67, and HR, 2.28; 95% CI, 1.05-4.94 for children whose mothers smoked 10 or more cigarettes per day; p= 0.084). In contrast, maternal smoking was associated with a lower risk of acute lymphocitic leukemia (ALL) (HR, 0.73; 95% CI, 0.58-0.91).

A meta-analysis reported no association between exposure to maternal tobacco smoke during pregnancy and leukemia based on 8 studies (RR,1.05; 95% CI, 0.82-1.34) [149]. Results from the UKCCS involving 1630 leukemia cases also showed no association between paternal or maternal smoking during preconception and leukemia in offspring [139]. A hospital-based case-control study in Italy, including 183 cases of leukemias and non-Hodgkin's lymphomas and 307 controls, showed no association between paternal smoking up to a child's birth and acute lymphocytic leukemia (ALL) and acute nonlymphocytic leukemia (ANLL), and no statistically significantly increased risk with ANLL (OR, 2.0; 95% CI, 0.8-4.8) for ever maternal smoking up to a child's birth [132]. A large case-control study in the USA, including 517 AML cases and 1914 ALL cases, reported that parental smoking during pregnancy or exposure to cigarette smoke shortly after birth did not contribute to the risk of childhood of ALL and AML [156].

A multicenter case-control study in France, including 280 incident cases and 288 hospital controls aged under 15, also reported that childhood leukemia was not related to exposure to maternal smoking during pregnancy or parental smoking before or after index child's birth [157]. However, an increased risk of acute leukemia was observed with increasing pack-years smoked by a father before conception (OR, 2.4; 95% CI, 1.1-5.6 for 5 or more pack-years; p=0.02) in a Chinese study based on 166 cases [138]. When the analysis was stratified by subtypes, an increased risk of ALL only was observed in fathers who smoked for 5 or more pack-years before conception (OR, 3.8; 95% CI, 1.3-12.3; p=0.03). Using data from a Children Cancer Group case-control study, based on 320 leukemia cases at 18 months of age or younger and 558 controls, showed an elevated risk of ALL from paternal smoking one month prior to pregnancy with OR of 1.56 (95% CI, 1.03-2.36) [158]. However, the study revealed that maternal smoking during pregnancy was negatively associated with infant leukemia risk (OR, 0.66; 95% CI, 0.46-0.94 for total leukemia and OR, 0.45; 95%CI, 0.21-0.96 for AML) [158].

A study, including 491 ALL cases and 491 controls, was conducted in Canada using case-control and case-only analyses [159]. Results showed that prenatal maternal smoking, but not postnatal smoking, was associated with small increases in risk of ALL in the offspring. The effect of parental smoking could be modified by variant alleles in the CYP1A1 gene [159]. Another study, including 219 leukemia cases and 105 controls in France, also examined childhood leukemia, polymorphisms of metabolism enzyme genes, and interaction with maternal tobacco smoking during pregnancy using both case-control and case-only analyses [160]. The study did not support an increased in risk of childhood leukemia related to maternal smoking during pregnancy, but an interaction was observed in the case-only analysis with CYP1A1*2A variant allele (OR, 2.2; 95% CI, 1.0-4.9) and with GSTM1 deletion (OR, 2.3; 95% CI, 1.2-2.4) [160].

Lymphomas

A large cohort study in Swedish children showed that maternal smoking was associated with an increased risk of children' lymphoma (HR, 1.25; 95% CI, 0.76-2.04) [155]. Whereas, A case-control study in China reported an increased risk of lymphomas by exposure to paternal smoking (OR, 4.0; 95% CI, 1.3-12.5) [138]. The risk increase was observed with increased smoking pack-years by a father before conception (OR, 4.5; 95%CI, 1.2-16.8 for 5 or more smoking pack-years; p=0.07) and after birth (OR, 5.0; 95% CI, 1.2-22.4 for 5 or more smoking pack-years, p=0.08), based on 87 cases in four strata. A large case-control study in Germany observed an elevated risk of non-Hodgkin's lymphoma (NHL) [154]. The OR was 5.2 (95% CI, 1.2-22.4) for heavy maternal smoking (>20 cigarettes per day) during pregnancy. A hospital-based case-control study in Italy, based on 17 cases and 228 controls, reported that fathers' smoking up to child's birth was associated with NHL (OR, 6.7; 95%CI, 1.0-43.4) [132]. However, a nested case-control study based on 1.7 million live births in Sweden from the Swedish Medical Birth Registry did not show a risk for developing childhood NHL by maternal and perinatal smoking (including 168 cases) [161]. No association was found from paternal and maternal cigarette smoking in preconception to childhood lymphoma, based on 351 cases in UKCCS [139].

Other Cancers

Results from the UKCCS, involving 28 cases reported a statistically significant increased risk of hepatoblastoma in children whose mothers smoked preconception (OR, 2.68; 95% CI, 1.16-6.21; p=0.02) and strongest for both parents smoking (OR, 4.74; 95% CI, 1.68-13.35; p=0.003) [139]. Another national case-control study from the Oxford Survey of Childhood Cancers (OSCC) in the UK, based on parents of 43 children who died with hepatoblastoma, showed a statistically significant association between smoking by both parents and hepatoblastoma (RR, 2.28; 95%CI, 1.02-5.09) [162].

A large population-based case-control study by the Children's Oncology Group in The USA, involving 274 children (under age 15) with Germ Cell Tumours (GCT), reported childhood GCT was not effected by parental smoking before pregnancy, during index pregnancy and the nursing period, and maternal passive smoking [163]. No risk of bone tumour and soft tissue sarcoma was found by maternal smoking during pregnancy and paternal smoking before pregnancy in a Germany study [154].

Exposure to ETS During Childhood

Exposure to ETS in Childhood and Lung Cancer

The evidence for an association between lung cancer and childhood exposure to ETS is less consistent than that for exposure in adulthood. The IARC concluded that there was no clear indication of lung cancer risk in later life associated with exposure to ETS in Childhood [3].

Findings from a large European Prospective study of EPIC indicated that the increased risk of lung cancer related to ETS exposure during childhood, particularly among those who had never smoked (RR, 3.63; 95% CI, 1.19-11.11 for daily exposure of many hours) [18]. Correspondingly, a meta-analysis in children exposure to ETS indicated that the detected association between postnatal exposures to ETS and hemoglobin adducts suggested a 30% increased level of biologically effective dose [124]. A hospital-based case-control study in non-smoking Taiwanese women (including 268 cases and 445 controls) reported that patients in childhood exposed to passive smoking had 2.2-fold risk (95% CI, 1.4-3.4) for developing lung cancer, compared with non-exposed women [164]. Another hospital-based case-control study based on 104 cases (aged 0-14) and 74 hospital controls also reported a significantly increased risk of female lung cancer associated with childhood exposure to ETS at home. The risk increased with increased exposure level (gram/day) [165]. However, a meta-analysis by Boffetta et al [149] from 11 studies did not provide evidence of exposure to ETS in childhood and the risk of lung cancer in adulthood (RR, 0.91; 95% CI, 0.80-1.05).

In addition, an analysis of tobacco-specific lung carcinogen (4-methylnitrosamino)-1-(3-pyridyl)-1-butanone (NNK) in Moldovan children showed a considerable uptake of tobacco smoke constituents, nicotine and the NNK, by some children [166]. Although there is no clear evidence of association between childhood exposure to ETS and development of lung cancer later in life, NNK uptake by some children involved in this study is comparable with that of nonsmoking adults for whom this association has already been estimated [166].

Exposure to ETS in Childhood and Other Cancers

A review by Okasha, et al [39] concluded that there is little evidence for an association between ETS in early life and breast cancer. A cohort study by Wartenberg, et al [49] found no relationship between ETS exposure and breast cancer mortality and little evidence for an association between ETS exposure in early life and breast cancer risk. No association between exposure to ETS in childhood and breast cancer was found in case-control studies [47,59,167]. In addition, exposure to ETS during childhood to parents' smoking increased a child's risk of leukemia and lymphoma during adulthood [168].

CONCLUSION

In summary, recent findings added more evidence of ETS and lung cancer [18, 20, 21, 25, 34-36], in which a causal association was established [3]. More recently epidemiologic studies have reported exposure to ETS and the risk of other cancers in adults, in particular, breast cancer based on studies using menopausal status [44,45]. The California Evironmental Protection Agency concluded that epidemiologic studies provided evidence consistent with a causal association between ETS exposure and breast cancer in younger primary premenopausal women [169]. The Surgeon General concluded that the evidence was suggestive but not sufficient to infer a causal relationship between ETS and breast cancer [170]. Further research is needed to clarify the associations between ETS and the risk of other cancers, including breast cancer.

Epidemiologic studies have indicated that offspring of mothers whose active or passive exposure to smoke might be at greater risk for developing cancer in later life [129-133,155]. Recently, results from two large prospective studies of 1.4 million Swedish children support a role for maternal smoking during pregnancy in the etiology of childhood cancer, which included brain tumours and leukemia and lymphoma [133,155]. Increased levels of biomarkers of genetic damage in newborns could have important implications for adverse health effects on exposure to ETS in utero [124]. Results from a toxicology study on exposure to ETS of pregnant mice further demonstrated the results from epidemiological studies [135]. The evidence is suggestive but not sufficient to infer a causal relationship between prenatal and postnatal exposure to secondhand smoke and childhood cancer [170]. Further study is required in the field to clarify ETS exposure and the risk of cancer at sites in children.

Epidemiological studies and biomarker monitoring of ETS exposure provided evidence of health hazards in humans exposed to ETS from foetus to childhood and adulthood. Avoiding exposure to ETS is one of the important strategies in cancer prevention. Tobacco smoke is a modifiable risk factor. Exposure to ETS is a significant and preventable cause of morbidity and mortality of cancer among adults [170] in non-smokers and children [6,171]. Eliminating exposure to ETS is a public health priority.

A number of conclusions are highlighted in the current literature. For example, smoke-free policies in workplaces and public places can be a very effective way to protect the public from the known risks of cancers associated with ETS (3, 19-26). It is suggested that prevention of passive exposure to cigarette smoke be considered as a part of a large framework of smoking prevention, especially among the young [173,174]. Comprehensive tobacco control programs (to reduce the prevalence of smoking in the total population) are likely to be the most effective and sustainable option for increasing the prevalence of smoke-free homes [175]. Moreover, interventions encouraging smokers to make their homes smoke-free would have the additional benefits of protecting their families and helping themselves gain greater control over their dependence, thus facilitating cessation attempts [176]. Health promotion campaigns as well as health education programs are important approaches for smoking cessation interventions [177].

REFERENCES

[1] Stewart, B. W. and Kleihues, P. World Cancer Report. Lyon, France, *IARC* Press, 2003.

[2] IARC. *IARC monographs on the evaluation of carcinogenic risk to humans, Vol. 38*, Tobacco Smoking. Loyon, France: IARC Press; 1986.

[3] IARC. *IARC monographs on the evaluation of carcinogenic risk to humans, Vol. 83*, Tobacco smoke and involuntary smoking. Lyon, France: *IARC* Press; 2004.

[4] Nelson, E (2001). The miseries of passive smoking. *Hum Exp Toxicol*, 20, 61-83.

[5] Dhala, A., Pinsker, K., Prezant, D. J (2006). Respiratory health consequences of environmental tobacco smoke. *Clin. Occup. Environ. Med*, *5*, 139-156.

[6] Hofhuis, W. M., de-Jongste, J. C., Merkus, P. J (2003). Adverse health effects of prenatal and postnatal tobacco smoke exposure on children. *Arch. Dis. Cild, 88*, 1086-1090.

[7] Pirkle, J. L., Flegal, K. m., Bernert, J. T., Brody, D. J., Etzel, R. A., Maurer, K. R (1996). Exposure of the US population to environmental tobacco smoke: the Third National Health and Nutrition Examination Survey, 1988 to 1991. *J. Am. Med. Assoc, 275*, 1233-1240.

[8] Wells, A. J (1988). An estimate of adult mortality in the United States from passive smoking. *Environ. Int, 14*, 382-385.

[9] Dubois, G (2005). Prevention of air pollution by indoor tobacco smoke in France. *Bull. Acad. Natl. Med, 189*, 803-812.

[10] Jaakkola, M. S (2002). Environmental tobacco smoke and health in the elderly. *Eur. Respir. J, 19*, 172-181.

[11] Nurminen, M. M., Jaakkola, M. S (2001). Mortality from occupational exposure to environmental tobacco smoke in Finland. *J. Occup. Environ. Med, 43*, 687-693.

[12] Das, S. K (2003). Harmful health effects of cigarette smoking. *Mol. Cell. Biochem, 253*, 159-165.

[13] Schick, S and Glantz, S (2005). Philip Morris toxicological experiments with fresh sidestream smoke: more toxic than mainstream smoke. *Tob. Control, 14*, 396-404.

[14] Hirayama, T (1981). Non-smoking wives of heavy smokers have a higher risk of lung cancer : A study from Japan. *Br. Med. J, 282*, 183-185.

[15] Trichoopoulos, D., Kalandidi, A., sparos, L. and MacMahon, B (1981). Lung cancer and passive smoking. *Int. J Cancer, 27*, 1-4.

[16] Tredaniel, J., Boffetta, P., Saracci, R., Hirsch, A (1993). Environmental tobacco smoke and the risk of cancer in adults. *Eur. J. Cancer, 29A*, 2058-2068.

[17] Hecht, S. S (2004). Carcinogen derived biomarkers: applications in studies of human exposure to secondhand tobacco smoke. *Tob. Control, 13 Suppl 1*: 148-156.

[18] Vineis, P., Airoldi, L., Veglia, P., Olgiati, L., Pastorelli, R., Autrup, H., et al (2005). Environmental tobacco smoke and risk of respiratory cancer and chronic obstructive pulmonary disease in former smokers and never smokers in the EPIC prospective study. *BMJ, 330*, 277-280.

[19] Boffetta, P (2002). Involuntary smoking and lung cancer. *Scand. J. Work Environ. Health, 28 Suppl* 2, 30-40.

[20] Brennan, P., Buffler, P. A., Reynolds, P., Wu, A. H., Wichmann, H. E., Agudo, A., et al (2004). Secondhand smoke exposure in adulthood and risk of lung cancer among never smokers: a pooled analysis of two large studies. *Int. J. Cancer, 109*, 125-31.

[21] Hedley, A. J., McGhee, S. M., Repace, J. L., Wong, L. C., Yu, M. Y. S., Wong, T. W., et al (2006). Risk for heart disease and lung cancer from passive smoking by workers in the catering industry. *Toxicological Sciences, 90*: 539-548.

[22] Lopez, M. J., Nebot, M., Juarez, O., Ariza, C., Salles, J., Serrahima, E (2006). Estimation of the excess of lung cancer mortality risk associated to environmental tobacco smoke exposure of hospitality works. *Med. Clin, 126*, 13-14.

[23] Siegel, M (1993). Involuntary smoking in the restaurant workplace. A review of employee exposure and health effects. *JAMA, 270*, 490-493.

[24] Siegel, M., Skeer, M (2003). Exposure to secondhand smoke and excess lung cancer mortality risk among workers in the "5 B's": bars, bowling alleys, billiard halls, betting establishments, and bingo parlours. *Tob. Control, 12*, 333-338.

[25] Tulunay, O. E., Hecht, S. S., Carmella, S. G., Zhang, Y., Lemmonds, C., Murphy, S., et al (2005). Urinary metabolites of a tobacco-specific lung carcinogen in nonsmoking hospitality workers. *Cancer Epidemiol Biomarkers Prev, 14,* 1283-1286.

[26] Anderson, K. E., Kliris. J., Murphy. L., Carmella, S. G., Han, S., Link, C., et al (2003). Metabolites of a tobacco-specific lung carcinogen in nonsmoking casino patrons. *Cancer Epidemiol Biomarkers Prev, 12*, 1544-1546.

[27] Hammond, E. C., Seidman, H (1980). Smoking and cancer in the United States. *Prev Med, 9*, 169-174.

[28] De Andrade, M., Ebbert, J. O., Wampfler, J. A., Miller, D. L., Marks, R. S., Croghan, G. A., et al (2004). Environmental tobacco smoke exposure in women with lung cancer. *Lung Cancer, 43*, 127-134.

[29] Yang, M., Pyo, M. Y (2005). Molecular epidemiology of lung cancer in female passive smokers. *J. Environ. Sci. Health C Environ. Carcinog. Ecotoxicol .Rev, 23*, 75-97.

[30] Flora, S. D., Balansky, R,. M., D'Agostini, F., Izzotti, A., Bennicelli, C., et al (2003). Molecular alteration and lung tumors in p53 mutant mice exposed to cigarette smoke. *Cancer Res, 63*, 793-800.

[31] Husgafvel-Pursiainen, K., Boffetta, P., Kannio, A., Nyberg, F., Pershagen, G., Mukeria, A, et al (2000). P53 Mutations and exposure to environmental tobacco smoke in a multicenter study on lung cancer. *Cancer Res, 60*, 2906-2911.

[32] Gealy, R., Zhang, L., Siegfried, J. M., Luketich, J. D., Keohavong, P (1999). Comparison of mutations in the p53 and –ras genes in lung carcinomas from smoking and non-smoking women: cancer epidemiology. *Biomarkers, 8*, 297-302.

[33] Husgafvel-Pursiainen, K (2004). Genotoxicity of environmental tobacco smoke: a review. *Mutat. Res, 567*, 427-425.

[34] Wenzlaff, A. S., Cote, M. L., Bock, C. H., Land, S. J., Schwartz, A. G (2005). GSTM1, GSTT1 and GSTP1 polymorphisms, environmental tobacco smoke exposure and risk of lung cancer among never smokers: a population-based study. *Carcinogenesis, 26*, 395-401.

[35] Wenzlaff, A. S., Cote, M. L., Bock, C. H., Land, S. J., Santer, S. K., Schwartz, D.R., et al (2005). CYP1A1 and CYP1B1 polymorphisms and risk of lung cancer among never smokers: a population-based study. *Carcinogenesis, 26*, 2207-2212

[36] Cohet, C., Borel, S., Nyberg, F., Mukeria, A., Bruske-Hohlfeld, I., Constantinescu, V., et al (2004). Exon 5 polymorphisms in the O^6-alkylguanine DNA alkyltransferase gene and lung cancer risk in non-smokers exposed to second-hand smoke. *Cancer Epidemiol. Biomarkers Prev, 13*, 320-323.

[37] Morabia, A (2002). Smoking (active and passive) and breast cancer: epidemiologic evidence up to June 2001. *Environ. Mol. Mutagen, 39*, 89-95.

[38] Terry, P. D., Rohan, T. E (2002). Cigarette smoking and the risk of breast cancer in women: a review of the literature. *Cancer Epidemiol. Biomarkers Prev, 11*, 953-971.

[39] Okasha, M., McCarron, P., Gunnell, D., Smith, G. D (2003). Exposures in child, adolescence and early adulthood and breast cancer risk: a systematic review of the literature. *Breast Cancer Res. Treat, 78*, 223-276.

[40] Kropp, S., Chang-Claude, J (2002). Active and passive smoking and risk of breast cancer by age 50 years among German women. *Am. J. Epidemiol, 156,* 616-626.

[41] Millikan, R. C., Pitman, G. S., Newman, B., Tse, C-K. J., Selmen, O., Rockhill, B., et al (1998). Cigarette smoking, N-acetyltrasferases1 and 2 and breast cancer risk. *Caner Epidemiol. Biomarkers Prev, 7*, 371-378.

[42] Lee, P.N (2002). Environmental tobacco smoke and cancer of sites other than the lung in adult non-smokers. *Food Chem. Toxicol, 40*, 747-766.

[43] Coyle, Y. M (2004). The effect of environment on breast cancer risk. *Breast Cancer Res. Treat, 84*, 273-288.

[44] Hanaoka, T., Yamamoto, S., Sobue, T., Sasaki, S., Tsugane, S (2005). Active and passive smoking and breast cancer risk in middle-aged Japanese women. *Int. J. Cancer, 114*, 317-322.

[45] Johnson, K. C (2005). Accumulating evidence on passive and active smoking and breast cancer risk. *Int. J Cancer, 117*, 619-628.

[46] Reynolds, P., Hurley, S., Goldberg, D. E., Anton-Culver, H., Bernstein, L., Deapen, D (2004). Active smoking, household passive smoking, and breast cancer: evidence from the California Teachers Study. *J. Natl. Cancer Inst, 96*, 29-37.

[47] Bonner, M. R., Nie, J., Han, D., Vena, J. E., Rogerson, P., Muti, P., et al (2005). Secondhand smoke exposure in early life and the risk of breast cancer among never smokers (United States). *Cancer Causes Control, 6*: 683-689.

[48] Woo, C., Davis, D., Gravitt, P., Skinner, H., Ward, C., White, J. E (2000). A prospective study of passive cigarette smoke exposure and breast cancer (Abstract (SER)). *Am. J. Epidemiol, 151 (Suppl.)*, S72.

[49] Wartenberg, D., Calle, E. E., Thun, M. J., Heath, C.W. Jr., Lally, C., Woodruff, T (2000). Passive smoking exposure and female breast cancer mortality. *J. Natl. Cancer Inst, 92*, 1666-1673.

[50] Egan, K.M., Stampfer, M. J., Hunter, D., Hankinson, S., Rosner, B. A., Holmes, M., et al (2002). Active and passive smoking in breast cancer: prospective results from the Nurses' Health Study. *Epidemiology, 13*, 138-145.

[51] Jee, S. H., Ohrr, H., Kim, I. S (1999). Eeffects of husbands' smoking on the incidence of lung cancer in Korean women. *Int. J. Epidemiol, 28*, 824-828.

[52] Hirayama, T (1987). Passive smoking and cancer: an epidemiology review. *GANN Monograph on Cancer Research, 33*, 127-135.

[53] Nishino, Y., Tsubono, Y., Tsuji, I., Komatsu, S., Kanemura, S., Nakatsuka, H., Fukao, A., Satoh, H., Hisamichi, S (2001). Passive smoking at home and cancer risk: a population-based prospective study in Japanese non-smoking women. *Cancer Causes Control, 12*, 797-802.

[54] Sander, D. P., Everson, R. B., Wilcox, A. J (1985). Passive smoking in adulthood and cancer risk. *Am. J. Epidemiol, 121*, 37-48.

[55] Gammon, M., Eng, S. M., Teitelbaum, S. L., Britton, J. A., Kabat, G. C., Hatch, M., et al (2004). Environmental tobacco smoke and breast cancer incidence. *Environ. Res, 96*, 176-185.

[56] Lash, T. L., Aschengrau, A (2002). A null association between active or passive cigarette smoking and breast cancer risk. *Breast Cancer Res. Treat, 75*, 181-184.

[57] Lash, T. L., Aschengrau, A (1999). Active and passive cigarette smoking and the occurrence of breast cancer. *Am-J-Epidemiol, 149*, 5-12.

[58] Delfino, R.J., Smith, C., West, J. G., Lin, H. J., White, E., Liao, S.Y., et al (2000). Breast cancer, passive and active cigarette smoking and N-acetyltransferase 2 genotype. *Pharmacogenetics, 10*, 461-469.

[59] Johnson, K.C., Hu, J., Mao, Y and The Canadian Cancer Registries Epidemiology Research Group (2000). Passive and active smoking and breast cancer risk in Canada, 1994-97. *Cancer Causes Control, 11*, 211-221.

[60] Smith, S. J., Deacon, J. M., Chilvers, C. E. D (1994). Alcohol, smoking, passive smoking and caffeine in relation to breast cancer risk in young women. *Br. J. Cancer,* 70, 112-119.

[61] Morabia, A., Bernstein, M., Heritier, S., Khatchatrian, N (1996). Relation of breast cancer with passive and active exposure to tobacco smoke. *Am. J. Epidemiol, 143*, 918-928.

[62] Lissowska, J., Brinton, L. A., Zatonski. W., Blair, A., Bardin-Mikolajczak, A., Peplonska, B., et al (2006). Tobacco smoking, NAT2 acetylation genotype and breast cancer risk. *Int. J. Cancer* [Epub ahead of print].

[63] Hirose, K., Tajima, K., Hamajima, N., Inoue, M., Takezaki, I., Kuroishi, T., et al (1995). A large-scale, hospital-based case-control study of risk factors of breast cancer according to menopausal status. *Japanese J. Cancer Res, 86*, 146-154.

[64] Liu, L., Wu, K., Lin, X., Yin, W., Zheng, X., Tang, X., et al (2000). Passive smoking and other factors at different period of life and breast cancer risk in Chinese women who have never smoked-A case-control study in Chongqing, Peple's Republic of China. *Asian Pac. J. Cancer Prev, 1,* 131-137.

[65] Shrubsole, M. J., Gao, Y. T., Dai, Q., Shu, X.O., Ruan, Z. X., Jin, F., et al (2004). Passive smoking and breast cancer risk among non-smoking Chinese women. *Int. J.Cancer, 110*, 605-609.

[66] Key, T. J., Verkasalo, P. K., Banks, E (2001). Epidemiology of breast cancer. *Lancet Oncol, 2*, 133-140.

[67] Li, D., Wang, M., Firozi, P. F., chang, P., Zhang, W., Baer-Dubowska, W., et al (2002). Characterization of a major aromatic DNA adduct detected in human breast tissues. *Environ. Mol. Mutagen, 39*, 193-200.

[68] Fizozi, P. F., Bondy, M. L., Sahin, A. A., Chang, P., Lukmanji, F., Singletary, E. S., et al (2002). Aromatic DNA adducts and polymophisms of CYPA1, NAT2, and GSTM1 in breast cancer. *Carcinogenesis, 23*, 301-306.

[69] Chang-Claude, J., Kropp, S., Jager, B., Bartsch, H., Risch, A (2002). Differential effect of NAT2 on the association between active and passive smoke exposure and breast cancer risk. *Cancer Epidemiol. Biomarkers Prev, 11*, 698-704.

[70] Lash, T.L., Bradbury, B. D., Wilk, J. B., Aschengrau, A (2005). A case-only analysis of the interaction between N-acetyltransferase 2 haplotypes and tobacco smoke in breast cancer etiology. *Breast Cancer Res, 7*, 385-393.

[71] Lilla, C., Risch, A., Kropp, S., Chang-Claude, J (2005). SULT1A1 genotype, active and passive smoking, and breast cancer risk by age 50 years in a German case-control study. *Breast Cancer Res, 7*, R229-237.

[72] Ryan, P., Lee, M. W., North, B., McMichael, A. J (1992). Risk factors for tumours of the brain and meninges: results from the Adelaide Adult Brain Tumor Study. *Int. J. Cancer, 51*, 20-27.

[73] Mills, P. K., Preston-Martin, S., Annegers, J. F., Beeson, W. L., Phillips, R. L., Fraser, G. E (1989). Risk factors for tumours of the brain and cranial meninges in Seventh-Day Adventists. *Neuroepidemiology, 8*, 266-275.

[74] Zheng, T., Cantor, K. P., Zhang, Y., Chiu, B. C. H., Lynch, D. F (2001). Risk of brain glioma not associated with cigarette smoking or use of other tobacco products in Iowa. *Cancer Epidemiol. Biomarkers Prev, 10*, 413-414.

[75] Hurley, S. F., McNeil, J. J., Donnan, G. A., Forbes, A., Salzberg, M., Giles, G. G (1996). Tobacco smoking and alcohol consumption as risk factors for glioma: a case-control study in Melbourne, Australia. *Epidemiol. Community Health, 50*, 442-446.

[76] Navarro Silvera, S., A., Miller, A. B., and Rohan, T. E (2006). cigarette smoking and risk of glioma: A prospective study. *Int. J. Cancer, 118,* 1848-1851.

[77] Efird, J. T., Friedman, G. D., Sidney, S., Klatsky, A., Habel, L. A., Udaltsova, N. V., Van den Eeden, S., Nelson, M (2004). The risk for malignant primary adult-onset glioma in a large, multiethnic, managed-care cohort: cigarette smoking and other lifestyle behavious. *J. Neurooncol, 68*, 57-69.

[78] Phillips, L. E., Longstreth, W. T., Koepsell, T., Custer, B. S., Kukull, W. A., van Belle, G (2005). Active and passive cigarette smoking and risk of intracranial meningioma. *Neuroepidemiology, 24*, 117-122.

[79] Hu, J., Little, J., Xu, T., Zhao, X., Guo, L. H., Jia, X. Y., Huang, G., Bi, D. Z., Liu, R. Z (1999). Risk factors for meningioma in adults: a case-control study in northeast China. *Int. J. Cancer, 83*, 299-304.

[80] Hirayama, T (1984). Cancer mortality in non-smoking women with smoking husband based on a large cohort study in Japan. *Preventive Medicine, 13*, 680-690.

[81] Benninger, M. S (1999). The impact of cigarette smoking and environmental tobacco smoke on nasal and sinus disease: a review of the literature. *Am. J. Rhinol, 13*, 435-438.

[82] Fukuda, K., Shibata, A (1990). Exposure-response relationships between woodworking, smoking or passive smoking, and squamous cell neoplasms of the maxillary sinus. *Cancer Causes Control, 1*, 165-168.

[83] Zheng, W., McLaughlin, J. K., Chow, W. H., Chien, H. T. C., Blot, W. J (1993). Risk factors for cancers of the nasal cavity and paranasal sinuses among white men in the United States. *Am J Epidemiol, 138*, 965-972.

[84] Parkin, D. M., Whelan, S. L., Ferlay, J., Teppo, L., and Thomas, D. B. *Cancer Incidence in Five Continents. Vol. VIII*, IARC Scientific Publications, No. 155, Lyon, France, 2002.

[85] Cheng, Y. J., Hildesheim, A., Hsu, M. M., Chen, I. H., Brinton, L. A (1999). Cigarette smoking, alcohol consumption and risk of nasopharyngeal carcinoma in Tawan. *Cancer Causes Control, 10*, 201-207.

[86] Yu, M. C., Garabrant, D. H., Huang, T. B., Henderson, B. E (1990). Occupational and other non-dietary risk factors for nasopharyngeal carcinoma in Guangzhou, China. *Int. J. Cancer, 45*, 1033-1039.

[87] Armstrong, R. W., Imrey, P. B., Lye, M. S., Aemstrong, M. J., Yu, M. C., Sani, S (2000). Nasopharyngeal carcinoma in Malaysian Chinese: occupational exposure to particles, formaldehyde and heat. *Int. J. Epidemiol, 29*, 991-996.

[88] Yuan, J. M., Wang, X. L., Xiang, Y. B., Gao, Y. T., Ross, R. K., Yu, M. C (2000). Non-dietary risk factors for nasopharyngeal carcinoma in Shanghai, China. *Int. J. Cancer, 85*, 364-369.

[89] Zhang, Z. F., Morgenstern, H., Spitz, M. R., Tashkin, D. P., Yu, G. P., Hsu, T. C., et al (2000). Environmental tobacco smoking, mutagen sensitivity, and head and neck squamous cell carcinoma. *Cancer Epidemiol. Biomarkers Prev, 9*, 1043-1049.

[90] Tan, E. H., Adelstein, D. J., Droughton, M. L. T., van Kirk, M. A., Lavertu, P (1997). Squamous cell head and neck cancer in non-smokers. *Am. J. Clinical Oncology, 20*, 146-150.

[91] Tredaniel, J., Boffetta, P., Buiatti, E., Saracci, R., Hirsch, A. (1997). Tobacco smoking and gastric cancer. Review and meta-analysis. *Int. J. Cancer, 72*, 565-573.

[92] Mao, Y., Hu, J., Semenciw, R., White, K and the Canadian-Cancer-Registries-Epidemiology-Research-Group (2002). Active and passive smoking and the risk of stomach cancer, by subsite, in Canada. *Eur. J. Cancer Prev, 11*, 27-38.

[93] Malfertheiner, P., Schutte, K (2006). Smoking--a trigger for chronic inflammation and cancer development in the pancreas. *Am. J. Gastroenterology, 101*, 160-162.

[94] Wittel, U. A., Pandey, K. K., Andrianifahanana , M., Johasson, S, L., Cullen, D, M., Akhter, M. P., Brand, R. E., Prokopczyk, B., Batra, S. K (2006). Chronic pancreatic inflammation induced by environmental tobacco smoke inhalation in rats. *Am. J. Gastroenterology, 101*, 148-159.

[95] Villeneuve, P. J., Johnson , K. C., Mao, Y., Hanley, A. J., Canadian Cancer Registries Research Group (2004). Environmental tobacco smoking and the risk of pancreatic cancer: findings from a Canadian population based case-control study. *Can. J. Public Health, 95*, 32-37.

[96] Sander,R. S., Sander, D. P., Comstock, G. W., Helsing, K. J., Shore, D. J (1988). Cigarette smoking and the risk of colorectal cancer in women. *J. Nat. Cancer Inst, 80*, 1329-1333.

[97] Slattery, M. L., Edwards, S., Curtin, K., Schaffer, D., Neuhausen, S (2003). Associations between smoking, passive smoking, GSTM-1, NAT2, and rectal cancer. *Cancer Epidemiol Biomarkers Prev, 12*, 882-889.

[98] Lilla, C., Verla-Tebit, E., Risch, A., Jager, B., Hoffmeister, M., Brenner, H, et al (2006). Effect of NAT1 and NAT2 genetic polyphisms on colorectal cancer risk associated with exposure to tobacco smoke and meat consumption. *Cancer Epidemiol. Biomarkers Prev, 15*, 99-107.

[99] Kreiger, N., Marrett, L. D., Dodds, L., Hilditch, S., Darlington, G. A (1993). Risk factors for renal cell carcinoma: results of a population-based case-control study. *Cancer Causes Control, 4*, 101- 110.

[100] Hu. J., Ugnat, A. M., and The Canadian Cancer Registries Epidemiology Research Group (2005). Active and passive smoking and risk of renal cell carcinoma in Canada. *Eur. J. Cancer, 41*, 770-778.

[101] Castelao, J. E., Yuan, J. M., Skipper, P. L., Tannenbaum, S. R., Gago-Dominguez, M., Ross, R. K., et al (2001). Gender-and smoking-related bladder cancer risk. *J. Natl. Cancer Inst, 93*, 538-545.

[102] Zeegers M. P., Goldbohm, R. A., van den Brandt, P. A (2002). A prospective study on active and environmental tobacco smoking and bladder cancer risk (The Netherlands). *Cancer Causes Control, 13*, 83-90.

[103] Kabat, G. C., Dieck, G.S., Wender, E. L (1986). Bladder cancer in nonsmokers. *Cancer, 57*, 362-367.

[104] Burch, J. D., Rohan, T. E., Howe G. R., Hill G. B., Steele, R., Miller, A. B (1989). Risk of bladder cancer by source and type of tobacco exposure: a case-control study. *Int. J. Cancer, 44*, 622-628.

[105] Chen, Y. C., Su, H. J., Guo, Y. L., Houseman, E, A., Christian, D. C (2005). Interaction between environmental tobacco smoke and arsenic methylation ability on the risk of bladder cancer. *Cancer Causes Control, 16*, 75-81.

[106] Skipper, P. L., Tannenbaum, S. R., Ross, R. K., Yu, M. C (2003). Nonsmoking-related arylammine exposure and bladder cancer risk. *Cancer Epidemiol Biomarkers Prev, 12*, 503-507.

[107] Trimble, C. L., Genkinger, J. M., Burke, A. E., Hoffman, S. C., Helzlsouer, K. J., Diener-West, M., et al (2005). Active and passive cigarette smoking and the risk of cervical neoplasia. *Obstet Gynecol, 105*, 174-181.

[108] Wu, M. T., Lee, L. H., Ho, C. K., Liu, C. L., Wu, T. N., Wu, S. C., et al (2003). Lifetime exposure to environmental tobacco smoke and cervical intraepithelial neoplasms among nonsmoking Taiwanese women. *Arch. Environ. Health, 58*, 353-359.

[109] Slattery, M. L., Robison, L. M., Schuman, K. L., French, T. K., Abbort, T, M., Overall, J. C, Jr., Gardner, J. W (1989). Cigarette smoking and exposure to passive smoking are risk factors for cervical cancer. *JMJA, 261*, 1593-1598.

[110] Coker, A., L., Rosenberg, A. J., McCann, M. F., Hulka, B. S (1992). Active and passive cigarette smoke exposure and cervical intraepithelial neoplasia. *Cancer Epidemiol. Biomarkers Prev, 1*, 349-356.

[111] Tay, S. K., Tay, K. J (2004). Passive smoking is a risk factor in cervical neoplasia. *Gynecol. Oncol, 93*, 116-120.

[112] Coker, A. L., Bond, S. M., Williams, A.., Gerasimova, T., Pirisi, L (2002). Active and passive smoking, high-risk human papillomaviruses and cervical neoplasia. *Cancer Detect. Prev, 26*, 121-128.

[113] Sobti, R. C., Kaur, S., Kaur, P., Singh, J., Gupta, I., Jain, V., Nakahara, A (2006). Interaction of passive smoking with GST (GSTM1, GSTT1, and GSTP1) genotypes in the risk of cervical cancer in India. *Cancer Genet. Cytogenet, 166*, 117-123.

[114] Baker, J. A., Odunuga, O. O., Rodabaugh, K. J., Reid, M. E., Menezes, R. J., Moysich, K. B (2006). Active and passive smoking and risk of ovarian cancer. *Int. J. Gynecol Cancer,* Suppl *1*, 211-218.

[115] Goodman, M. T., Tung, K. H (2003). Active and passive tobacco smoking and the risk of borderline and invasive ovarian cancer (United States). *Cancer Causes Control, 14*, 569-577.

[116] Kasim, K., Levallois, P., Abdous, B., Auger, P., Johnson, K. C and Canadian Cancer Registries Epidemiology-Research-Group (2005). Environmental tobacco smoke and risk of adult leukemia. *Epidemiology, 16*, 672-680.

[117] Kasim, K., Levallois, P., Abdous, B., Auger, P., Johnson, K. C (2005). Lifestyle factors and the risk of adult leukemia in Canada. *Cancer Causes Control, 16*, 489-500.

[118] Randall, S (2006). Children and secondhand smoke: not just a community issue. *Paediatr. Nurs, 18*, 29-31.

[119] Turka, p., Wielosz, M., Zatonski, W (2002). Exposure to environmental tobacco smoke and children health. *Int. J. Occup. Med. Environ. Health, 15*, 325-335.

[120] Kukla, L., Hruba, D., Tyrlik, M (2004). Influence of prenatal and postnatal exposure to passive smoking on infants' health during the first six months of their life. *Cent. Eur. J. Public Health, 12*, 157-160.

[121] Andres, R. L., Day, M. C (2000). Perinatal complications associated with maternal tobacco use. *Semin. Neonatol, 5,* 231-241.

[122] Perera, F. P., Tang, D., Tu, Y. H., Cruz, L. A., Borjas, M., Bernert, T., Whyatt, R. M (2004). Biomarkers in maternal and newborn blood indicate heightened fetal susceptibility to procacinogenic DNA damage. *Environ. Health Perspect, 112*, 1133-1136.

[123] Pichini, S., Basagana, X. B., Pacifici, R., Garcia, O., Puig, C., Vall, O., et al (2000). Cord serum cotinine as a biomarker of fetal exposure to cigarette amoke at the end of pregnancy. *Environ. Health Perspect, 108*, 1079-1083.

[124] Neri, M., Ugolini, D., Bonassi, S., Fucic, A., Holland, N., Knudsen, L. E., Sram, R. J., Ceppi, M., Bocchini, V., Merlo, D. F (2006). Children's exposure to environmental pollutants and biomarkers of genetic damage. II. Results of a comprehensive literature search and meta-analysis. *Mutat. Res, 612*, 14-39.

[125] Manuel, J. S (2000). Sins of the father. Parental smoking and childhood cancer. *Environ Health Perspect, 108*, A30

[126] Preston-Martin, S. Epidemiological studies of perinatal carcinogenesis. In Napalkov, N. P., Rice, J. M., Tomatic, L., Yamasaki, H. Perinatal and Multigenerational carcinogesis. *IARC Sci. Publ,* PP 289-314, Lyon, France, 1989.

[127] Tredaniel, J., Boffetta, P., Little, J., Saracci, R., Hirsch, A (1994). Exposure to passive smoking during pregnancy and childhood, and cancer risk: the epidemiological evidence. Paediatr. *Perinat. Epidemiol, 8*, 233-255.

[128] Sasco, A. J., Vainio, H (1999). From in utero and childhood exposure to parental smoking to childhood cancer: a possible link and the need for action. *Hum Exp. Toxicol, 18,*192-201.

[129] Filippini, G., Farinotti, M., Lovicu, G., Maisonneuve, P., Boyle, P (1994). Mothers' active and passive smoking during pregnancy and risk of brain tumours in children. *Int. J. Cancer, 57*, 769-774.

[130] Filippini, G., Farinotti, M., Ferrarini, M (2000). Active and passive smoking during pregnancy and risk of central nervous system tumours in children. *Paediatr. Perinat. Epidemiol, 14,* 78-84.

[131] Schuz, J., Kaletsch, U., Kaatsch , P., Meinert, R., Michaelis, J (2001). Risk factors for pediatric tumors of the central nervous system: results from a German population-based case-control study. *Med. Pediatr Oncol, 36,* 274-282.

[132] Magnani, C., Pastore, G., Luzzatto, L., Terracini, B (1990). Parental occupational and other environmental factors in the etiology of leukemias and non-Hodgkin's lymphomas in Childhood: a case control study. *Tumori, 76*, 413-419.

[133] Books, D. R., Mucci, L. A., Hatch, E. E., Cnattingius, S (2004). Maternal smoking during pregnancy and risk of brain tumours in the offspring. A prospective study of 1.4 million Swedish births. *Cancer Causes Control, 15*, 997-1005.

[134] Grant, S. G (2005). Quantitatively and qualitatively similar effects of active and passive maternal tobacco smoke exposure on the utero mutagenesis at HPRT locus. *BMC Pediatr, 29*, 5-20.

[135] Ng, P., Silverstone, A. E., Lai, Z.W., Zelikoff, J.T (2006). Effects of prenatal exposure to cigarette smoke on offspring tumour susceptibility and associated immune mechanisms. *Toxicol. Sci., 89*, 135-144.

[136] Sorahan, T., Prior, P., Lancashire, R. J., Faux, S. P., Hulten, M. A., Peck, I. M., Stewart, A. M (1997). Childhood cancer and parental use of tobacco: deaths from 1971 to 1976. *Br. J. Cancer, 76*, 1525-1531.

[137] Sorahan, T., McKinney, P. A., Mann, J. R., Lancashire, R. J., Stiller, C. A., Birch, J. M., et al (2001). Childhood cancer and parental use of tobacco: findings from the inter-regional epidemiological study of childhood cancer (IRESCC). *Br. J. Cancer, 84*, 141-146.

[138] Ji BT, Shu XO, Linet MS, Zheng W, Wacholder S, Gao YT, Ying DM, Jin F (1997). Paternal cigarette smoking and the risk of childhood cancer among offspring of non-smoking mothers. *J. Natl. Cancer Inst, 89*, 238-244.

[139] Pang, D., McNally, R., Birch, J. M (2003). Parental smoking and childhood cancer: results from the United Kingdom Childhood Cancer Study. *Br. J. Cancer, 88*, 373-381.

[140] Kuijten, R. R., Bunin, G. R., Nass, C. C., Meadows, A. T (1990). Gestational and familial risk factors for childhood astrocytoma: results of a case-control atudy. *Cancer Res, 50*, 2608-2612.

[141] Norman, M. A., Holly, E. A., Ahn, D. K., Preston-Martin, S., Mueller, B. A., Bracci, P.M (1996). Prenatal exposure to tobacco smoke and childhood brain tumors: results from the United States West Coast childhood brain tumour study. *Cancer Epidemiol. Biomarkers Prev, 5,* 127-133.

[142] John, E. M., Savitz, D. A., Sandler, D. P (1991). Prenatal exposure to parents' smoking and childhood cancer. *Am. J. Epidemiol, 133*,123-132.

[143] Gold, E. B., Leviton, A., Lopez, R., Gilles, F.H., Hedley-Whyte, E. T., Kolonel, L.N., et al (1993). Parental smoking and risk of childhood brain tumours. *Am. J. Epidemiol, 137*, 620-628.

[144] Filippini, G., Maisonneuve, P., McCredie, M., Peris-Bonet, R., Modan, B., Preston-Martin, S., et al (2002). Relation of childhood brain tumors to exposure of parents and children to tobacco smoke: the SEARCH international case-control study. Surveillance of Environmental Aspects Related to Cancer in Humans. *Int. J. Cancer, 100*, 206-213.

[145] Bunin, G. R., Buckley, J. D., Boesel, C. P., Rorke, L. B., Meadows, A. T (1994). Risk factors for astrocytic glioma and primitive neuroectodermal tumour of the brain in young children: a report from the children's Cancer Group. *Cancer Epidemiol. Biomarkers prev, 3*, 197-204.

[146] Hu, J., Mao, Y., Ugnat, A-M (2000). Parental cigarette smoking and hard liquor consumption and the risk of childhood brain tumours: a case-control study in northeast China. *Acta Oncol, 39*, 979-984.

[147] Howe, G. R., Burch, J. D., Chiarelli, A. M., Risch, H. A., Choi, B. C. K (1989). An exploratory case-control study of brain tumors in children. *Cancer Res, 49*, 4349-4352.

[148] Cordier, S., Iglesias, M. J., Le Goaster, C., Guyot, M. M., Mandereau, L., hemon, D (1994). Incidence and risk factors for childhood brain tumours in the Ile de France. *Int. J. Cancer, 59*, 776-782.

[149] Boffetta, P., Tredaniel, J., Greco, A (2000). Risk of childhood cancer and adult lung cancer after childhood exposure to passive smoke: A meta-analysis. *Environ. Health Perspect, 108*, 73-82.

[150] Huncharek, M., Kupelnick, B., Klassen, H (2001). Maternal smoking during pregnancy and the risk of childhood brain tumors: results of a meta-analysis. *In Vivo,* 15, 535-541.

[151] Parkin, D. M., Kramarova, E., Draper, G. J., Masuyer, J., Michaelis, J., Neglia, J., et al. *International Incidence of Childhood Cancer. IARC* scientific publications, No. 144. Lyon, France, 1998.

[152] Levi, F., La Vecchia, C., Lucchini, F., Negri, E., Boyle, P (1992). Patterns of childhood cancer incidence and mortality in Europe. *Eur. J. Cancer, 28A*, 2028-2049.

[153] Pershagen. G., Ericson, A., Otterblad-Olausson. P (1992). Maternal smoking in pregnancy: does it increase the risk of childhood cancer? *Int. J. Epidemiol, 21*, 1-5.
[154] Schuz, J., Kaatsch, P., Kaletsch, U., Meinert, R., Michaelis, J (1999). Association of childhood cancer with factors related to pregnancy and birth. *Int. J. Epidemiol, 28*, 631-639.
[155] Mucci, L. A., Granath, F., Cnattingius, S (2004). Maternal smoking and childhood leukemia and lymphoma risk among 1,440,542 Swedish children. *Cancer Epidemiol. Biomarkers Prev, 13*, 1528-1533.
[156] Brondum, J., Shu, X. O., Steinbuch, M., Severson, R. K., Potter, J. D., Robison, L. L (1999). Parental cigarette smoking and the risk of acute leukemia in children. *Cancer, 85*, 1380-1388.
[157] Menegaux F, Steffen C, Bellec S, Baruchel A, Lescoeur B, Leverger G, et al (2005). Maternal coffee and clcohol consumption during pregnancy, parental smoking and risk of childhood acute leukemia. *Cancer Detect. Prev, 29*, 487-493.
[158] Shu, X. O., Ross, J. A., Pendergrass, T. W., Reaman, G. H., Lampkin, B.,Robison, L. L (1996). Parental alcohol consumption, cigarette smoking, and risk of infant leukemia: a Children's Cancer Group Study. *J. Natl. Cancer Inst, 88*, 24-33.
[159] Infante-Rivard, C., Krajinovic, M., Labuda, D., Sinnett, D (2000). Parental smoking, CYP1A1 genetic polymorphisms and childhood leukemia (Quebec, Canada). *Cancer Causes Control, 11*, 547-553.
[160] Clavel, J., Bellec, S., Rebouissou, S., Menegaux, F., Feunteun, J., Bonaiti-Pellie, C., et al (2005). Childhood leukaemia, polymorphisms of metabolism enzyme genes, and interactions with maternal tobacco, coffee and alcohol consumption during pregnancy. *Eur. J. Cancer Prev, 14*, 531-540.
[161] Adami, J., Glimelius, B., Cnattingius, S., Ekbom, A., Zahm, S. H., Linet, M, et al (1996). Maternal and perinatal factors associated with non-Hodgkin's lymphoma among children. *Int. J. Cancer, 65*, 774-777.
[162] Sorahan, T., Lancashire, R. J (2004). Parental cigarette smoking and chidhood risk of hepatoblastoma: OSCC data. *Br. J. Cancer, 90*, 1016-1018.
[163] Chen, Z., Robison, L., Gliller, R., Krailo, M., Davies, S., Gardner, K., et al (2005). Risk of childhood germ cell tumors in association with parental smoking and drinking. *Cancer, 103*, 1064-1071.
[164] Lee, C. H., Ko, Y. C., Goggins, W., Huang, J. J., Huang, M. S., Kao, E. L., Wang, H. Z (2000). Lifetime environmental exposure to tobacco smoke and primary lung cancer of non-smoking Taiwanese women. *Int. J. Epidemiol, 29*, 224-231.
[165] Wang, F. L., Love, E. J., Liu, N., Dai, X. D (1994). Childhood and adolescent passive smoking and the risk of female lung cancer. *Int. J. Epidemiol, 23*, 223-230.
[166] Stepanov I, Hecht SS, Duca G, Mardari I (2006). Uptake of the tobacco-specific lung carcinogen 4-(methylnitrosamino)-1-(3-pyridyl)-1-butanone by Moldovan children. *Cancer Epidemiol. Biomarkers Prev, 15*, 7-11.
[167] Sander, D. P., Everson, R. B., Wilcox, A. J (1985). Cancer risk in adulthood from early life exposure to parents' smoking. *Am. J. Public Health, 75*, 487-492.
[168] Etzel, R. A (1997). Active and passive smoking: hazards for children. *Cent. Eur. J. Health, 5*, 54-56.

[169] California Environmental Protection Agency, Air Resources Board. Proposed identification of environmental tobacco smoke as a toxic air contaminant. Part B: Health effects. Chapter 7: Carcinogenic effects. Sacramento, California EPA, 2003. Available at: *www.arb.ca.gov/toxics/ets/dreport/dreport.htm.*

[170] Department of Health and Human Services (2006). The Health Consequences of Involuntary Exposure to Tobacco Smoke, A Report of the Surgeon General. http://www.cdc.gov/tobacco. Executive summary 1-27.

[171] Byers, T., Barrera E, Fontham ET, Newman LA, Runowicz CD, Sener SF, et al (2006). A midpoint assessment of the American Cancer Society challenge goal to halve the U.S. cancer mortality rates between the years 1990 and 2015. *Cancer.* [Epub ahead of print]

[172] Alligne, C. W., Stoddard, J. j (1997). Tobacco and Children: An economic evaluation of the medical effects of parental smoking. *Arch. Pediatr. Adolescent Med, 151*, 648-653.

[173] Tredaniel, J., Savinelli, F., Vignot, S., Bousquet, G., Lemaignan, C., Misset, J. L (2006). The sequences of passive smoking in adults. *Rev. Mal. Respir,* Suppl *2*, 67-73.

[174] The GTSS Collaborative Group (2006). A cross-country comparison of exposure to secondhand smoke among youth. *Tob. Control, 15,* 4-19.

[175] Thompson, G., Wilson. N., Howden-Chapman, P (2006). Population level policy options for increasing the prevalence of smokefree homes. *J. Epidemiol. Community Health, 60*, 298-304.

[176] Borland, R., Yong, H. H., Cummings, K. M., Hyland, A., Anderson, S., Fong, G. T (2006). Determinants and consequences of smoke-free homes: findings from the International Tobacco Control (ITC) Four Country Survey. *Tob. Control, 15*, 42-50.

[177] Nishi, N., Ocuri, S., Onoda, T., Nohara, M., Inoue, H., Okayama, A (2005). Knowledge of smoking-related risk and opinions on tobacco control by smoking status and education level in Japan. *Nippon Koshu Eisei Zasshi, 52*, 962-970.

In: Cancer Research Perspectives
Editor: Larissa S. Pereira, pp. 167-189
ISBN 978-1-60021-980-1

Chapter V

Gene Expression in Lymphomas and Immunodeficiencies Provides New Insights into B-Lymphocyte Development

***Jessica M. Lindvall*[1,3], *K. Emelie M. Blomberg*[1], *Birger Christensson*[2], *Birgitta Sander*[2,*1] *and C. I. Edvard Smith*[1,*]**

[1] Clinical Research Center, [2] Department of Laboratory Medicine, Division of Pathology, Karolinska Institutet, Karolinska University Hospital Huddinge, SE 141 86 Stockholm, Sweden

[3] Current address: Department of Informatics, University of Oslo, PO Box 1080 Blindern, NO-0316 Oslo, Norway

Abstract

Advances in molecular genetics have provided a wealth of information relevant to the understanding of the mechanisms underlying both primary immunodeficiency diseases and lymphomas. This information provides the research community with insights into the different lymphocyte developmental stages. In this chapter we discuss expression profiling in lymphomas and primary immunodeficiencies affecting the B-cell lineage. In particular mantle cell lymphomas, chronic lymphocytic leukemias/small lymphocytic lymphomas and X-linked agammaglobulinemia (Btk deficiency) are discussed.

There is considerable hope that the microarray technology will lead to a better understanding of different disease processes. The results of a multitude of gene expression studies in malignant lymphomas clearly suggest that the vast majority of B-cell lymphomas emanate from antigen experienced cells or memory B-cells and not from

[1]*Corresponding authors, e-mail address: *edvard.smith@ki.se* Telephone: +46-8-58583651. Fax: +46-8-58583650 and *birgitta.sander@ki.se* Telephone: +46-8-58587843. Fax: +46-8-58581005.

naïve B-cells. These findings, together with preferential use of certain V heavy chain gene conformations, points to a role for antigen at some stages in lymphoma development. This seems to be of particular relevance as to the discussion of cell-of-origin for low-grade lymphomas such as B-cell chronic lymphocytic leukemia, mantle cell lymphoma and marginal zone lymphoma.

The gene expression studies conducted in primary immunodeficiencies have foremost been helpful to better understand the basic biology of the disease. Microarray analysis has also been used as an exploratory tool to study gene expression in immunodeficiency diseases of unknown cause. For X-linked agammaglobulinemia, the technique has provided better understanding of the genes influenced by Btk.

Keywords: B-lymphocyte, B-cell development, gene expression profiling, Primary immunodeficiency (PID), X-linked agammaglobulinemia (XLA), Bruton tyrosine kinase (Btk), Mantle cell lymphoma (MCL), B-cell chronic lymphocytic leukemia (B-CLL), Cyclin D1 mRNA splice variants.

INTRODUCTION

Improved definition of the B-lymphocyte developmental pathway is profoundly aided by the analysis of lymphomas and antibody deficiencies. The human genome consists of 20,000-25,000 protein-coding genes [1] and post-translational modifications allow for even greater diversity. In addition there are non-protein-coding genes, many of which influence developmental process. Also, in a given cell not all genes are expressed simultaneously. As an example, using transcriptional profiling, the total number of different transcripts in a B-lymphocyte is in the range of 5,000 [2]. Many of these genes are house-keeping genes, but even among this population of genes there can be characteristic, developmental differences [3]. Important steps in B-cell development that are vulnerable and susceptible to dysregulations causing immunodeficiencies and malignant lymphoma have been identified using gene expression profiling. In tumors the accumulation of transformed cells highlights populations of cells for which the normal counter parts are rare and therefore difficult to study. Although useful, malignant cells are also characterized by both gain- and loss-of-function genetic alterations, which may result in a phenotype distinguishing the lymphoma cells from their non-malignant counterparts. A diverse array of genetic events from the stem cell and onward has now been elucidated in B lineage malignancies. Gene expression profiling of lymphomas has provided evidence for the existence of tumor types not previously recognized and the genetic signatures indicate molecular pathways of importance for pathogenesis of both small B-cell lymphomas and aggressive lymphomas [4, 5].

Conversely, in PIDs different inherited mutations are manifested as characteristic blocks at distinct developmental stages resulting in specific phenotypes. As for the primary immunodeficiency area, the application of gene expression profiling has allowed a better understanding of these disorders at a molecular level [2, 6-9]. There is also an example where the affected gene was first identified through microarray analysis, namely the CD3δ-chain deficiency [10]. Thus, expression profiling may be used to hunt for the primary cause of a PID.

In the following sections we will summarize recent findings in studies of lymphomas and PIDs with emphasis of the low-grade B-cell lymphomas, B-cell chronic lymphocytic leukemia (B-CLL)/small lymphocytic lymphoma (SLL), mantle cell lymphoma (MCL) and marginal zone lymphoma (MZL) and of the antibody deficiency disease, X-linked agammaglobulinemia (XLA).

We will also discuss how recent insights into B-lymphocyte development may increase the understanding of lymphoma development and antibody deficiencies. Results obtained using gene expression profiling are brought to light and summarized below. In figure 1 we have outlined B-lymphocyte development with special emphasis on the stages where these diseases are manifested.

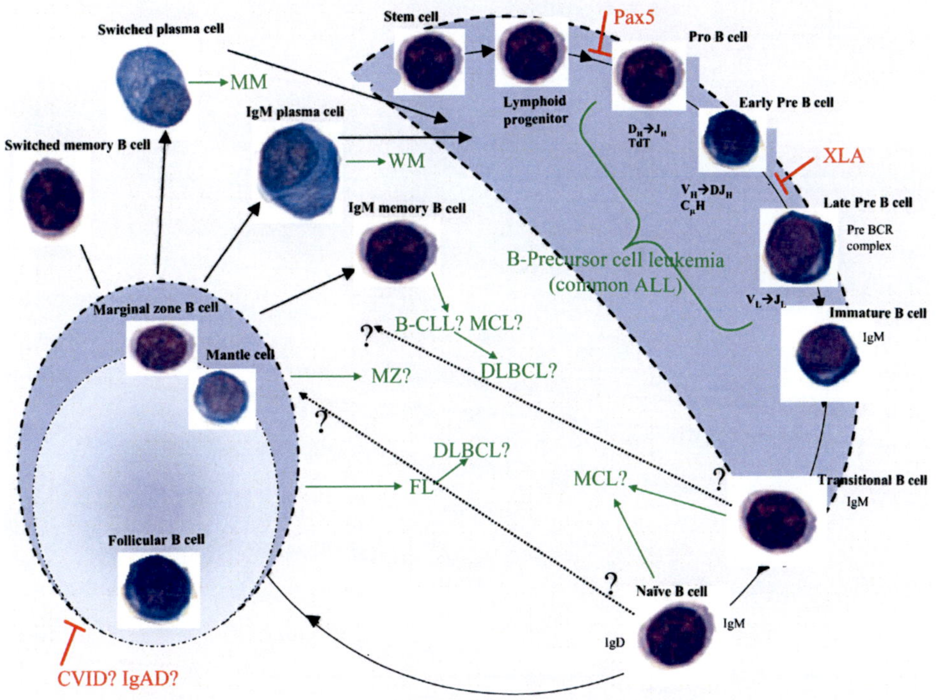

Figure 1. B-cell development and differentiation with related immunodeficiencies and B-cell lymphomas. B-cells develop from lymphoid progenitors to transitional B-cells in the bone marrow. A key regulator of B-cell development is Pax5, which when absent will cause a block after the early pro B-cell stage (shown in red). B-cells leave the bone marrow as transitional B-cells and travel into the peripheral lymphoid organs. Naïve B-cells can be recruited either to the B-cell follicle or differentiate through extra follicular pathways. Both switched plasma cells, derived from the follicular pathway, and IgM plasma cells will return to the bone marrow. The different immunodeficiencies are presented in red and the B-cell lymphomas are shown in green. MCL; mantle cell lymphoma, FL; follicular lymphoma, MZL; marginal zone lymphoma, MM; multiple myeloma, WM; Waldenstroms macroglobulinemia, DLBCL; diffuse large B cell lymphoma, B-CLL; B-cell chronic lymphocytic leukemia, ALL; acute lymphocytic leukemia.

B-Lymphocyte Development and Differentiation

Haematopoietic stem cells are thought to progress through an irreversible cascade of differentiation steps as they commit to a particular cell lineage. This is a very complex process that depends on a number of B-cell intrinsic factors that need to be expressed as well as extrinsic components found in the local environment at the time of commitment. B- and T-lymphocytes provide long-term immunological memory and highly specific effector functions in the immune defence to foreign antigens. For that purpose they carry antigen-specific receptors, the ligation of which regulates diverse responses such as proliferation, differentiation and cell death depending on their developmental stage and the microenvironmental context. For B-cells, there are two major phases of development; an initial phase that is antigen independent, in which a diverse repertoire of antigen specific B-cells develops in the bone marrow. The second phase occurs when B-cells are stimulated by antigen to undergo clonal expansion in the peripheral lymphoid system. During B-lymphocyte development in the bone marrow, each B-cell randomly rearranges its Ig gene segments to form one complete, productive heavy-chain gene and one complete, productive light-chain gene. This is to ensure that all B-cell antigen receptors (BCRs) on a single B-cell have the same antigen-binding site, whereas the total population of generated B-lymphocytes has a diverse repertoire of antigen-specific antibodies.

During the second phase of B-lymphocyte development, taking place in the peripheral lymphoid organs, the immature B-cell that recognizes self-antigen initiates strong BCR signaling resulting in receptor editing or apoptosis. The next step is for the transitional B-cells (T1 and T2) to differentiate into mature circulating B-cells. These transitional B-cells must then pass through multiple checkpoints before entering the mature B-cell pool. Thus, before becoming mature B-lymphocytes, the transitional B-cells are either selected to the follicle or the mantle zone. The follicular B lineage cells recirculate continuously. At the same time they are being enriched for specificities common to T-dependent antigens. Mantle zone B-cells, on the other hand, are static and are enriched for specificities common to T-independent antigens. The mature B-lymphocytes circulate throughout the body and encounter foreign antigens.

In addition to activating B-cell immune effector functions, signaling through the BCR also regulates B-cell development, proliferation, survival and elimination of auto-reactive B-cells. Signal transduction through the BCR is an absolute requirement for the selection and development of B-lymphocytes at multiple checkpoints. How can the BCR on one hand provide survival and differentiation and on the other hand induce cell death? The outcome depends on the maturation state of the B-cell, the level and duration of the BCR signal and also on signals from other receptors such as CD19 and CD40.

The initiation of BCR signaling follows upon antigen cross-linking causing the cytoplasmic domains of Igα and Igβ to become phosphorylated on their respective immunoreceptor tyrosine-based motifs (ITAMs). When phosphorylated, these motifs recruit and activate Src family tyrosine kinases. This alone is sufficient to commence the BCR signaling. One of the prevailing models is that BCRs exist as monomers on the surface of B-lymphocytes and that antigen binding to the receptor causes the BCRs to cluster allowing the Src family kinases to phosphorylate tyrosine residues on nearby BCRs and by this create binding sites for other kinases [11]. Once the BCR is activated, a cascade of proteins becomes phosphorylated, activating downstream components of the BCR signaling pathway. In contrast to this "clustering" view, an alternative model is that many receptors exist as pre-formed multimeric complexes. Binding of the ligand forces the complex to reorganise and by these means allow initiation of signaling downstream. This model has also been suggested for e.g. the tumor necrosis factor receptors and the erythropoietin receptor [12, 13]. Yet another model suggests that BCRs, before antigen binding, also exist as oligomeric complexes [14]. Here, within the same oligomer, BCR associated Src kinases continually phosphorylate ITAMs on other BCRs. This allows the recruitment of other cytoplasmic kinases to the complex and further activation of downstream signaling. The major signaling pathways activated by BCR are controlled by PI3K, PLC-γ2 and the Ras, Rac GTPases (reviewed in [15]). A key feature of all of these signaling pathways is the recruitment of cytosolic signaling proteins to the plasma membrane. These interactions among molecules in the plasma membrane, promote the assembly of different complexes resulting in the activation of downstream targets (reviewed in e.g. [16]).

The Microarray Technology for Detection of Gene Expression at the mRNA Level

In contrast to the traditional molecular technologies, where only a limited number of genes are analyzed in one assay, the microarray method allows a global view of gene expression. The overall gene expression profile provides a snapshot of the average expression of genes in the cell populations contained in the analysis. The microarray technology has been widely used in studies of lymphomas and solid tumors, drug response studies as well as basic research in immunology [4, 7, 17-19].

Currently, one of the most used gene expression profiling methods is the Affymetrix™ technique where arrays of probes are synthesized directly on glass chips using photolithography. However, nowadays there is an "array of arrays" on the market, all widely used by the scientific community. For instance, one of the most commonly used arrays is the cDNA array, which uses full-length cDNA clones spotted either on filters or on specially coated glass slides. This approach requires simultaneous analysis of two biological samples, a test and a control, each labelled with a different fluorescent dye, Cy3 (green) and Cy5 (red). Of particular interest is the Lymphochip, a gene chip specially designed for the analysis of lymphoid cells. Many studies using the Lymphochip focused on finding the molecular mechanisms causing human lymphoid malignancies.

Current densities of commercially available Affymetrix™ arrays allow measurements of up to 40,000 probe-sets or transcripts on one single array for a particular species. These arrays contain both known genes and so-called expressed sequence tags (ESTs). Almost all the publicly available EST sequences can be monitored in either human or mouse samples relatively easily by *in silico* analysis.

Oncogenic Events in B-CLL and MCL

Small B-cell lymphomas comprise approximately one-third of non-Hodgkin lymphomas of B-cell type. This group includes such entities as B-cell chronic lymphocytic leukemia/small lymphocytic lymphoma (B-CLL/SLL), mantle cell lymphoma (MCL), marginal zone lymphoma (MZL) and follicular lymphoma (FL). It is important to distinguish these lymphoma entities since their clinical characteristics with respect to therapy and survival are different. Based mainly on morphology and growth pattern, these specific lymphoma entities have been named after their proposed normal B-cell counterparts, indicating possible cells-of-origins. Thus, FL in many instances has a follicular growth pattern that imitates reactive B-cell follicles.

However, in other types of small cell lymphomas such as B-CLL/SLL and MCL the normal B-cell counterpart has not yet been well defined. It is well established that B-cells in the germinal centre of the B-cell follicle are induced to proliferate in response to stimulatory signals from antigen and co-stimulatory T-cell help. During this follicular response, affinity maturation and Ig heavy chain class switching also occurs. Following introductions of mutations in the antigen combining regions of the B-cell receptor genes, B-cells ending up with increased antigen binding capacity are positively selected. The presence or absence of somatic mutations in immunoglobulin genes has thus been considered indicative of whether a B-cell has passed through germinal centre differentiation or not. The mutational status of the immunoglobulin genes in malignant lymphoma has therefore been used, together with the expression of activation markers, to indicate whether a particular lymphoma entity has emanated from "pre-germinal", possibly naïve B-cells or from "post-germinal" B-lymphocytes. Since MCL in the majority of cases has non-mutated IgVH genes it was hypothesized that this lymphoma stems from naïve B-cells. In B-CLL/SLL on the other hand approximately 60% of the tumors have evidence for somatic mutation in the immunoglobulin genes and could therefore possibly stem from post-germinal B-cells. Recent work, however, has suggested that in some instances somatic mutation might also occur outside germinal centers, such as in the splenic red pulp [20, 21]. Therefore, it might be informative to use other tools, such as gene expression profiling to compare the various normal B-cell populations with the lymphoma entities in order to clarify possible cells of origin. The rationale for this approach is that normal B-cell populations exhibit specific gene expression signatures that in part are preserved in the malignant lymphomas. In addition, oncogenic events such as chromosomal translocations, chromosomal- or gene- amplifications and deletions affect proliferation, cell survival and differentiation and can possibly also be identified by specific gene expression profiles.

MCL is characterized by a chromosomal translocation where the cyclin D1 gene on chromosome 11 becomes translocated to the immunoglobulin heavy chain locus on chromosome 14, the t(11;14)(q13;q32). This translocation results in increased expression of cyclin D1 protein and disturbed cell cycle regulation. Detailed studies of the translocation breakpoints can provide information concerning at what time-point in B-cell differentiation the breaks occur. Such studies have suggested that the t(11;14)(q13;q32) occurs mainly during the Ig gene rearrangement process in B-precursor cells in the bone marrow, during which one D- and one J segment of the Ig locus are joined [22, 23]. The translocation breakpoint in MCL would therefore suggest that the t(11:14) translocation is an early event in MCL pathogenesis which takes place at the pre-B-cell stage and is followed by other oncogenic and selective events (see below) later on during tumorigenesis.

In B-CLL there is not a specific gene translocation. Instead, in this lymphoma there are certain patterns of genomic aberrations such as chromosome gains and deletions that provide prognostic information, such as deletion of chromosome 11q14 or 17p13 and trisomy 12 that are associated with short survival time [24-26]. Gene expression profiling of these subgroups in B-CLL have shown different gene expression profiles that only in part can be explained by a gene dosage effect provided by genes located in the aberrant chromosomal regions [27]. Apart from translocations and numeric changes there are additional genetic changes that in part are common between B-CLL and MCL. Both in MCL and CLL mutations of the ataxia telangiectasia gene (ATM) is frequently seen as well as TP53 aberrations. However, the molecular mechanisms causing B-CLL and MCL are largely unknown as is the progenitor cell(s) for the two diseases.

It has long been assumed that B-CLL and MCL are derived from human B-cell subsets constituting counterparts of the mouse B-1 subset. Moreover, since both MCL and B-CLL express the CD5 molecule it has been suggested that they arise from a B-cell population similar to the B-1a cells in the mouse. In mice at least four subpopulations of mature B-cells have been defined namely, recirculating follicular B-cells (B-2 cells), marginal zone B-cells (MZ), enriched in the marginal zones surrounding the lymphoid follicles and B-1 lymphoid cells that are divided in B-1a cells expressing CD5 and B-1 cells that are CD5 negative (reviewed in [28, 29]). The mouse B-1 cells produce polyreactive antibodies preferentially recognising self-antigens and human B-cells suggestively corresponding to B-1 cells are found in increased levels in some autoimmune diseases such as rheumatoid arthritis. The repertoire of the B1-cells is restricted and there is limited, or no, somatic hypermutation of their immunoglobulin genes. Often microbial antigens are recognized, which suggests that these cells provide the natural antibodies. Since B-CLL and MCL express CD5 and since a substantial fraction of these lymphomas have non-mutated immunoglobulin variable heavy chain genes (IgVH) it has been hypothesised that the normal counterpart for these lymphomas is a human B-lymphocyte similar to mouse B-1a cells.

Experiments, using transgenic mice expressing self-antigens, points to a role for surface immunoglobulin signaling, either during the precursor stage or later during differentiation or expansion, for generating B-1 cells [30, 31]. Importantly, the development of B-1a cells is dependent on the specificity of the antigen receptor. Thus, it seems that if a precursor B-cell expresses immunoglobulin receptors which bind self-antigens or T-independent antigens, this precursor B-cell could mature into a B-1a cell (reviewed in [28, 29]). This B-1a cell does not pass germinal centres or exhibit a high degree of somatic hypermutation in the variable region of the heavy chain of the immunoglobulin gene (VH gene).

Like B-1a cells, approximately 40% of B-CLL and the majority of MCL have do not show hypermutation in the variable region (non-mutated VH genes) and could thus be considered "antigen-naïve". However, there are several lines of evidence that point to a role of antigen also in CLL and MCL with non-mutated VH genes. During VDJ recombination one out of approximately 52 functional VH family genes is stochastically used to join the previously formed DJ complex. In both mutated and non-mutated B-CLL and MCL certain

VH genes are reported to be "over-represented" as compared to normal peripheral blood B-cells. However, there is very limited knowledge as to actual frequencies of VH gene usage in normal individuals at different ages. One can thus not with any higher degree of certainty state that some VH genes are "over-represented". Still, there is undoubtedly a marked accumulation of certain VH genes such as VH1-69 that has been associated with non-mutated B-CLL [32-34]. Similarly, VH3-21 was detected among mutated B-CLL cases [35]. Intriguingly, detailed analysis of the B-cell receptor genes reveals that in a substantial number of cases with a particular VH gene usage also the hypervariable regions are highly similar between cases [36-38]. Moreover, also a restricted immunoglobulin light chain usage has been found. Taken together, these findings strongly point towards a role for antigen in the development of CLL and MCL.

In humans the IgM+, IgD+, CD27+ B-cells in blood are responsible for T-cell independent immune reactions, such as rapid responses to encapsulated bacteria [39]. In contrast CD27- B-cells that have non-mutated immunoglobulin genes have been considered antigen naive. Recently, it was suggested that the blood IgM+, IgD+, CD27+ cells correspond to circulating splenic marginal zone B-cells that are rapidly activated during T independent immune responses [39]. Intriguingly, this population, that was detected in small children and has mutated immunoglobulin genes already at one year of age, was selected and underwent further hypermutation during immunization with vaccines against encapsulated bacteria [39]. Gene expression analysis showed that this cell-population, in comparison with B-cells lacking IgD and/or CD27, expressed CD1d and CD1c that are involved in presenting lipid antigens.

It thus appears that memory B-cells of IgM type carrying limited somatic mutations in immunoglobulin genes may be generated by a, possibly T-cell independent extra follicular pathway.

Gene Expression Profiling in B-Cll, MCL and MZL

Gene expression profiling has recently been used to compare the transcriptomes in mouse B-1a cells and conventional B-2 cells. Among genes differentially expressed in B-1a cells compared to splenic B-2 cells were CD72, and CD1 [40]. By gene expression profiling, CD72 has been found to be highly expressed in human mantle zones [41] but down regulated in MCL compared to normal B-cells [42]. CD1a was reported as under expressed in MCL [42] while CD1d was highly expressed [19]. It thus seems that there are some features in common between human B-CLL and MCL on the one hand and murine B-1a cells on the other.

Gene Expression of B-CLL Shows Higher Similarities to Memory B-Cells than to Naïve B-Cells or CD5+ B-Cells from Cord Blood

Approximately 60% of B-CLL has mutations in the IgVH gene and the mutational state has been found to provide new prognostic information [34, 43]. B-CLL patients without evidence of somatic mutation in the highly variable regions of the immunoglobulin heavy chain genes (>98% homology to germ line) have a more malignant course than those with mutated IgVH.

Based on recent microarray studies of gene expression, zeta associated protein-70 (ZAP-70) expression has been found to be a marker for IgVH mutational status in B-CLL [44, 45]. The tyrosine kinase ZAP-70 is part of the CD3 receptor-signaling complex in T-lymphocytes. Recent studies have shown an increased B-cell receptor signaling both in ZAP-70+, IgVH non-mutated B-CLL and also in the rare IgVH mutated cases that express ZAP-70 [46].

Among other genes that have been reported to be differentially expressed in IgVH mutated and non-mutated cases are FGFR1, gravin, dystrofin, PAK1 and BCL-7 [44] as well as PAX5 and TCF1, which are a downstream targets in the Wnt pathway [47]. PAX5 is a key regulator of B-cell differentiation (Figure 1). Thus, mice with a mutationally inactivated Pax5 gene lack B-lymphocytes [48]. In early lymphoid development, Notch and Pax5 have opposing effects, Notch expression being a signature of T-cell lineage differentiation, while Pax5 is essential for B lineage commitment and maintenance [49, 50].

It was hypothesised that B-CLL with non-mutated IgVH genes would represent malignant transformation of naïve B-cells, while Ig-gene mutated cases would stem from memory B-cells. However, results from gene expression profiling using the Affymetrix U95A chip or the Lymphochip appears not to support this hypothesis, since a large overlap in the transcriptomes between IgVH-mutated and non-mutated cases was shown [44, 51]. Importantly, both IgVH-mutated and non-mutated B-CLL have gene expression profiles that are more similar to CD27+ memory B-cells than to CD27-, naïve B-cells [51] or CD5+ B-cells isolated from cord blood [44, 51].

Gene Expression in B-Cell Compartments of Normal Lymphoid Organs Compared to MCL

Different strategies have been used to analyse gene expression in B-cell lymphomas. In most publications concerning B-CLL, tumor cells have been isolated from peripheral blood and there are only few reports of gene expression in the solid tumor counterpart, the small lymphocytic lymphoma (SLL). By the use of pure tumor cell populations subtle changes in gene expression that otherwise could have been masked by infiltrating normal cells can be detected. However, in the majority of published investigations, for other lymphoma subtypes whole tumor tissue has been used. This enables analysis also of the stromal compartment and the infiltrating normal cells. The gene expression in the tumor tissue has been compared to reactive lymphoid tissue or to purified subpopulations of B-lymphocytes. The latter approach facilitates the comparison with putative cells-of-origin. However, since the stromal compartment is not represented, important information might be lost.

An alternative approach would be to microdissect areas representing naïve, activated and memory B-cells from normal lymphoid organs in such a way that both the B-cells residing in these areas as well as the stromal compartment could be analyzed. Such an approach has recently been reported by Shen *et al.* [41]. Gene expression in different compartments of human peripheral lymphoid organs has been investigated; the germinal center, the mantle zone and the marginal zone. The mantle zone contains B-cells with non-mutated immunoglobulin genes, high expression of surface IgD and negativity for CD27. In this area generally very few T-cells reside. Most marginal zone B-cells in adults are high in expression of surface IgM, low in IgD and are CD27+ memory-like cells.

Shen *et al.* found that the cells in the normal marginal zone expressed specific cytokines and cytokine receptors that were not highly expressed in the other compartments [41]. There was for instance a high expression of lymphotoxin, IL-11 and receptors for IL-17 and IL-7. Furthermore, the cannabinoid receptor type 2 (CNR2) that is involved in immune regulation was highly expressed in the marginal zone but not in the other B-cell compartments investigated. In germinal centres there was a high expression of genes involved in proliferation, DNA repair and replication. Also in this compartment there was a differential expression of certain genes such as RGS13 that regulate migration and chemokine response.

While the cells in the marginal zone expressed low levels of proliferation-associated genes the mantle zone cells had highly variable expression of these genes – not as high as seen in germinal centers, but substantially higher than in marginal zones [41]. Interestingly, cyclin G2 was highly expressed in the mantle zone. This gene has been associated to suppression of proliferation [52].

How do the gene expression profiles of the microdissected normal B-cell compartments compare to what is known for mantle cell lymphoma? Mantle cell lymphoma gene expression profiling [5, 19, 53, 54] as well as other studies [55] have revealed high expression of genes involved in proliferation and cell division. In the normal mantle zone, very few proliferating cells are detected by immunohistochemical staining, while gene expression profiling has suggested that there is a slightly elevated expression of genes involved in replication and cell division when compared to the marginal zone [41]. The high expression of cyclin G2 in the mantle zone was suggested to counter-act the proliferative signals [41, 52] and it could therefore be hypothesized that dysregulated cyclin G2 could be part of the pathogenesis in mantle cell lymphoma as has been suggested for thyroid carcinoma [56]. Cyclin G2 has indeed been reported as an under-expressed gene in mantle cell lymphoma compared to sorted B-cell subpopulations [42], suggesting that dysregulation of cyclin G2 could be a new oncogenic event in MCL.

Enhanced Proliferation and Differences in Genes Involved in G-Protein Coupled Signaling in MCL

Most MCL exhibit non-mutated IgVH genes and the proportion of cases with mutated IgVH genes is lower than in B-CLL, varying between 15-30% in different recent series [57-60]. MCL has therefore been considered to arise from naïve B-cells. In gene expression profiling of a small series of MCL a heterogenous pattern of clustering was found; with 4 out of 7 MCL clustering together with sorted populations of resting naïve or memory B-cells [42].

As in B-CLL, MCL is characterized by a biased use of IgVH genes that seems to correlate with prognosis [57-59]. There is an over-representation of the VH3-21 gene also in MCL. However, in contrast to B-CLL, in MCL these cases show no evidence of somatic mutations in the IgVH genes. Moreover, MCL cases using VH3-21 are associated with a better prognosis. As of today there is limited information on differences in gene expression associated with mutational status of the Ig receptor in MCL. However, in a recent report a few genes such as EGR2, SMARCA5 and replication protein A1 were found to be differently expressed in mutated cases [61].

In MCL there is generally higher expression of genes involved in proliferation compared to B-CLL/SLL [5, 19, 51, 55]. In addition to cyclin D1, some mantle cell lymphomas express high levels of genes such as topoisomerase IIA, CDK4, PCNA, BUB1. These genes are highly expressed in germinal centres in normal lymph nodes, but in the context of MCL they characterize the highly proliferative tumors with adverse prognosis [5, 62]. We have shown that many of these highly proliferative MCL cases express a more stable, truncated cyclin D1 transcript, lacking the 3′UTR region of the mRNA [5, 19] [62]. Further studies of this MCL variant has revealed that the short, stable cyclin D1 mRNA isoform is associated with 3.4 times higher levels of cyclin D1 mRNA coding region and higher cyclin D1 protein levels [62]. These MCL tumors have high expression of a number of cell cycle regulating genes such as cyclin A1 and cyclin B1 leading to further disturbances of cell cycle regulation, increased cell proliferation and a more aggressive disease.

We have recently shown that genes encoding proteins involved in G-protein mediated signaling are differentially regulated in MCL compared to reactive lymphoid tissue [19]. Regulator of G protein signaling 13 (RGS13) and other RGS proteins have an important role in regulating chemokine-induced cell migration and germinal center reactions [63-65]. Especially RGS13 is localized to germinal centers [63] and was absent in mantle cell lymphoma while highly expressed in reactive tonsils and lymph nodes [19]. By gene expression profiling we and others found that the G-protein coupled receptor, cannabinoid receptor type I (CB1), which is highly expressed in brain and is involved in regulation of food-intake, is significantly expressed in MCL [19, 42]. Recent data suggest that the CB1 gene also is expressed in B-CLL with 11q22-q23 deletions [27]. Also the cannabinoid receptor 2 is highly expressed in MCL [19]. In normal lymphoid tissue this gene seems to be preferentially expressed in the mantle/marginal zones [41, 66, 67] and has immunoregulatory functions. We have investigated the functional importance of high cannabinoid receptor expression in MCL and found that targeting of cannabinoid receptors impair proliferation and induce cell death [68] in MCL. The cannabinoid system could thus be considered as a new therapeutic target, originally defined by array screening of the mRNA pool.

Marginal Zone Lymphoma is a Heterogenous Tumor that Can Be Distinguished from other Small Cell Lymphomas by Gene Expression Profiling

The lymphoma entity, marginal zone lymphoma (MZL), seem to contain several different subtypes with different genomic alterations, some of which are preferentially seen in MZL located at distinct anatomical sites [69-74]. While most MZL exhibit somatic mutations of IgVH genes, non-mutated cases are associated with a worse prognosis [75].

The MZL entity displays a highly variable immunohistochemical profile [76] that in some instances overlaps with other lymphoma entities. It is therefore very interesting that by gene expression profiling a small set of genes could be used to differentiate MZL from CLL or MCL in a study containing 37 marginal zone lymphomas [77]. In addition to a large MZL cluster corresponding to genes characteristic for "spleen" there was another MZL cluster specifically associated with the marginal zone signature [77] irrespectively of which organ was affected by the lymphoma. This cluster contained genes involved in intracellular signaling or transcription such as AKT1 and the transcription factor TPCP2. Also genes for many S100 proteins were highly expressed.

Apart from this study by Thieblemont *et al.* [77] not much is known concerning global gene expression profiles in MZL. In this study, as few as 44 genes grouped in 4 clusters could differentiate between SLL, MCL and MZL with a high degree of certainty. Although these findings have to be confirmed in other studies, the results are very promising indeed and clearly indicates that microarray analysis might have an important role not only in research but also in diagnostic practice.

Primary Immunodeficiency Disorders

B-lymphocytes at different developmental stages express distinct sets of important signaling components. Diseases associated with constitutively active, non-functional states of these genes highlight their importance. This is true not only for lymphomas but also for PIDs. In the decade that has passed since the molecular basis of XLA was identified, mutated genes in more than 100 PIDs have been described in the literature.

The PIDs are characterized by defects of specific functions of the immune system, most often manifested by increased susceptibility to infections. The disorders, although rare, provide a wide spectrum of defects, including antibody deficiencies, cellular immune deficiencies, combined immune deficiencies, phagocytic defects and complement defects [78-83], where antibody deficiencies represent the most common types of PIDs in humans [84].

These disorders involve components of both the adaptive and innate immune system, including T- and B-lymphocytes, NK cells, phagocytic cells and various complement proteins. In general, the T-cell deficiencies are clinically more severe than those associated with antibody deficiency disorders. In the absence of treatment, those affected by defective cellular immunity, rarely survive beyond infancy or childhood. As with the T-cell immune deficiencies, the spectrum of antibody deficiency disorders is broad, ranging from the most severe type, with next to absent B-cells and immunoglobulins, to patients having selective Ig isotype defects, to those with almost normal immunoglobulins in the serum.

In B-cell deficiencies, the symptoms often do not appear until 9-12 months of age, since the patient has acquired protective levels of Ig from the mother. In addition to a high susceptibility to infections certain antibody deficiency disorders are associated with other features in their clinical presentation, e.g. autoimmunity and malignancies. Many of the genes involved in antibody deficiencies have now been identified and this has led to a better understanding and elucidation of the B-lymphocyte development and the differentiation pathways. However, it is important to consider the various stages of B-lymphocyte differentiation and development in order to understand the abnormal mechanisms underlying the different antibody immunodeficiencies. PIDs affect several subsets of cells. In Figure 1 the effects on B-cell development and differentiation is shown. This figure also summarizes the developmental stages where different immunodeficiencies and lymphomas are suggested to occur.

XLA (X-Linked Agammaglobulinemia)

X-linked agammaglobulinemia (XLA) was reported in 1952 by Dr. Ogden C. Bruton [80]. In 1993, two independent laboratories cloned the gene responsible for XLA [85, 86]. The gene was named Bruton tyrosine kinase (*BTK*) after Dr. Bruton's discovery of the disease. XLA patients present a vast number of distinct mutations in the *BTK* gene [78, 87, 88] all of which affects their B-cell development and differentiation [89, 90]. For several years the existence of a genotype-phenotype correlation remained elusive. However, it was recently demonstrated that there in fact exists such a correlation, since missense mutations are highly restricted in XLA with only certain residues being sensitive [91]. This phenomenon is particularly evident for CpG sites, which are frequently mutated and where certain codons cause XLA upon non-sense mutations, while amino acid substitutions seem to be tolerated. It is likely that certain forms of splice site mutations result in a milder form of the disease. However, such patients have not been described to date.

Approximately 1 in every 380,000 males is affected with XLA [92]. The onset of infections occurs during the later part of the first year of life, when maternal antibodies are reduced below protective levels [83, 93]. There is an almost total absence, or a marked deficiency, of serum Igs in patients affected with XLA. The percentage of circulating B-cells is reduced or extremely low. However, pro-B-cells numbers in the bone marrow are normal or even increased in number [89, 90]. The defect is B-cell intrinsic not affecting T-lymphocytes and other lymphoid subpopulations, which appear in normal numbers. Lymphoid tissues show absence of plasma cells, lymphoid follicles and germinal centers. The treatment for XLA remains the same as the one Dr. Bruton himself introduced in the 1950s, a combination of gammaglobulin substitution and antibiotics and most patients have few severe infections with this regular treatment.

SIgAD (Selective IgA Deficiency)

SIgAD is the most common form of PID in the Western world and affects approximately 1 in every 600 individuals [84]. Patients affected with SIgAD have markedly reduced or absent serum IgA levels but normal IgM and IgG concentrations. Many individuals with SIgAD are clinically asymptomatic but those patients with symptoms display respiratory tract infections and involvement of the gastrointestinal tract with giardiasis and nodular lymphoid hyperplasia [94]. The genes encoding the α heavy chain genes are intact [95], whereas abnormalities lies in isotype switching have been found [96]. A number of abnormalities in the cytokine network have been observed in SIgAD but no mutation in cytokine genes have been found to date [97]. For this reason a relevant animal model has not been created for SIgAD and therefore primary peripheral blood B-cells or Epstein-Barr Virus (EBV) transformed B-cells from patients are commonly used as the research tool in molecular biology.

CVID (Common Variable Immunodeficiency)

Common variable immunodeficiency (CVID), also called acquired hypogammaglobulinemia, adult-onset hypogammaglobulinemia or dysgammaglobulinemia, is a heterogenous group of disorders involving both B- and T-cell immune function. Patients present with recurrent bacterial infections, decreased serum Ig levels and deficient antibody production. The wide spectrum of CVID phenotypes is also reflected in the age of onset of the disease, which ranges from early childhood to young adults with an average age of onset of around 25 years. Variability is also found in the degree and type of hypogammaglobulinemia and the patients may also suffer from chronic inflammatory and autoimmune conditions [98]. Several mechanisms have been proposed to explain the immune abnormalities in patients with CVID such as B-cell defects, excessive T-suppressor cell activity [99], deficient T-cell helper function [100], cytokine deficiency [101, 102] and suboptimal T- and B-cell interactions through the CD40 ligand [103]. The clinical variability of CVID is likely to be a reflection of a complex multigene involvement of the disease. The concept that more than one gene is responsible for the disease is supported by the involvement of one or more genes within the MHC region on chromosome 6 in the pathogenesis for both SIgAD and CVID [104-106]. Recently, mutations in the ICOS as well as the TACI genes were found to cause a rare form of CVID [107, 108].

ICF (Immunodeficiency, Centromeric Region Instability and Facial Anomalies)

ICF is an autosomal recessive disease caused by mutations in the DNA methyltransferase 3B gene (*DNMT3B*). The disease is a rare chromosome instability syndrome and is the only disease shown to be associated with mutations in a DNA methyltransferase gene [109]. In this syndrome the immunodeficiency is characterized by agammaglobulinemia in the presence of B-cells. DNA rearrangements are targeted to the centromere-adjacent heterochromatic region of chromosomes 1, 16, and sometimes 9 in mitogen-stimulated lymphocytes. Immune-related problems in ICF patients are generally, but not always, severe. Many patients exhibit low *in vitro* stimulation indices for B- or T-cells upon exposure to mitogens or antigens. ICF is usually diagnosed in the early years [110, 111], and these patients often die in infancy or childhood [110, 112-114]. The cause of death in these patients is usually infection.

Gene Expression Profiling in PIDs

With regards to immunodeficiency diseases, analysis with the microarray technology has been conducted in two ways. First, it has been used to study gene expression in patients with known defects in order to better understand the basic biology and pathophysiology of the disease [7, 8, 115]. Second, microarray analysis can be used as an exploratory tool to study differential gene expression in immunodeficiency diseases of unknown cause, such as CVID or SIgAD [9].

Depending on the type of immunodeficiency disease, patients may have low numbers of circulating lymphocytes. An example is XLA, where the patients essentially lack antibody producing B-lymphocytes. This makes it hard, next to impossible, to do research on primary B-cells from XLA patients. A way to circumvent this is to immortalize B-cells from these individuals by EBV transformation. In CVID and SIgAD, where circulating B-cells usually are found, peripheral blood mononuclear cells have been used for gene expression profiling.

Both cDNA spotted filter arrays as well as Affymetrix™ high-density oligonucleotide arrays have been used in order to study the influence of Btk in cellular signaling [7]. EBV transformed B-cells from healthy individuals were used in comparison to XLA patients. The profile revealed a number of genes differentially expressed between healthy controls and patients. These genes included those expressed in haematopoietic cells including genes from groups corresponding to receptors, kinases, transcription factors and cofactors. Several interesting genes such as *FYN*, *HCK* and *CYP1B1* were more highly expressed in the XLA patient compared to the normal control. One EST and eight complementary DNA clones with unknown function were down-regulated in the XLA patient cell line. In addition to these results, the B-cell specific OCT binding factor-1 was found to be up-regulated in the cell lines from the XLA patient in comparison to the healthy control. The study clearly demonstrated that the influence of Btk mutations can be detected by the use of microarrays, and that this type of analysis can infer potential roles for genes with both unknown and known function. Furthermore, primary splenic B-cells from *Xid* and Btk KO mice were analyzed and compared to normal splenic B-cells from healthy mice of the same genetic background [2]. The authors found approximately 40 genes differing between the Btk defective B-cells compared to healthy controls. Amongst these 40 genes, microsomal epoxide hydrolase (mEH), CD9 and ionized calcium-binding adaptor molecule 1 (Iba1) were found to be affected by the Btk defect.

Other immunodeficiency disorders that have been studied using gene expression profiling are the related immunodeficiency diseases, CVID and SIgAD, as well as the rare ICF syndrome. [109, 116, 117]. In a recent study Qin *et. al.* show [9] that the gene expression pattern from both the CVID and the SIgAD patients gave similar results with some skew-ness towards the Th1 pathway. The results found in both patient groups were in agreement with the observed clinical phenotype. Gene expression microarrays have also been used to analyse EBV transformed B-cell lines from ICF patients [8]. The aim was to identify dysregulation of gene expression that might explain the symptoms of ICF. Genes, such as *RGS1*, *GU-CY1B3* and *F13A1*, which are known to play an important role in the immune function, were identified. The result also suggests that mutations in the gene *DNMT3B* cause lymphogenesis-associated gene dysregulation by indirect effects on gene expression that interfere with normal lymphocyte signaling, maturation and migration.

Conclusion

During development cells differentiate from precursors, starting with the fertilized egg. Numerous markers, such as cell surface proteins, characterize different developmental stages. These processes have best been studied in model organisms with *C. elegans* being the prototype for multicellular species. The adult worm consists of 959 somatic cells compared to approximately 10^{14} in humans. It is considered that *C. elegans* is formed by 10 to 12 different cell types and the corresponding number in humans has been estimated to roughly 250. However, a key issue is what distinguishes one cell type from another.

Analysis of gene transcription of B cell lymphomas and PID has widened our understanding of normal B cell differentiation in addition to identifying new disease entities. Array based expression analysis will certainly continue to provide crucial information in both clinical and experimental medicine. Identifying specific transcriptional profiles in malignant lymphomas can also be used to better define from which normal B-cell subset the malignant cells have originated and thus provide new insights in the pathogenesis of the disease. Using transcriptome and proteome analysis in combination with more assays of gene function will allow more precise definition of developmental stages with important biological characteristics.

Acknowledgements

This work was supported by the Swedish Science Council, the Wallenberg Foundation, the Swedish Cancer Foundation, the Magnus Bergvall´s foundation, European union grant

EURO-POLICY-PID, the Stockholm County Council, the Gunnar Nilsson's Cancer foundation and the Cancer Society of Stockholm.

REFERENCES

[1] Consortium, I.H.G.S., Finishing the euchromatic sequence of the human genome. *Nature, 2004.* 431(7011): p. 931-45.

[2] Lindvall, J.M., et al., Gene expression profile of B cells from Xid mice and Btk knockout mice. *Eur J Immunol, 2004.* 34(7): p. 1981-91.

[3] Oltz, E.M., et al., A novel regulatory myosin light chain gene distinguishes pre-B cell subsets and is IL-7 inducible. *Embo J, 1992.* 11(7): p. 2759-67.

[4] Alizadeh, A.A., et al., Distinct types of diffuse large B-cell lymphoma identified by gene expression profiling. *Nature, 2000.* 403(6769): p. 503-11.

[5] Rosenwald, A., et al., The proliferation gene expression signature is a quantitative integrator of oncogenic events that predicts survival in mantle cell lymphoma. *Cancer Cell, 2003.* 3(2): p. 185-97.

[6] Fruman, D.A., et al., Phosphoinositide 3-kinase and Bruton's tyrosine kinase regulate overlapping sets of genes in B lymphocytes. *Proc Natl Acad Sci U S A, 2002.* 99(1): p. 359-64.

[7] Islam, T.C., et al., Expression profiling in transformed human B cells: influence of Btk mutations and comparison to B cell lymphomas using filter and oligonucleotide arrays. *Eur J Immunol, 2002.* 32(4): p. 982-93.

[8] Ehrlich, M., et al., DNA methyltransferase 3B mutations linked to the ICF syndrome cause dysregulation of lymphogenesis genes. *Hum Mol Genet, 2001.* 10(25): p. 2917-31.

[9] Qin, H., et al., Tracking gene expression in primary immunodeficiencies. *Curr Opin Allergy Clin Immunol, 2003.* 3(6): p. 437-42.

[10] Dadi, H.K., A.J. Simon, and C.M. Roifman, Effect of CD3delta deficiency on maturation of alpha/beta and gamma/delta T-cell lineages in severe combined immunodeficiency. *N Engl J Med, 2003.* 349(19): p. 1821-8.

[11] Reth, M. and J. Wienands, Initiation and processing of signals from the B cell antigen receptor. *Annu Rev Immunol, 1997.* 15: p. 453-79.

[12] Chan, F.K., et al., A domain in TNF receptors that mediates ligand-independent receptor assembly and signaling. *Science, 2000.* 288(5475): p. 2351-4.

[13] Livnah, O., et al., Crystallographic evidence for preformed dimers of erythropoietin receptor before ligand activation. *Science, 1999.* 283(5404): p. 987-90.

[14] Schamel, W.W. and M. Reth, Monomeric and oligomeric complexes of the B cell antigen receptor. *Immunity, 2000.* 13(1): p. 5-14.

[15] Gold, M.R., To make antibodies or not: signaling by the B-cell antigen receptor. *Trends Pharmacol Sci, 2002.* 23(7): p. 316-24.

[16] Dal Porto, J.M., et al., B cell antigen receptor signaling 101. *Mol Immunol, 2004.* 41(6-7): p. 599-613.

[17] Clarke, P.A., R.T. Poele, and P. Workman, Gene expression microarray technologies in the development of new therapeutic agents. *Eur J Cancer, 2004*. 40(17): p. 2560-91.

[18] Villeneuve, D.J. and A.M. Parissenti, The use of DNA microarrays to investigate the pharmacogenomics of drug response in living systems. *Curr Top Med Chem, 2004*. 4(13): p. 1329-45.

[19] Islam, T.C., et al., High level of cannabinoid receptor 1, absence of regulator of G protein signalling 13 and differential expression of Cyclin D1 in mantle cell lymphoma. *Leukemia, 2003*. 17(9): p. 1880-90.

[20] William, J., et al., Evolution of autoantibody responses via somatic hypermutation outside of germinal centers. *Science, 2002*. 297(5589): p. 2066-70.

[21] Weller, S., et al., CD40-CD40L independent Ig gene hypermutation suggests a second B cell diversification pathway in humans. *Proc Natl Acad Sci U S A, 2001*. 98(3): p. 1166-70.

[22] Welzel, N., et al., Templated nucleotide addition and immunoglobulin JH-gene utilization in t(11;14) junctions: implications for the mechanism of translocation and the origin of mantle cell lymphoma. *Cancer Res, 2001*. 61(4): p. 1629-36.

[23] Stamatopoulos, K., et al., Molecular analysis of bcl-1/IgH junctional sequences in mantle cell lymphoma: potential mechanism of the t(11;14) chromosomal translocation. *Br J Haematol, 1999*. 105(1): p. 190-7.

[24] Stilgenbauer, S., et al., Genetics of chronic lymphocytic leukemia: genomic aberrations and V(H) gene mutation status in pathogenesis and clinical course. *Leukemia, 2002*. 16(6): p. 993-1007.

[25] Fegan, C., et al., Karyotypic evolution in CLL: identification of a new sub-group of patients with deletions of 11q and advanced or progressive disease. *Leukemia, 1995*. 9(12): p. 2003-8.

[26] Juliusson, G., et al., Prognostic information from cytogenetic analysis in chronic B-lymphocytic leukemia and leukemic immunocytoma. *Blood, 1985*. 65(1): p. 134-41.

[27] Haslinger, C., et al., Microarray gene expression profiling of B-cell chronic lymphocytic leukemia subgroups defined by genomic aberrations and VH mutation status. *J Clin Oncol, 2004*. 22(19): p. 3937-49.

[28] Berland, R. and H.H. Wortis, Origins and functions of B-1 cells with notes on the role of CD5. *Annu Rev Immunol, 2002*. 20: p. 253-300.

[29] Martin, F. and J.F. Kearney, B1 cells: similarities and differences with other B cell subsets. *Curr Opin Immunol, 2001*. 13(2): p. 195-201.

[30] Hardy, R.R., C.J. Wei, and K. Hayakawa, Selection during development of VH11+ B cells: a model for natural autoantibody-producing CD5+ B cells. *Immunol Rev, 2004*. 197: p. 60-74.

[31] Hayakawa, K., et al., Positive selection of anti-thy-1 autoreactive B-1 cells and natural serum autoantibody production independent from bone marrow B cell development. *J Exp Med, 2003*. 197(1): p. 87-99.

[32] Kipps, T.J., et al., Developmentally restricted immunoglobulin heavy chain variable region gene expressed at high frequency in chronic lymphocytic leukemia. *Proc Natl Acad Sci U S A, 1989*. 86(15): p. 5913-7.

[33] Fais, F., et al., Chronic lymphocytic leukemia B cells express restricted sets of mutated and unmutated antigen receptors. *J Clin Invest, 1998*. 102(8): p. 1515-25.

[34] Hamblin, T.J., et al., Unmutated Ig V(H) genes are associated with a more aggressive form of chronic lymphocytic leukemia. *Blood, 1999*. 94(6): p. 1848-54.

[35] Tobin, G., et al., Somatically mutated Ig V(H)3-21 genes characterize a new subset of chronic lymphocytic leukemia. *Blood, 2002*. 99(6): p. 2262-4.

[36] Tobin, G., et al., Subsets with restricted immunoglobulin gene rearrangement features indicate a role for antigen selection in the development of chronic lymphocytic leukemia. *Blood, 2004*.

[37] Ghia, P., et al., Geographical patterns and pathogenetic implications of IGHV gene usage in chronic lymphocytic leukemia: the lesson of the IGHV3-21 gene. *Blood, 2004*.

[38] Messmer, B.T., et al., Multiple distinct sets of stereotyped antigen receptors indicate a role for antigen in promoting chronic lymphocytic leukemia. *J Exp Med, 2004*. 200(4): p. 519-25.

[39] Weller, S., et al., Human blood IgM "memory" B cells are circulating splenic marginal zone B cells harboring a pre-diversified immunoglobulin repertoire. *Blood, 2004*.

[40] Kretschmer, K., et al., Antibody repertoire and gene expression profile: implications for different developmental and functional traits of splenic and peritoneal B-1 lymphocytes. *J Immunol, 2003*. 171(3): p. 1192-201.

[41] Shen, Y., et al., Distinct gene expression profiles in different B-cell compartments in human peripheral lymphoid organs. *BMC Immunol, 2004*. 5(1): p. 20.

[42] Ek, S., et al., Mantle cell lymphomas express a distinct genetic signature affecting lymphocyte trafficking and growth regulation as compared with subpopulations of normal human B cells. *Cancer Res, 2002*. 62(15): p. 4398-405.

[43] Damle, R.N., et al., Ig V gene mutation status and CD38 expression as novel prognostic indicators in chronic lymphocytic leukemia. *Blood, 1999*. 94(6): p. 1840-7.

[44] Rosenwald, A., et al., Relation of gene expression phenotype to immunoglobulin mutation genotype in B cell chronic lymphocytic leukemia. *J Exp Med, 2001*. 194(11): p. 1639-47.

[45] Wiestner, A., et al., ZAP-70 expression identifies a chronic lymphocytic leukemia subtype with unmutated immunoglobulin genes, inferior clinical outcome, and distinct gene expression profile. *Blood, 2003*. 101(12): p. 4944-51.

[46] Chen, L., et al., Expression of ZAP-70 is associated with increased B-cell receptor signaling in chronic lymphocytic leukemia. *Blood, 2002*. 100(13): p. 4609-14.

[47] Ferrer, A., et al., Different gene expression in immunoglobulin-mutated and immunoglobulin-unmutated forms of chronic lymphocytic leukemia. *Cancer Genet Cytogenet, 2004*. 153(1): p. 69-72.

[48] Busslinger, M., Transcriptional control of early B cell development. *Annu Rev Immunol, 2004*. 22: p. 55-79.

[49] Hoflinger, S., et al., Analysis of Notch1 function by in vitro T cell differentiation of Pax5 mutant lymphoid progenitors. *J Immunol, 2004*. 173(6): p. 3935-44.

[50] Tagoh, H., et al., Epigenetic silencing of the c-fms locus during B-lymphopoiesis occurs in discrete steps and is reversible. *Embo J, 2004*. 23(21): p. 4275-85.
[51] Klein, U., et al., Gene Expression Profiling of B Cell Chronic Lymphocytic Leukemia Reveals a Homogeneous Phenotype Related to Memory B Cells. *J. Exp. Med., 2001*. 194(11): p. 1625-1638.
[52] Horne, M.C., et al., Cyclin G2 is up-regulated during growth inhibition and B cell antigen receptor-mediated cell cycle arrest. *J Biol Chem, 1997*. 272(19): p. 12650-61.
[53] Ek, S., et al., Increased expression of Ki-67 in mantle cell lymphoma is associated with de-regulation of several cell cycle regulatory components, as identified by global gene expression analysis. *Haematologica, 2004*. 89(6): p. 686-95.
[54] Schmechel, S.C., et al., Identification of genes whose expression patterns differ in benign lymphoid tissue and follicular, mantle cell, and small lymphocytic lymphoma. *Leukemia, 2004*. 18(4): p. 841-55.
[55] Korz, C., et al., Evidence for distinct pathomechanisms in B-cell chronic lymphocytic leukemia and mantle cell lymphoma by quantitative expression analysis of cell cycle and apoptosis-associated genes. *Blood, 2002*. 99(12): p. 4554-61.
[56] Ito, Y., et al., Decreased expression of cyclin G2 is significantly linked to the malignant transformation of papillary carcinoma of the thyroid. *Anticancer Res, 2003*. 23(3B): p. 2335-8.
[57] Walsh, S.H., et al., Mutated VH genes and preferential VH3-21 use define new subsets of mantle cell lymphoma. *Blood, 2003*. 101(10): p. 4047-54.
[58] Kienle, D., et al., VH mutation status and VDJ rearrangement structure in mantle cell lymphoma: correlation with genomic aberrations, clinical characteristics, and outcome. *Blood, 2003*. 102(8): p. 3003-9.
[59] Camacho, F.I., et al., Molecular heterogeneity in MCL defined by the use of specific VH genes and the frequency of somatic mutations. *Blood, 2003*. 101(10): p. 4042-6.
[60] Orchard, J., et al., A subset of t(11;14) lymphoma with mantle cell features displays mutated IgVH genes and includes patients with good prognosis, nonnodal disease. *Blood, 2003*. 101(12): p. 4975-81.
[61] Martinez, N., et al., The molecular signature of mantle cell lymphoma reveals multiple signals favoring cell survival. *Cancer Res, 2003*. 63(23): p. 8226-32.
[62] Sander, B., et al., Mantle cell lymphomas with low levels of cyclin D1 long mRNA transcripts are highly proliferative and can be discriminated by elevated cyclin A2 and cyclin B1. *Int. J. Cancer, 2005*. 117(3): p. 418-30.
[63] Shi, G.X., et al., RGS13 regulates germinal center B lymphocytes responsiveness to CXC chemokine ligand (CXCL)12 and CXCL13. *J Immunol, 2002*. 169(5): p. 2507-15.
[64] Shi, G.X., et al., Toll-like receptor signaling alters the expression of regulator of G protein signaling proteins in dendritic cells: implications for G protein-coupled receptor signaling. *J Immunol, 2004*. 172(9): p. 5175-84.
[65] Moratz, C., K. Harrison, and J.H. Kehrl, Regulation of Chemokine-Induced Lymphocyte Migration by RGS Proteins. *Methods Enzymol, 2004*. 389: p. 15-32.

[66] Rayman, N., et al., Distinct expression profiles of the peripheral cannabinoid receptor in lymphoid tissues depending on receptor activation status. *J Immunol, 2004*. 172(4): p. 2111-7.

[67] Galiegue, S., et al., Expression of central and peripheral cannabinoid receptors in human immune tissues and leukocyte subpopulations. *Eur J Biochem, 1995*. 232(1): p. 54-61.

[68] Flygare J, G.K., Kimby E, Christensson B, Sander B., Cannabinoid receptor ligands mediate growth inhibition and cell death in mantle cell lymphoma. *FEBS Lett, 2005*. 579(30): p. 6885-9.

[69] Sanchez-Izquierdo, D., et al., MALT1 is deregulated by both chromosomal translocation and amplification in B-cell non-Hodgkin lymphoma. *Blood, 2003*. 101(11): p. 4539-46.

[70] Remstein, E.D., et al., Primary pulmonary MALT lymphomas show frequent and heterogeneous cytogenetic abnormalities, including aneuploidy and translocations involving API2 and MALT1 and IGH and MALT1. *Leukemia, 2004*. 18(1): p. 156-60.

[71] Streubel, B., et al., T(14;18)(q32;q21) involving IGH and MALT1 is a frequent chromosomal aberration in MALT lymphoma. *Blood, 2003*. 101(6): p. 2335-9.

[72] Morgan, J.A., et al., Breakpoints of the t(11;18)(q21;q21) in mucosa-associated lymphoid tissue (MALT) lymphoma lie within or near the previously undescribed gene MALT1 in chromosome 18. *Cancer Res, 1999*. 59(24): p. 6205-13.

[73] Dierlamm, J., et al., The apoptosis inhibitor gene API2 and a novel 18q gene, MLT, are recurrently rearranged in the t(11;18)(q21;q21)p6ssociated with mucosa-associated lymphoid tissue lymphomas. *Blood, 1999*. 93(11): p. 3601-9.

[74] Akagi, T., et al., A novel gene, MALT1 at 18q21, is involved in t(11;18) (q21;q21) found in low-grade B-cell lymphoma of mucosa-associated lymphoid tissue. *Oncogene, 1999*. 18(42): p. 5785-94.

[75] Algara, P., et al., Analysis of the IgV(H) somatic mutations in splenic marginal zone lymphoma defines a group of unmutated cases with frequent 7q deletion and adverse clinical course. *Blood, 2002*. 99(4): p. 1299-304.

[76] Camacho, F.I., et al., Nodal marginal zone lymphoma: a heterogeneous tumor: a comprehensive analysis of a series of 27 cases. *Am J Surg Pathol, 2003*. 27(6): p. 762-71.

[77] Thieblemont, C., et al., Small lymphocytic lymphoma, marginal zone B-cell lymphoma, and mantle cell lymphoma exhibit distinct gene-expression profiles allowing molecular diagnosis. *Blood, 2004*. 103(7): p. 2727-37.

[78] Vihinen, M., et al., Mutations of the human BTK gene coding for bruton tyrosine kinase in X-linked agammaglobulinemia. *Hum Mutat, 1999*. 13(4): p. 280-5.

[79] Bonilla, F.A. and R.S. Geha, *12*. Primary immunodeficiency diseases. *J Allergy Clin Immunol, 2003*. 111(2 Suppl): p. S571-81.

[80] Bruton, O.C., Agammaglobulinemia. *Pediatrics, 1952*. 9: p. 722-27.

[81] Buckley, R.H., Primary cellular immunodeficiencies. *J Allergy Clin Immunol, 2002*. 109(5): p. 747-57.

[82] Chinen, J. and W.T. Shearer, Basic and clinical immunology. *J Allergy Clin Immunol, 2003*. 111(3 Suppl): p. S813-8.

[83] Ochs, H.D. and C.I. Smith, X-linked agammaglobulinemia. A clinical and molecular analysis. *Medicine (Baltimore), 1996*. 75(6): p. 287-99.

[84] Ochs, H.D., C.I.E. Smith, and J.M. Puck, *Primary Immunodeficiency Diseases: A Molecular and Genetic Approach. 2007*: Oxford University Press.

[85] Vetrie, D., Isolation of the defective gene in X linked agammaglobulinaemia. *J Med Genet, 1993*. 30(6): p. 452-3.

[86] Tsukada, S., et al., Deficient expression of a B cell cytoplasmic tyrosine kinase in human X-linked agammaglobulinemia. *Cell, 1993*. 72(2): p. 279-90.

[87] Vihinen, M., et al., BTKbase: a database of XLA-causing mutations. International Study Group. *Immunol Today, 1995*. 16(10): p. 460-5.

[88] Vihinen, M., et al., BTKbase, mutation database for X-linked agammaglobulinemia (XLA). *Nucleic Acids Res, 1997*. 25(1): p. 166-71.

[89] Campana, D., et al., Phenotypic features and proliferative activity of B cell progenitors in X-linked agammaglobulinemia. *J Immunol, 1990*. 145(6): p. 1675-80.

[90] Noordzij, J.G., et al., Composition of precursor B-cell compartment in bone marrow from patients with X-linked agammaglobulinemia compared with healthy children. *Pediatr Res, 2002*. 51(2): p. 159-68.

[91] Lindvall, J.M., et al., Bruton's tyrosine kinase: cell biology, sequence conservation, mutation spectrum, siRNA modifications, and expression profiling. *Immunol Rev, 2005*. 203: p. 200-15.

[92] Winkelstein, J.A., et al., X-linked agammaglobulinemia: report on a United States registry of 201 patients. *Medicine (Baltimore), 2006*. 85(4): p. 193-202.

[93] Sideras, P. and C.I. Smith, Molecular and cellular aspects of X-linked agammaglobulinemia. *Adv Immunol, 1995*. 59: p. 135-223.

[94] Gryboski, J.D., et al., Selective immunoglobulin A deficiency and intestinal nodular lymphoid hyperplasia: correction of diarrhea with antibiotics and plasma. *Pediatrics, 1968*. 42(5): p. 833-7.

[95] Hammarstrom, L., G.G. de Lange, and C.I. Smith, IgA2 allotypes determined by restriction fragment length polymorphism in IgA deficiency. Re-expression of the silent A2m(2) allotype in the children of IgA-deficient patients. *J Immunogenet, 1987*. 14(4-5): p. 197-201.

[96] Islam, K.B., et al., Molecular analysis of IgA deficiency. Evidence for impaired switching to IgA. *J Immunol, 1994*. 152(3): p. 1442-52.

[97] Briere, F., et al., Interleukin 10 induces B lymphocytes from IgA-deficient patients to secrete IgA. *J Clin Invest, 1994*. 94(1): p. 97-104.

[98] Cunningham-Rundles, C. and C. Bodian, Common variable immunodeficiency: clinical and immunological features of 248 patients. *Clin Immunol, 1999*. 92(1): p. 34-48.

[99] Waldmann, T.A., et al., Role of suppressor T cells in pathogenesis of common variable hypogammaglobulinaemia. *Lancet, 1974*. 2(7881): p. 609-13.

[100] Reinherz, E.L., et al., Immunodeficiency associated with loss of T4+ inducer T-cell function. *N Engl J Med, 1981*. 304(14): p. 811-6.

[101] Eisenstein, E.M., K. Chua, and W. Strober, B cell differentiation defects in common variable immunodeficiency are ameliorated after stimulation with anti-CD40 antibody and IL-10. *J Immunol, 1994*. 152(12): p. 5957-68.

[102] Sneller, M.C. and W. Strober, Abnormalities of lymphokine gene expression in patients with common variable immunodeficiency. *J Immunol, 1990*. 144(10): p. 3762-9.

[103] Farrington, M., et al., CD40 ligand expression is defective in a subset of patients with common variable immunodeficiency. *Proc Natl Acad Sci U S A, 1994*. 91(3): p. 1099-103.

[104] Ashman, R.F., et al., Genetic and immunologic analysis of a family containing five patients with common-variable immune deficiency or selective IgA deficiency. *J Clin Immunol, 1992*. 12(6): p. 406-14.

[105] Olerup, O., C.I. Smith, and L. Hammarstrom, Different amino acids at position 57 of the HLA-DQ beta chain associated with susceptibility and resistance to IgA deficiency. *Nature, 1990*. 347(6290): p. 289-90.

[106] Olerup, O., et al., Shared HLA class II-associated genetic susceptibility and resistance, related to the HLA-DQB1 gene, in IgA deficiency and common variable immunodeficiency. *Proc Natl Acad Sci U S A, 1992*. 89(22): p. 10653-7.

[107] Grimbacher, B., et al., Homozygous loss of ICOS is associated with adult-onset common variable immunodeficiency. *Nat Immunol, 2003*. 4(3): p. 261-8.

[108] Salzer, U., et al., Mutations in TNFRSF13B encoding TACI are associated with common variable immunodeficiency in humans. *Nat Genet, 2005*. 37(8): p. 820-8.

[109] Xu, G.L., et al., Chromosome instability and immunodeficiency syndrome caused by mutations in a DNA methyltransferase gene. *Nature, 1999*. 402(6758): p. 187-91.

[110] De Ravel, T.J., et al., The ICF syndrome: new case and update. *Genet Couns, 2001*. 12(4): p. 379-85.

[111] Smeets, D.F., et al., ICF syndrome: a new case and review of the literature. *Hum Genet, 1994*. 94(3): p. 240-6.

[112] Sawyer, J.R., et al., Chromosome instability in ICF syndrome: formation of micronuclei from multibranched chromosomes 1 demonstrated by fluorescence in situ hybridization. *Am J Med Genet, 1995*. 56(2): p. 203-9.

[113] Fasth, A., et al., Fragility of the centromeric region of chromosome 1 associated with combined immunodeficiency in siblings. A recessively inherited entity? *Acta Paediatr Scand, 1990*. 79(6-7): p. 605-12.

[114] Brown, D.C., et al., ICF syndrome (immunodeficiency, centromeric instability and facial anomalies): investigation of heterochromatin abnormalities and review of clinical outcome. *Hum Genet, 1995*. 96(4): p. 411-6.

[115] Feske, S., et al., Gene regulation mediated by calcium signals in T lymphocytes. *Nat Immunol, 2001*. 2(4): p. 316-24.

[116] Cunningham-Rundles, C., et al., Lymphomas of mucosal-associated lymphoid tissue in common variable immunodeficiency. *Am J Hematol, 2002*. 69(3): p. 171-8.

[117] Hammarstrom, L., I. Vorechovsky, and D. Webster, Selective IgA deficiency (SIgAD) and common variable immunodeficiency (CVID). *Clin Exp Immunol, 2000*. 120(2): p. 225-31.

In: Cancer Research Perspectives
Editor: Larissa S. Pereira, pp. 191-218
ISBN 978-1-60021-980-1

Chapter VI

Fas-Resistance in Adult T-Cell Leukemia Lymphoma

Yasuaki Yamada* and Shimeru Kamihira
Division of Laboratory Medicine, Department of Translational Medical Sciences,
Nagasaki University Graduate School of Biomedical Sciences, Japan.

Abstract

Fas (APO-1/CD95) is a member of tumor necrosis factor (TNF)/nerve growth factor (NGF) receptor superfamily. Cross-linking of cell membrane Fas (mFas) by Fas ligand (FasL) transduces a death signal that results in a unique cell death, apoptosis, in which cells show chromatin condensation and nuclear fragmentation. One of the important biological roles of this system is the maintenance of immune homeostasis. Activated lymphocytes which express mFas are eliminated after appropriate immune reaction to avoid prolonged and surplus reaction. Interestingly, *lpr* and *gld* mice that show spontaneous dysfunctional mutations of Fas and (FasL), respectively, show autoimmune diseases with increased numbers of activated lymphocytes. The balance between death and survival is delicately controlled not only by the mFas expression but also by its isoform soluble Fas (sFas) and cytoplasmic apoptosis promotive and repressive molecules. Adult T-cell leukemia lymphoma (ATLL) is a unique neoplasm of activated mature T-cells caused by human T-cell leukemia virus type-1 (HTLV-1). Because of its activated T-cell nature, ATLL cells express abundant mFas. Nevertheless, ATLL cells vigorously proliferate escaping from the attack of FasL, which suggests that ATLL cells acquire strong apoptosis-resistant systems during their development. Here, we review the molecules involved in apoptosis resistance in ATLL and discuss their role in oncogenesis and their clinical significance.

* Correspondence concerning this article should be addressed to: Yasuaki Yamada, 1-7-1 Sakamoto, Nagasaki 852-8501 Japan; Tel: +81-95-849-7408. Fax: +81-95-849-7422; E-mail: y-yamada@ nagasaki-u.ac.jp.

1. Adult T-Cell Leukemia Lymphoma (ATLL)

ATLL is a neoplasm of mature helper/inducer T-cell origin (CD3+, CD4+, CD8-) [1,2]. Its activated cell nature is known by the constitutional expression of interleukin-2 receptor α chain (IL-2Rα: CD25) and HLR-DR[3]. Since ATLL is caused by a retrovirus HTLV-1[4-6], demonstration of the monoclonal integration of HTLV-1 proviral DNA by Southern blot is indispensable for its conclusive diagnosis especially when other peripheral T-cell neoplasms such as cutaneous T-cell lymphomas are suspected (Figure 1). There are approximately 1.2 million HTLV-1 carriers in Japan and the cumulative risk of the development of this disease among the carriers is 2.5~5% in their whole life. Since the prevalence of this virus infection is high in the southwestern districts of Japan, especially in the Kyushu, ATLL is clustered in this area [7]. Such a regional clustering of this disease is caused by mother-to-child transmission of the virus by breast-feeding in closed population groups [8,9]. Other clusters are found in the Caribbean islands, South America, tropical Africa, and Oceania. HTLV-1 is also known to cause a neurological disease named tropical spastic paraparesis (TSP)/HTLV-1-associated myelopathy (HAM) [10,11].

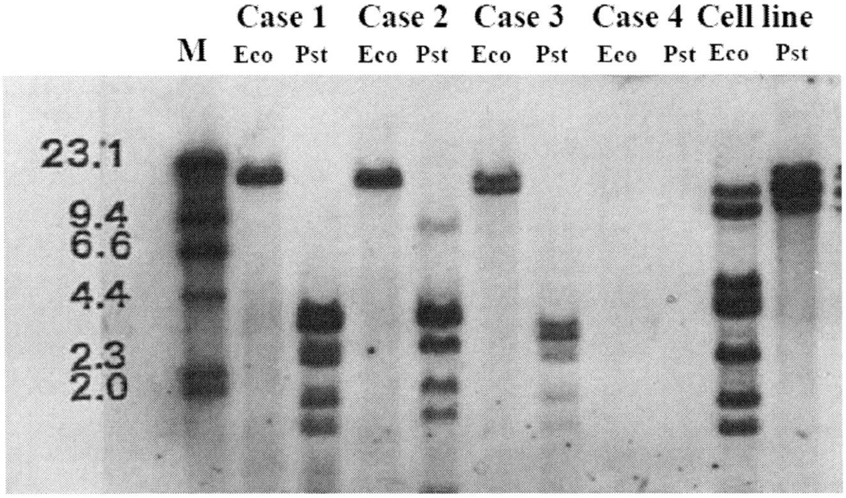

Figure 1. Southern blot analysis of HTLV-1 proviral DNA in primary leukemia samples. Cellular DNA was isolated from Case 1, 2, 3, 4 and our original ATLL cell line SO4, digested with *Eco*RI (Eco) or *Pst*I (Pst), and hybridized with an HTLV-1-probe. HTLV-1 does not have an *Eco*RI site but it has *Pst*I sites. Presence of single or two bands in *Eco*RI-digested DNA of cases 1, 2 and 3 indicate that there is a monoclonal population of HTLV-1 integrated cells. Case 4 is a peripheral blood sample from an Sèzary syndrome patient, the same neoplasm of mature CD4-positive T-cell origin having similar cell morphology and clinical manifestations to ATLL. This sample does not have the integration band and the diagnosis of ATLL is thus denied. There are multiple bands in long-term cultured ATLL cell line SO4 cells, which is the result of super infection of HTLV-1 in vitro.

ATLL patients show several characteristic clinical and laboratory features. They usually have abnormal lymphocytes with nuclear indentation (Figure 2); cells having multi-lobulated nuclei are called flower cells. In addition to the common feature of lymphoid neoplasms such as lymph node swelling and hepatosplenomegaly, up to 40% of the patients show hypercalcemia and skin lesions. Multi-organ involvement is frequent and lungs, liver, gastrointestinal tract, central nervous system and bone are affected [12-14]. Although ATLL is bundled as one clinical entity because of its etiological agent HTLV-1, this disease is quite heterogeneous clinically, and hence it is subclassified into four subtypes: acute type, lymphoma type, chronic type and smoldering type [15]. The prognosis of the aggressive subtypes, acute type and lymphoma type, is extremely poor and their median survival time is only 13 month even in our most recent protocol study [16]. In contrast, patients with indolent subtypes, chronic type and smoldering type, survive several years even without therapy.

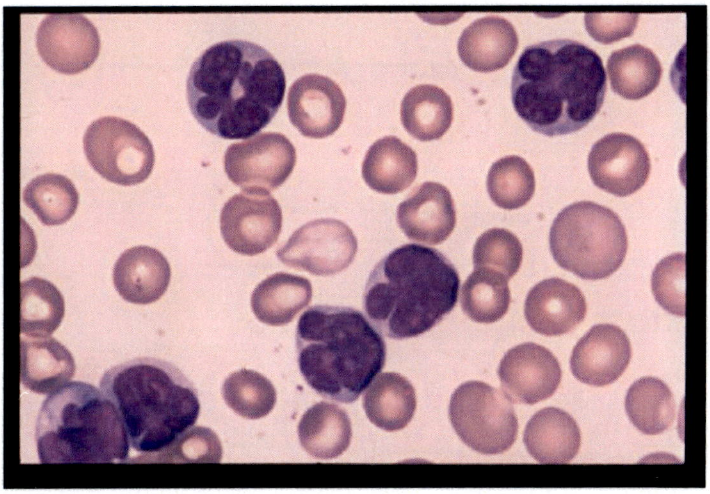

Figure 2. Peripheral blood ATLL cells. Typical ATLL cells with nuclear indentation are shown. Cells having multi-lobulated nuclei are called flower cells.

As the character of mature T-cells, ATLL cells express many kinds of functional receptors. In addition to IL-2R that is one of the marker molecules of activated T-cells, ATLL cells express other cytokine receptors such as IL-4R, IL-7R and IL-15R that all belong to the common-gamma receptor family and show proliferative response to these cytokines [17-19], which signals are supposed to be used in the early stage of ATLL development. The cause of nodal and extranodal involvement in this disease has recently been disclosed to be due to inclined chemokine receptor expression; increased CCR7 expression plays a role in lymphoid organ infiltration [20], and CCR4 expression is highly associated with skin invasion [21]. Peripheral blood T-cells are subdivided into two subpopulations according to antigen-activated status, $CD45RO^+$ memory T-cells and $CD45RO^-$ naive T-cells. $CD45RO^+$ memory T-cells preferentially express mFas [22]. Since ATLL cells are $CD45RO^+$, it is natural that ATLL cells express mFas, and they indeed express abundant mFas in common [23]. Nevertheless, ATLL cells proliferate without apparent sign of apoptosis suggesting that ATLL cells are endowed with an anti-apoptotic mechanism from their developmental phase. In this sense, ATLL provide us a good model to understand the participation of the abnormality of apoptosis signal transduction system in the development of common neoplasms. Strong chemo-resistance and poor prognosis in ATLL patients may be attributable to this deregulation.

2. Fas Gene and Its Transcripts

The Fas receptor, a 48-kDa (319 amino acids) transmembrane protein, mediates apoptosis signal when it is cross-linked by (FasL) or by agonistic IgM anti-Fas monoclonal antibodies [24]. The Fas gene consists of 9 exons encoding three regions, a N-terminal extracellular (EC) domain as the FasL binding site, a single transmembrane (TM) domain for cell membrane anchoring, and an intracytoplasmic (IC) domain for death signal transduction (Figure 3) [25].

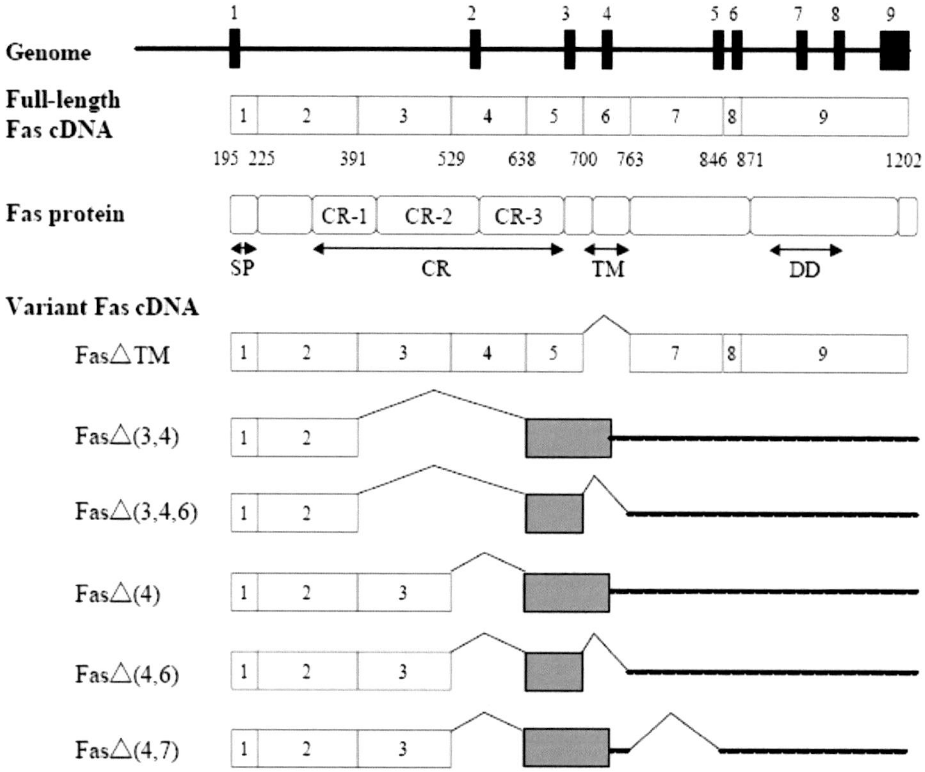

Figure 3. Fas gene structure and Fas isoforms. Full-length Fas cDNA contains nine exons encoding signal peptide (SP: exon 1), three cysteine rich extracellular domains (CR-1, CR-2 and CD-3: exons 2, 3, 4, 5), transmembrane domain (TM: exon 6), and intracellular domain (exons 7, 8, 9) with death domain (DD). There are many alternatively spliced Fas transcripts in human PBMCs. The representative variant cDNA are shown[26-29]. FasΔTM is the major variant and is generated by alternative splicing of the transmembrane domain. Others lack with various combinations of exon 3, 4, 6 and 7, in which the deletions result in different reading frame with premature termination codons. Numbered boxes indicate translated regions with the same reading frame as that of full-length Fas, gray boxes indicate altered reading frame, and dotted bold lines indicate untranslated regions.

The EC domain has three repeats of a cysteine-rich subdomain common to all members of the TNF receptor family, and the IC domain has death domain (DD) that is the most important part for apoptosis signal transduction. In addition to the full-length mRNA that is translated into mFas, activated normal peripheral blood mononuclear cells (PBMCs) express many shorter splicing variants (Figure 3) [26-29]. The major variant is FasΔTM that lacks

TM domain (exon 6), which is translated into soluble Fas (sFas). Differs from mFas, sFas is released from the cells and hence it does not transduce death signal. In most of the other variants, FasΔ(3,4), FasΔ(3,4,6), FasΔ(4), FasΔ(4,6), and FasΔ(4,7), the deletions result in a different reading frame with premature termination codons, thus producing smaller Fas proteins lacking IC domain. The proportion of these transcripts in normal T-cells is 60% in full-length and 40% in FasΔTM, and the others are quite small populations. Fairly high proportion of FasΔTM in normal T-cells suggests that this isoform is in charge of important physiological role of T-cells. Since all these variants have EC domain, they preserve a capacity to bind with FasL. It has been reported that intra-hepatic T-cells in the mouse show different sensitivity to apoptosis according to the level of sFas mRNA expression [30]. Accordingly, these variants seems to act as the decoy of mFas and inhibit Fas-mediated apoptosis signaling by interfering with ligation to FasL or by causing incomplete trimerization between intact mFas and variants. The similar competition has also been reported in TNF receptor system [31,32]. Of note, sera from patients with malignant B- and T-cell leukemias and lymphomas show increased level of sFas suggesting its role for tumor cells protection from the attack of FasL [33].

3. Fas-Mediated Apoptosis Signaling

When FasL binds to the Fas receptor, it causes trimerization of the receptor, and the resultant trimerized DD recruits pro-caspase-8 through a FADD adaptor, and forms a death-inducing signaling complex (DISC) (Figure 4) [34-36]. In addition to the DD, FADD has a death-effector domain (DED) capable of splicing pro-caspase-8 into its active form, caspase-8 [37]. The activated caspase-8 directly processes its downstream enzyme pro-caspase-3, a key enzyme for apoptosis induction, or indirectly processes it through mitochondria [38]. Caspase-8 cleaves BID into the functional C-terminal fragment tBID, which translocates to the mitochondria, permeabilize mitochondrial membrane and accelerates the releases of cytochrome C into the cytosol by Bax and Bak [39]. On the other hand, apoptosis inhibitors Bcl-2 and Bcl-xL inhibit the release of cytochrome C [40]. The released cytochrome C activates pro-caspase-9 together with apoptotic protease activating factor (Apaf-1), and then the mature caspase-9 activates caspase-3 [41]. Irrespective of the activation routes, the activated caspase-3 sets caspase-activated DNase (CAD) free to enter the nucleus by cleaving its inhibitor ICAD [42-44], and the CAD causes DNA fragmentation.

In addition to Bcl-2 and Bcl-xL, there are many other molecules known to inhibit apoptosis cascade (Figure 4). Fas-associated phosphatase-1 (FAP-1) interacts with the IC domain of Fas and inhibits Fas-mediated apoptosis [45]. FLICE-inhibitory proteins (FLIPs) contain two DED domains and inhibit the activation of caspase-8 by disturbing the formation of DISC [46]. Inhibitor of apoptosis proteins (IAP) is another family protein for apoptosis inhibition. X-linked inhibitor of apoptosis proteins (XIAP), one of the members of IAP, not only inhibits caspase-3, -7 and -9 directly, but also inhibits caspase-3 indirectly through Apaf-1 [47,48]. Survivin is also a member of IAP family and inhibits caspase-3 and -7 [49]. Since survivin is expressed in the G2/M phase of the cell cycle in a cycle-regulated manner, it is supposed that survivin counteract a default induction of apoptosis in G2/M phase [50].

Although survivin is undetectable in terminally differentiated adult tissues, it becomes prominently expressed in all the most common human cancers from various organs [51], indicating its general role in neoplasms. Thus, there are many apoptosis promotive and repressive molecules and apoptosis signaling is delicately controlled. Once any part of this pathway was disrupted, it is favorable for tumor cell proliferation.

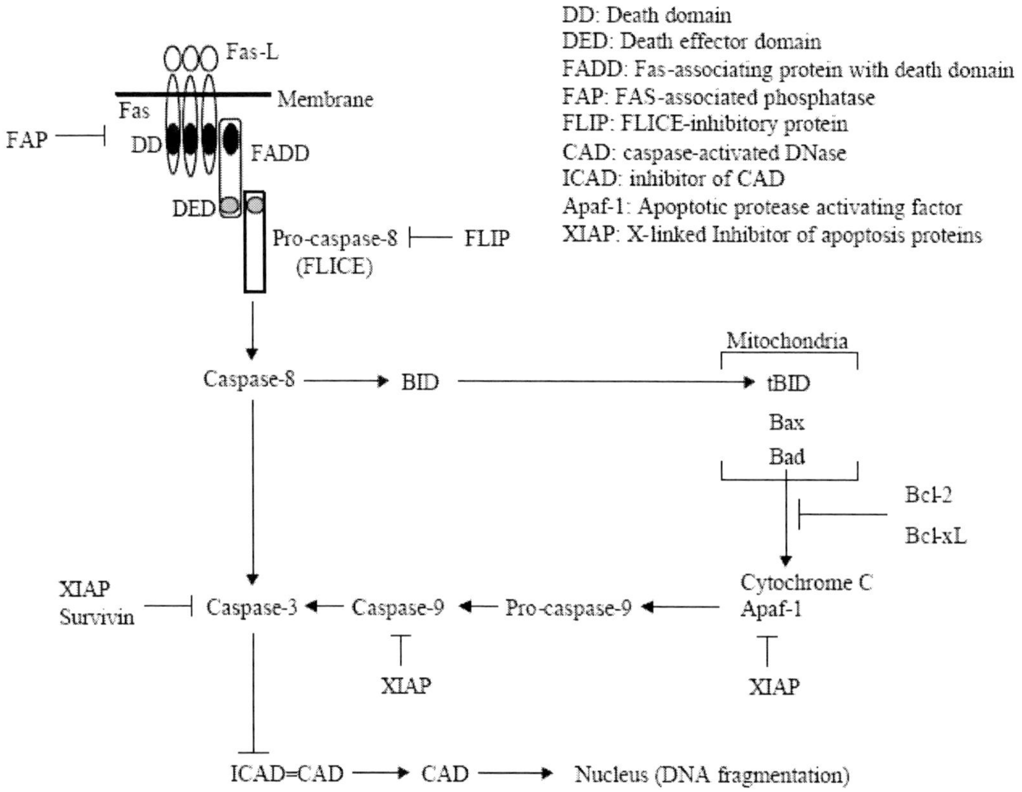

Figure 4. Schema of Fas-mediated apoptosis signal transduction. DD: Death domain, FADD: Fas-associating protein with death domain, DED: Death effector domain, FAP: Fas-associated phosphatase, FILP: FLICE(pro-caspase 8)-inhibitory protein, XIAP: X-linked inhibitor of apoptosis proteins, Apaf-1: Apoptotic protease activating factor, CAD: caspase-activated DNase, ICAD: inhibitor of CAD. Explanation of this figure is described in the text.

4. Fas Sensitivity of ATLL Cells

Expression of mFas and sensitivity to anti-Fas antibody in primary ATLL cells and HTLV-1-infected T-cell lines have firstly been reported by Debatin et al [52,53]. Among nine primary samples they examined, eight were sensitive to anti-Fas antibody and apoptosis was induced. However, one sample was fairly resistant despite abundant mFas expression suggesting the presence of intrinsic anti-apoptotic mechanism in ATLL cells. Indeed, ATLL cells prepare many devices to prevent apoptosis at multiple levels of apoptosis signaling cascade as we discuss in detail below.

4.1. mFas-Negative ATLL Patients

Most primary ATLL cells express abundant mFas by nature as the character of activated T-cells. However, some patients' cells scarcely express it (Figure 5). Among 81 ATLL patients we examined previously (8 smoldering, 14 chronic, 43 acute and 16 lymphoma), 10 patients (12.3%) showed less than 30% positivity (Figure 6A) [54].

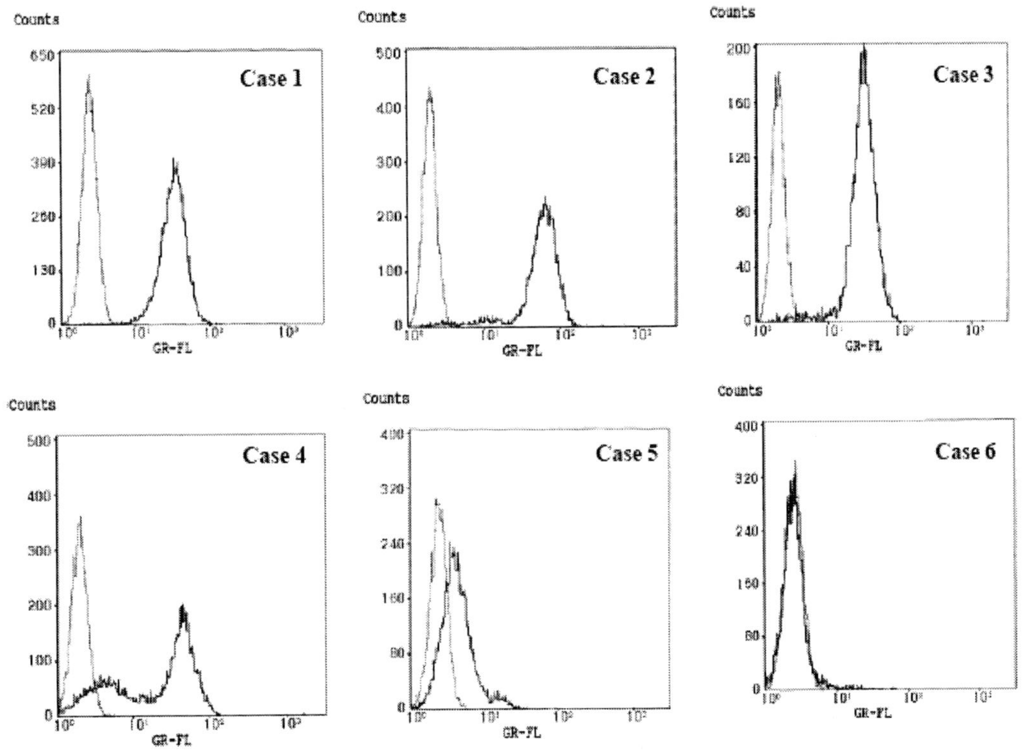

Figure 5. Flow cytometric analysis of mFas in primary samples. Thin lines indicate the cells treated with an isotype-matched control antibody, and bold lines indicate the cells treated with an anti-Fas antibody. Cells from cases 1, 2, 3, and 4 show abundant mFas, while case 5 shows scant expression, and case 6 is totally negative.

Naturally, ATLL cells of these Fas-negative patients are resistant to anti-Fas antibody [23]. mFas-negative patients are found irrespective of ATLL subtypes, and there is no correlation between mFas expression status and survival. mFas density per cell is measurable by converting the mean fluorescence intensity value of the positive cells into antibody binding capacity value (mFas^{ABC}). In normal peripheral blood lymphocytes, mFas is positive in 58% (range 50-66%) with a mFas^{ABC} value of 3,470 (range 2,519-5,950). The mFas^{ABC} values of mFas-negative patients are quite low and are all less than 600 (Figure 6B). When FasL is produced as the result of immune reaction against some pathogen *in vivo*, neighboring mFas-positive cells should undergo apoptosis and should be eliminated from the body. ATLL sometimes show spontaneous regression [55] that seems be due to apoptosis. mFas-negative cells have an advantage over mFas-positive cells for survival, and ATLL cells that do not have intrinsic anti-apoptotic mechanism may inevitably down-regulate mFas to evade from the attack of FasL, as the first step of the acquisition of Fas-resistance. Different from primary ATLL cells, all ATLL cell lines show high mFas positive rates and high mFas^{ABC} values without exception. This discordance may be interpreted that cell lines need not to evade from the attack of FasL, and hence they have returned to their original character as activated T-cells during culture.

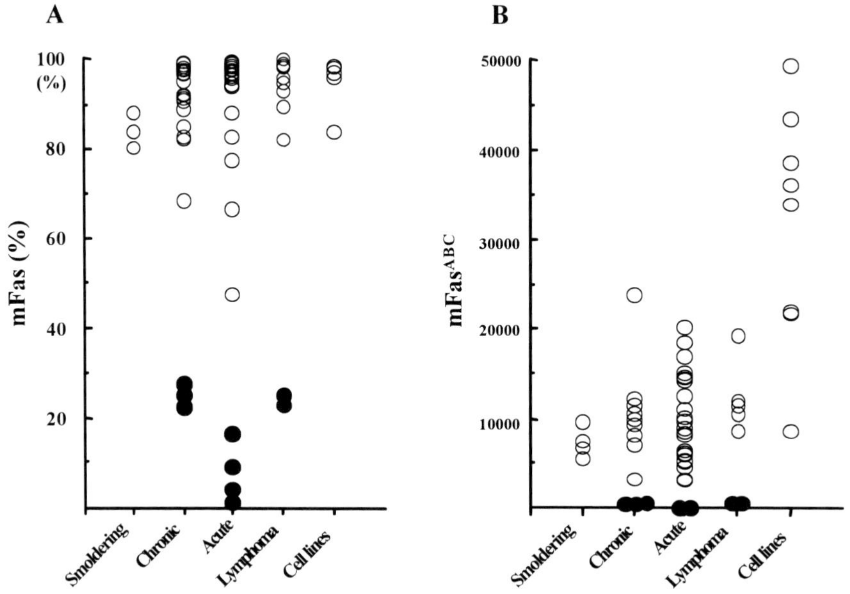

Figure 6. mFas positivity (mFas (%)) and anti-Fas antibody binding capacity (mFas^{ABC}) Ref. no. [54]. Eighty-one primary ATLL samples are examined by flow cytometry and the results are expressed as positive rate (A) or antibody binding capacity per cell (B). Ten samples show less than 30% positivity (closed circle) and the mFas^{ABC} values of these samples are quite low being less than 600. Both positive rates and mFas^{ABC} values are quite high in cell lines. There is no correlation between mFas expression status and clinical subtypes.

4.2. Production of sFas

When RT-PCR analysis for Fas transcripts is performed in normal PBMCs, at least two different sizes products are visualized, a full-length product correspond to mFas and a 63 bp shorter product correspond to sFas (Figure 7). Primary ATLL cells express both transcripts although the expression levels differ greatly patient-by-patient (Figure 7). In contrast, all ATLL cell lines completely lack sFas transcripts. This is also one of the characters of the cell lines, and cell lines may have down-regulated the expression because they need not to produce sFas in culture condition. Since sFas is released from cells, human sera contain certain levels of sFas, and it is possible to measure the concentration by an enzyme-linked immunosorbent assay (ELISA). Sera from ATLL patients contain significantly higher levels of sFas than those from healthy adults ($p<0.001$) [56], and the value is correlated with serum lactate dehydrogenase (LDH) activity, ATLL cell count in the peripheral blood and ATLL subtypes (Figure 8) [54].

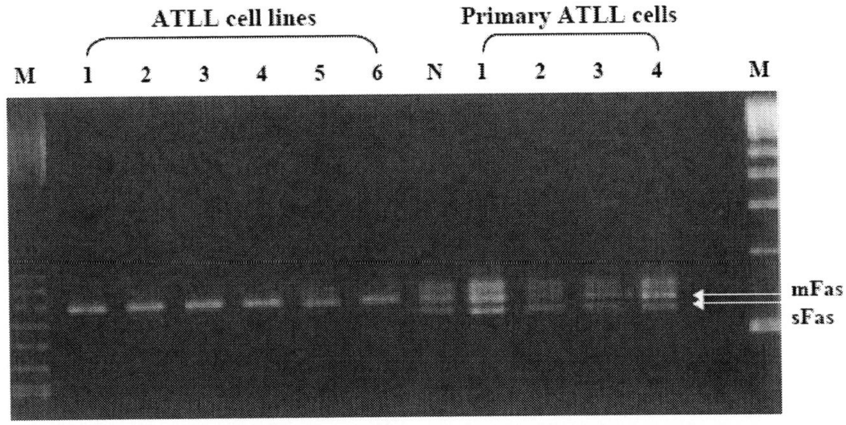

Figure 7. RT-PCR analysis of Fas transcripts (1) Ref. no. [56]. Two expected bands of 1,167-bp and 1,104-bp that correspond to mFas and sFas, respectively, are observed in normal PBMCs and primary ATLL cells. The band densities differ greatly in primary ATLL samples. Only mFas band is observed in ATLL cell lines indicating that cell lines lack sFas transcripts. N: normal PBMCs, M: size marker.

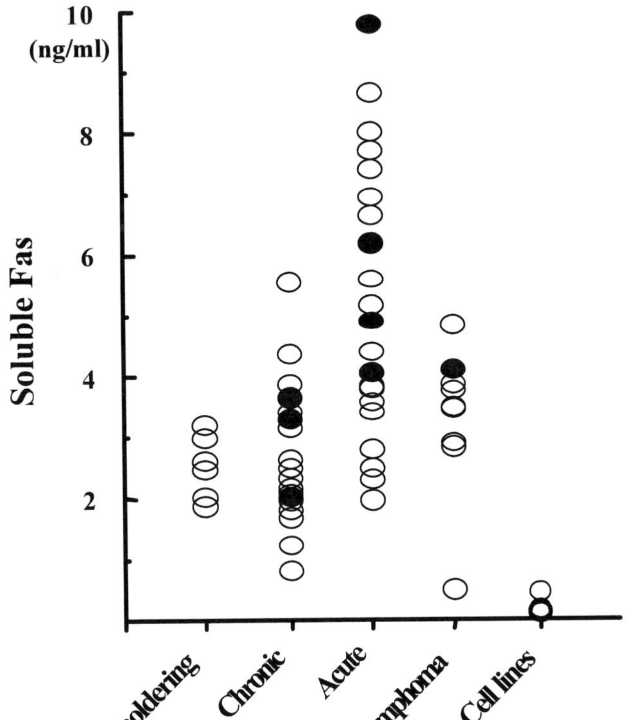

Figure 8. Serum sFas concentration Ref. no. [54]. sFas is detected in all patients with higher concentrations in acute subtype than in other subtypes. mFas-negative cases (closed circle) also show similar levels of sFas to mFas-positive patients (open circle). Coincident with the result of RT-PCR, culture supernatants of ATLL cell lines do not contain sFas.

Interestingly, there is no correlation between sFas concentration and mFas density indicating that the translation and/or transcription efficiencies of these isoforms are different in ATLL cells. A multivariate analysis by a Cox proportional hazards model indicates that serum sFas concentration is an independent factor associated with survival time. Patients with higher serum sFas (>4ng/ml) show significantly shorter survival than patients with lower serum sFas (<4ng/ml) (Figure 9). High serum sFas concentration has also been reported in other lymphoid neoplasms. Sera from patients with B- and T-cell leukemias contain increased levels of sFas compare to healthy donors [33]. In non-Hodgkin's lymphoma (NHL), complete remission rate, overall survival (OS) rate and disease-free survival (DFS) rate are all significantly decreased in the subgroup having high serum sFas levels [57].

More interestingly, breast cancer patients also show increased serum sFas concentration [58], although the source of the sFas is not identified. Patients with high-sFas have a worse prognosis than those with low-sFas for both OS and DFS, and a multivariate analysis confirmed that sFas level is an independent prognostic indicator in this disease also.

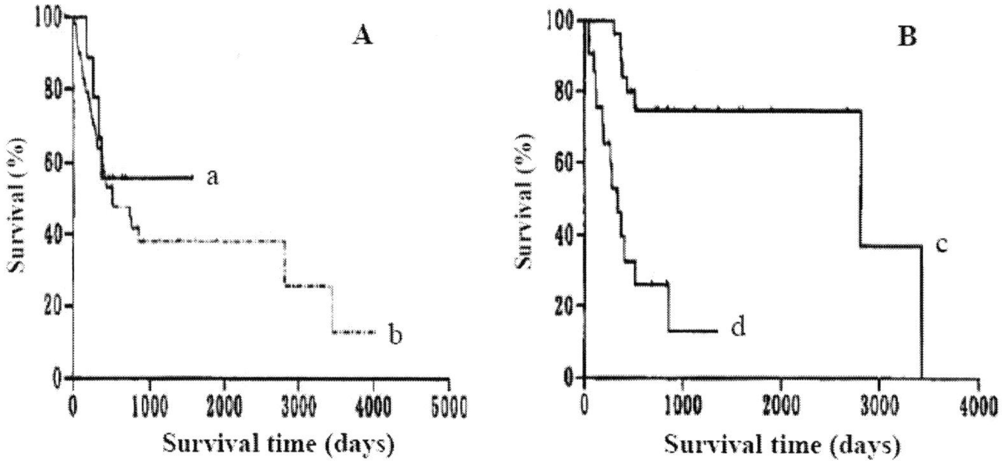

Figure 9. Overall survival curves of ATLL patients Ref. no. [54]. Patients are subdivided according to the mFas expression status (A) (a: mFas-negative cases, b: mFas-positive cases) or serum sFas concentration (B) (c: sFas <4ng/ml, d: sFas >4ng/ml). There is no difference in survival between mFas-positive cases and mFas-negative cases. In contrast, patients with high serum sFas show significantly shorter survival than the patients with low serum sFas (p<0.0001).

4.3. Diversity of Fas Transcripts

Fas gene expression is quite diverse in ATLL cells. In addition to the two main transcripts, full-length Fas and FasΔ(6), ATLL cells express many aberrantly spliced transcripts. The production ratio of such aberrant transcripts to full-length Fas is high in ATLL cells compare to normal PBMCs (Figure 10) [59]. All variants reported in normal PBMCs (Figure 3) are found in ATLL cells. In addition, ATLL cells express several unique variants that have not been reported in normal PBMCs (Figure 11) [59].

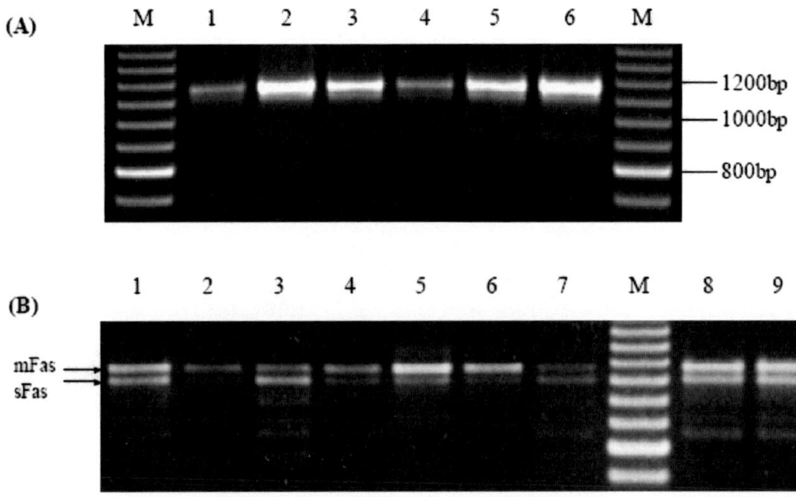

Figure 10. RT-PCR analysis of Fas transcripts (2) Ref. no. [59]. Results of normal PBMCs (A) and primary ATLL cells (B). In addition to the two main bands correspond to mFas and sFas, three to four faint bands smaller in size are visible in ATLL cells, especially in cases 3, 7, 8, and 9. M: size marker.

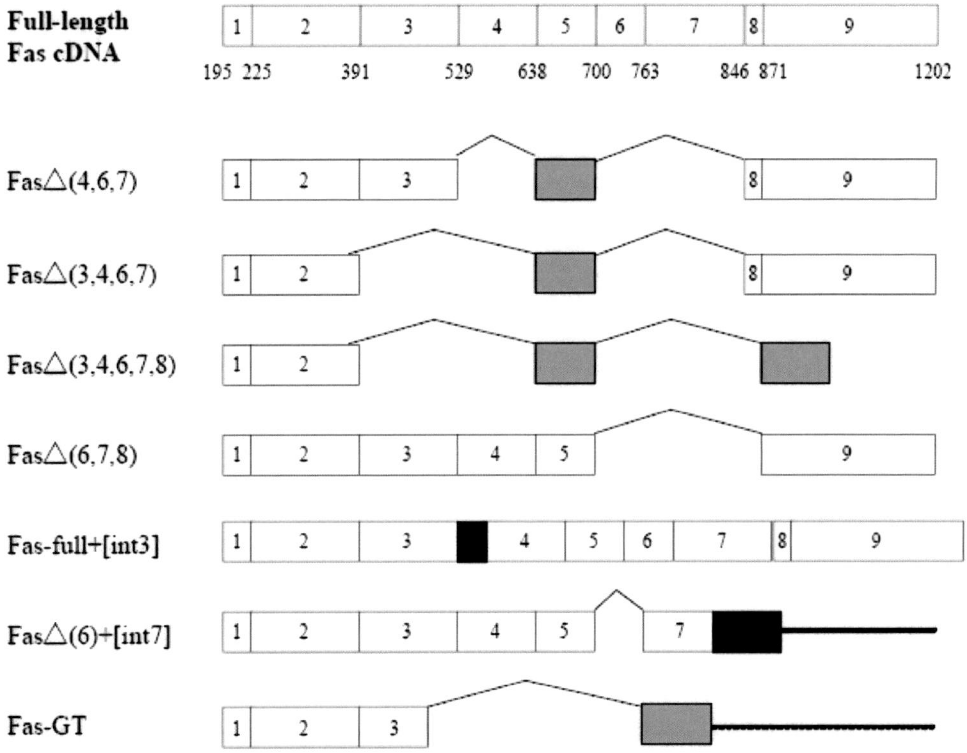

Figure 11. Novel Fas splicing variants Ref. no. [59]. Numbered boxes indicate translated regions with the same reading frame as that of full-length Fas, gray boxes indicate altered reading frame, closed boxes indicate the retained intronic sequences, and dotted bold lines indicate untranslated regions. Explanation of this figure is described in the text.

Among 7 such novel variants we found, FasΔ(4,6,7), FasΔ(3,4,6,7) and FasΔ(3,4,6,7,8) share the same altered reading frame of exon 5 and produce short sFas isoforms. FasΔ(3,4,6,7,8) also has an altered reading frame of exon 9 with a premature termination resulting in the loss of the DD. FasΔ(6,7,8) encodes the truncated Fas structure in which some of the central domains including TM are removed. In addition, two intron-retention forms due to splicing outside of the conventional exon/intron boundaries are also identified, which suggests abnormalities in the splicing process of Fas pre-mRNA in ATLL cells. Fas-full+[int3] retains 3' end (9 bp) of intron 3, and FasΔ(6)+[int7] retains 5' end (254 bp) of intron 7 that has a termination codon. In Fas-GT, 311 nucleotides between nt.452 (within exon3) and nt.764 (within exon 7) are deleted, which results in an altered reading frame of exon 7 with a premature termination. Interestingly, since most of these variants lack exon 6 and their protein products are released from the cells, they should participate in the protection of ATLL cells from the attack of FasL like sFas.

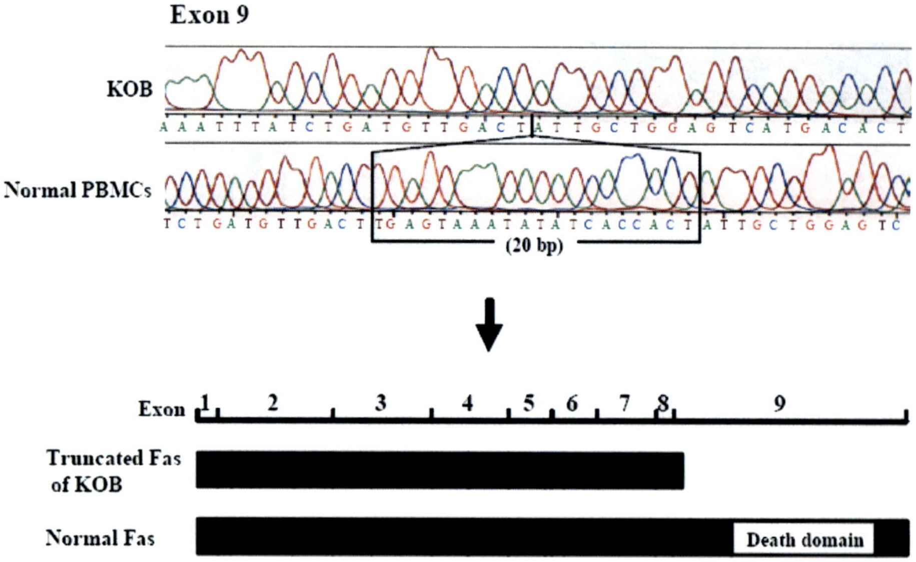

Figure 12. Sequence analysis of Fas transcripts of KOB cells Ref. no. [63]. In addition to full-length Fas transcript, KOB cells have an aberrant transcript that lacks 20 bp at exon 9. The frame shift caused by the deletion generates a premature stop codon, resulting in the production of truncated mFas lacking death domain.

4.4. Fas Gene Mutation

Fas gene mutation is responsible for lymphocyte proliferation in *lpr* mice, and the mice show the accumulation of a large number of nonmalignant T lymphocytes in the lymph nodes and spleen [60]. Its human counterpart, congenital autoimmune lymphoproliferative syndrome (ALPS), also shows lymphadenopathy [61,62]. Accordingly, when a function-ablating mutation of the Fas gene has occurred in malignant cells, it may cause surplus proliferation of tumor cells. We experienced such patient in ATLL [63]. The patient was admitted with systemic lymphadenopathy. After diagnosis of ATLL, he received ten cycles of combination chemotherapy and was discharged with a partial remission. Three months later, however, he was readmitted with massive ascites, and died of a multi-organ involvement of ATLL cells soon. ATLL cell line, KOB, was established from his ascites, which was resistant to anti-Fas antibody despite of abundant mFas expression. The KOB expressed two forms of Fas transcripts, the normal form and a truncated form. The truncated form lacked 20 bp at exon 9, resulting in a frame shift and the generation of a premature stop codon (Figure 12). The same mutation was detected in primary ascitic cells and peripheral blood cells but, surprisingly, not in lymph node cells although all these primary cells and KOB cell line are of the same clonal origin (Figure 13), which was confirmed by the integration pattern of HTLV-1 proviral DNA and TCR β chain gene rearrangement profile.

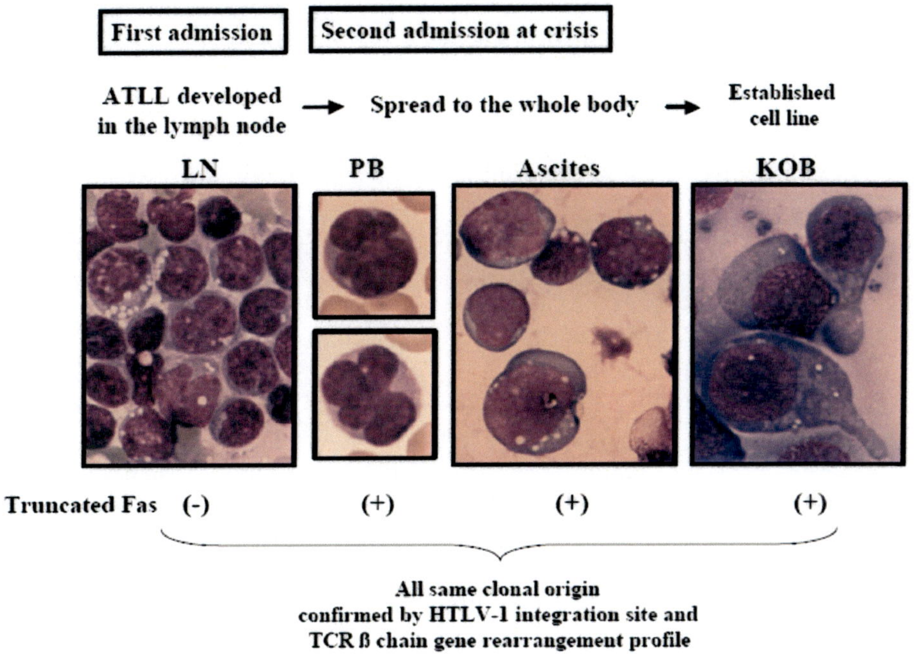

Figure 13. Origin of the truncated Fas Ref. no. [63]. The same truncated Fas is detected in peripheral blood ATLL cells and ascitic ATLL cells. However, no such product is detected in lymph node ATLL cells indicating that the mutation occurred after development of ATLL in the lymph node.

These results indicate that ATLL developed in the lymph node, acquired Fas gene mutation outside the lymph node, and then the subclone with the mutation spread to the whole body. Although KOB cells express normal mFas, IgM anti-Fas antibody does not induce apoptosis in this cell line. Since the trimerization of the death-signaling domain within the cytoplasmic region of Fas is essential for signal transduction, the truncated Fas of KOB may behave as a decoy and interfere with the trimerization of normal mFas in a competitive manner. We investigated this hypothesis using Jurkat cells that have normal mFas and are sensitive to IgM ant-Fas antibody. As expected, truncated Fas-transduced Jurkat cells become resistant to the antibody (Figure 14), supporting the theory that the truncated Fas inhibits Fas-mediated apoptosis signal by a dominant negative interference mechanism.

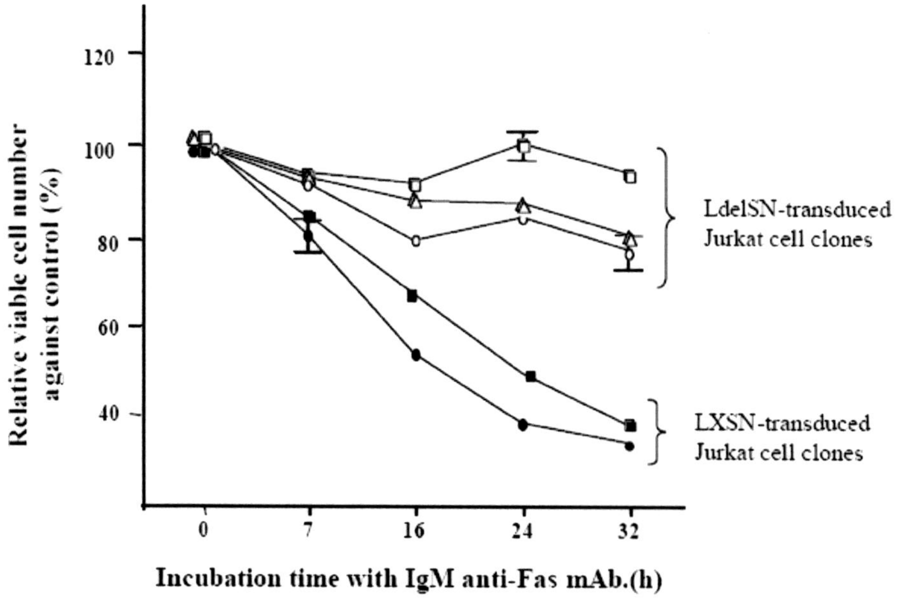

Figure 14. Acquisition of Fas resistance in the truncated Fas-transduced Jurkat cells Ref. no. [63]. Retroviral vector LdelSN that contains the truncated Fas cDNA was transduced into Jurkat cells. LdelSN-transduced Jurkat cell clones became resistant to anti-Fas antibody. In contrast, LXDN-transduced clones remained sensitive and apoptosis was induced.

The incidence of Fas gene mutation in ATLL differs by report depending on the method used. Among 47 patients examined by an RNase protection assay, three patients (6.4%) were identified to have mutations: a 5-bp deletion in exon 2, a 1-bp insertion in exon 2 and a loss of exon 4 [64]. In our study using RT-PCR followed by sequence analysis on seven low- or negative-mFas patients, the incidence was much higher and four patients (57.1%) showed mutations [59]. Two identical nucleotide substitutions, T297C and A416G, were found in two patients and normal control, which do not change the amino acid sequence and are supposed to be single nucleotide polymorphism. Substitution of G502A in exon3 was found in one patient, resulting in the amino acid substitution of 87Arg to Lys. Since this 87th Arg residue is one of the most important residues for the interaction between mFas and FasL [65], this mutation may cause mFas disable to bind with Fas-L. Two base pair deletions, Δ851A and Δ852G, were found in another patient that results in an altered reading frame in exon 8 with a premature termination. These products also should protect ATLL cells from the attack of FasL.

Other types of lymphoid malignancies such as NHL, myeloma, acute lymphoblastic leukemia, and chronic lymphocytic leukemia also show Fas gene mutations. Further more, solid tumors also show Fas gene mutation although the incidence is much smaller than that those observed in lymphoid malignancies. If these mutations play a role in tumor development and/or progression, they must be clustered in important regions for signal transduction. In fact, the majority of these mutations are located in the intracytoplasmic domain. Mutations are detected 89.5% in exons: 5.3% in exon2, 3.9% in exon 3, 3.9% in exon 4, 7.9% in exon 6, 2.6% in exon 7, 1.3% in exon 8, and 64.5% in exon 9, but only 10.5% in introns [66]. This high incidence in exon 9 is quite suggestive because it encodes death domain. Moreover, all mutations in introns occur at 5' or 3' splice sites and cause probably aberrant splicing, resulting in premature termination and production of truncated Fas. Thus, most of these mutations render mFas dysfunctional. We believe that this is not accidental but Fas gene mutations are closely involved in tumorigenesis. It is, however, unlikely that Fas gene mutation alone is enough to produce malignant phenotype because *lpr* mice usually do not develop malignancies. In this context, there is an interesting report. E mu L-myc/(lpr,lpr) mice that constitutively express the L-myc transgene in the lymphoid lineage show accelerated formation of T- and B-cell lymphoma when compared to normal E mu L-myc transgenics [67]. This report, together with our experience of an unique patient who acquired Fas gene mutation at his crisis phase, suggest that other event(s), besides the loss of mFas function, is required for the development of malignancies, and that Fas gene mutation is probably a late event for tumor progression.

4.5. Abnormality of Apoptosis Signaling Cascade

Even though cells have complete mFas, apoptosis signal is not transduced if there are any defects in the signal transduction pathway. Fas-associated phosphatase (FAP-1) interacts with the cytoplasmic domain of mFas and inhibits apoptosis signal [68]. FAP-1 expression is highest in tissues and cell lines that are relatively resistant to Fas-mediated cytotoxicity. It has been reported that HTLV-1 infected T cell lines derived from HAM patients show increased levels of FAP-1 expression compared to non-infected T cell lines and show Fas resistance [69]. However, our ATLL cell lines hardly express FAP-1 and the expression does not correlate with the Fas resistance [70]. In addition, since primary ATLL cells scarcely express FAP-1 transcript [71], it is unthinkable that FAP-1 renders Fas resistance in ATLL.

Pro-caspase-8 is an initiator of caspase cascade in Fas-mediated signal transduction. There are at least 7 alternatively spliced pro-caspase-8 isoforms beside intact pro-caspase-8 [35,72]. One of the isoforms Caspase-8L is generated by alternative splicing of intron 8, thereby carrying a 136-bp insertion and frame shift of the transcript resulting in a production of truncated pro-caspase-8 [72]. The caspase-8L keeps two repeats of DED but lacks proteolytic domain. Accordingly, it does not process pro-caspase-3 but rather inhibits the production of active caspase-8 by interfering with the binding of intact pro-caspasae-8 to FADD [73]. Since caspase-8L is predominantly produced in primary ATLL cells, the increased ratio of caspase-8L to intact pro-caspase-8 may indicate that it participates in the Fas-resistance mechanism of ATLL cells [74]. On the contrary, the ratios of caspase-8L to intact pro-caspase-8 are extremely low in ATLL cell lines, and ATLL cell lines hardly express caspase-8L. This discrepancy between primary cells and cell lines may be again interpreted that cell lines need not to produce caspase-8L anymore in culture condition, and hence they down regulated the expression.

Survivin, a member of IAP family, inhibits apoptosis by interfering with post-mitochondrial events. Although its expression is switched off during fetal development and is undetectable in terminally differentiated adult tissues, it becomes prominently expressed in all the most common human cancers of lung, colon, pancreas, prostate and breast [51], and hence it is believed that survivin plays an important role in oncogenesis. We examined survivin expression in 40 patients with ATLL and ATLL cell lines [71]. Survivin transcripts are found in all primary ATLL samples and ATLL cell lines but not in normal PBMC. The expression differs by ATLL subtypes and acute-type patients show significantly higher expression than chronic-type patients (Figure 15). Different from sFas and caspase-8L that are drastically down regulated in cell lines compare to primary cells, survivin expressions of ATLL cell lines are extremely high.

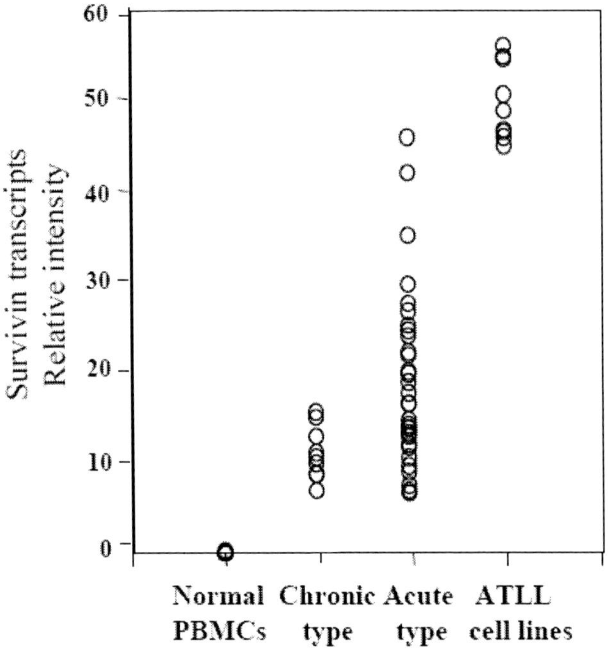

Figure 15. Semi-quantitative analysis of survivin transcripts in ATLL cells Ref. No. [71]. The level of the transcript is expressed as the relative value of amplified DNA per 10 μl of PCR reaction. Survivin is undetectable in normal PBMCs, variably detectable in ATLL samples with higher expression in acute-type ATLL than in chronic-type ATLL, and abundant expression in ATLL cell lines without exception.

The result suggests that survivin is needed not only for anti-apoptotic purpose but also for other unknown purpose as neoplastic cells such as cell division, because survivin localizes the mitotic apparatus. When patients are subdivided into two subgroups according to the survivin expression level, high expression group show significantly shorter survival times than low expression group (Figure 16). To evaluate its significance as an independent prognostic factor, we assessed several laboratory parameters including survivin that are known to be associated with prognosis by a Cox proportional hazards model. Consequently, the survivin expression remained as an independent prognostic factor. Prognostic significance of survivin expression has also been reported in other types of neoplasms. In the study of diffuse large B-cell lymphomas, the overall 5-year survival rate is significantly lower in patients with survivin expression than in those without [75]. A multivariate analysis identifies survivin expression as an independent predictive parameter on survival in this disease also. Because of its fixed expression in tumors, survivin may become a universal target for the treatment of malignancies. Resveratrol, a phytoalexin found in grapes and wine, is known to exhibit a wide range of pharmacological properties. It has been reported that resveratrol has cancer-chemopreventive activity (e.g., anti-initiation, anti-promotion, and anti-progression) and inhibits the growth of a number or cancer cell lines [76].

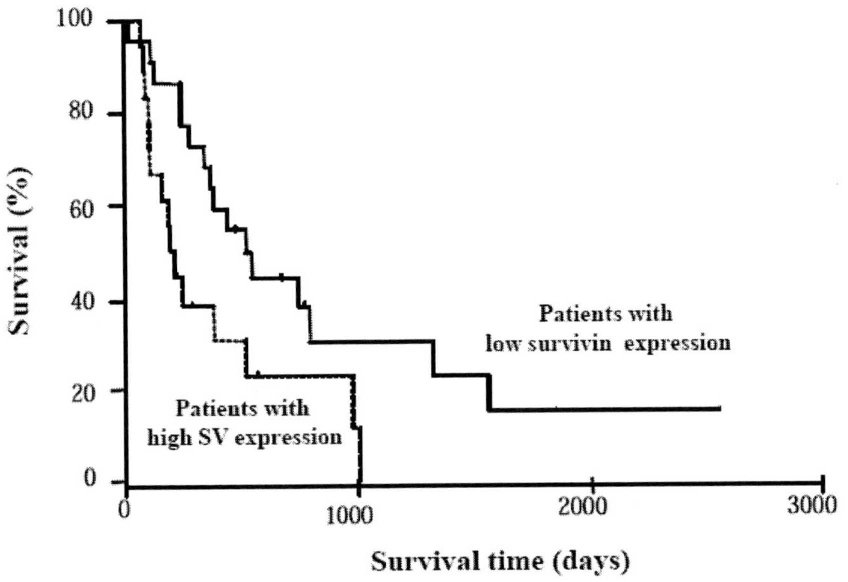

Figure 16. Overall survival curves of ATLL patients subdivided according to survivin expression status Ref. No. [71]. Patients with high survivin expression show significantly shorter survival times than patients with low survivin expression.

Indeed, resveratrol induces apoptosis in ATLL cell lines [77]. For understanding of its molecular mechanism, we chased the expression of several apoptosis modulators of ATLL cell lines after treatment with resveratrol. Resveratrol specifically decreased survivin expression, but other molecules such as Bcl-2, Bcl-xL, Bax and CIAP remained unchanged, indicating that survivin is required for ATLL cell survival and is one of the key targets of resveratrol. Since resveratrol is a common constituent of the human diet, it has little side effect at ordinary doses. Accordingly, resveratrol may become the best choice to prevent the development of ATLL from HTLV-1 carriers, although no such preventive trial has unfortunately been performed so far in Japan. Reinforcement of cellular antioxidant systems may also be attributable to the Fas-resistance in ATLL. In our study using ATLL cell lines, anti-Fas induces the formation of oxygen radicals in sensitive cell lines but not in resistant cell lines, and the resistant cell lines show increased concentrations of the intracellular antioxidant, glutathione, and the key enzyme for its synthesis, γ-glutamylcyteine synthetase [78]. Moreover, in the experiment using Fas-sensitive cell lines, addition of exogenous glutathione ester compound decreases the formation of 8-hydroxydeoxyguanosine, a biomarker of DNA damage caused by oxygen radicals.

4.6. Role of HTLV-1 in Apoptosis Resistance

HTLV-1 encodes an oncoprotein Tax, which is a potent deregulator of many kind cellular genes. Tax indirectly enhances the transcription of the genes for IL-2, IL-2R, IL-6, GM-CSF, PTHrP, *c-fos* etc. through cellular transcription factors such as CREB/ATF, NF-κB/Rel and SRF [79]. Tax, on the other hand, down-regulates the expression of DNA polymerase-β, a DNA repair enzyme, which event is probably related to the complex chromosomal abnormalities observed in primary ATLL cells. These mechanisms are supposed to be crucially involved in the development of ATLL. Tax also affects the expression of apoptosis modulators. It has been reported that Tax represses transcription of the Bax gene, a gene whose protein product induces apoptosis by accelerating the releases of cytochrome C from mitochondria into the cytosol [80]. In our study, however, Tax does not affect the expression of Bax [81], and there is no significant difference in the expression levels of Bax transcripts between primary ATLL ells and normal PBMCs denying the possibility of its role in ATLL cell survival [82]. Bcl-xL, in contrast to Bax, inhibits the release of cytochrome C and protects cells from apoptotic death. Bcl-xL promoter is transactivated by Tax, and Tax expressing T cell lines show higher levels of Bcl-xL transcripts than HTLV-1 negative T cell lines [81]. Moreover, primary ATLL cells express higher levels of Bcl-xL compared to normal PBMCs. In the study of retinoic acids (RAs)-induced apoptosis of ATLL cells, RAs specifically decreases Bcl-xL expression without affecting Bcl-2 expression [83], which indicates that Bcl-xL is important for ATLL cell survival and that apoptosis signal induced by RAs is transduced by the down regulation of Bcl-xL. The anti-apoptosis effect of tax is also studied in JPX-9 cells [84]. JPX-9 is a Jurkat cell subclone generated by the stable introduction of a tax expession-plasmid vector. It is possible to induce tax with CdCl2 treatment in this cell line. Tax-positive JPX-9 cells express apparently increased level of Bcl-xL than tax-negative JPX-9 cells. Moreover, tax-positive JPX-9 cells are more resistant to both receptor-mediated apoptosis signal (induced by anti-Fas and tumor necrosis factor-related apoptosis-inducing ligand) and chemical-induced apoptosis signal (induced by pyrrolidine dithiocarbamate, etoposide, and staurosporine) compare to tax-negative JPX-9 cells. These results further support the idea that Bcl-xL is one of the major factors producing apoptosis resistance in ATLL cells. In the study of gene expression profiles of HTLV-1-immortalized T cells using gene array, Harhaj et al. found that Tax deregulated a number of genes that modulate apoptosis signal [85]. Compare to normal PHA-activated T cells, nine apoptosis inhibitors are increased but three apoptosis inducers are decreased in HTLV-1-immortalized T cells. Especially, the level of I-309, a chemokine known to show autocrine anti-apoptotic stimulation of cultured ATLL cells [86], is 62.4-fold increased, and the level of IAP-1 is 20.7-fold increased. Another group performed similar study and disclosed that Bcl-2 was 4 to 7-fold increased in HTLV-1-infected cells compare to activated normal lymphocytes [87]

4.7. Proteasome Inhibitors Overcome Fas Resistance

It is possible to invalid Fas resistant mechanism in ATLL cells by proteasome inhibitors. Proteasome is responsible for the degradation of proteins with short half-lives such as transcription factors and cell cycle regulatory proteins. For instance, proteasome degradates phosphorylated and ubiquitinated NF-κB inhibitory protein IκBα, then the freed NF-κB migrates from the cytoplasm into the nucleus and plays its role as a transcription factor. We found that lactacystin (LC), a microbial metabolite known to specifically inhibits the proteasome [88], induced apoptosis in Fas-resistant ATLL cell lines [89]. Fas-resistant ATLL cell subclones RSO4 and RST1 are obtained from their parental Fas-sensitive cell lines SO4 and ST1 by a long-term culture in the presence of IgM anti-Fas monoclonal antibody (Figure 17).

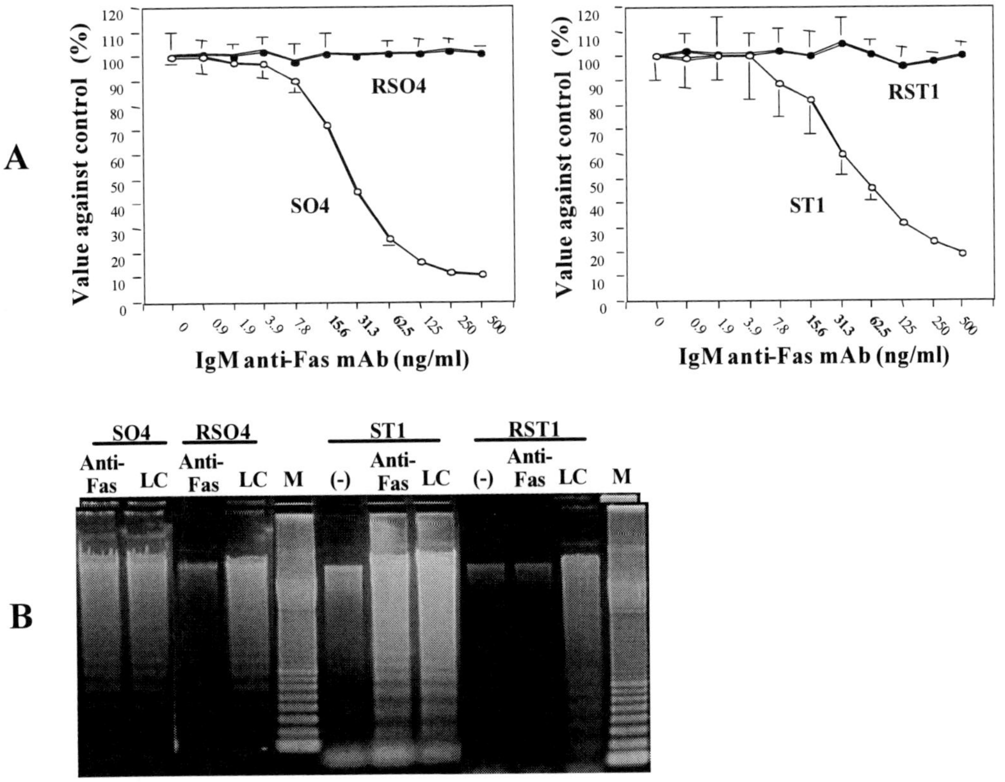

Figure 17. Sensitivity of Fas-resistant ATLL cell lines to proteasome inhibitor, lactacystin (LC) Ref. No. [88]. RSO4 and RST1 are Fas-resistant subclones of SO4 and ST1, respectively, and are hardly induced apoptosis by IgM anti-Fas monoclonal antibody (A). LC overcomes the resistance and induces DNA fragmentation in both sensitive and resistant cell lines (B).

LC and synthesized proteasome inhibitory peptide MG-115 (ZLLnV-CHO) induces the activation of pro-caspase-8, pro-caspase-3 and pro-caspase-6 in an identical manner to Fas-mediated apoptosis (Figure 18).

Thus, inhibition of the proteasome function may become a new strategy for the treatment of ATLL. Actually, a therapeutic potential of another proteasome inhibitor PS-341, an agent currently used for the treatment of multiple myeloma patients, has been tried in ATLL animal model. PS-341 prolongs the survival of ATLL tumor-bearing mice when used in combination with humanized anti-CD25 monoclonal antibody anti-Tac [90]. PS-341 decreases NF-κB DNA binding activity by preventing the degradation of IκBα, thereby probably inhibiting the production of anti-apoptotic molecules.

A

B

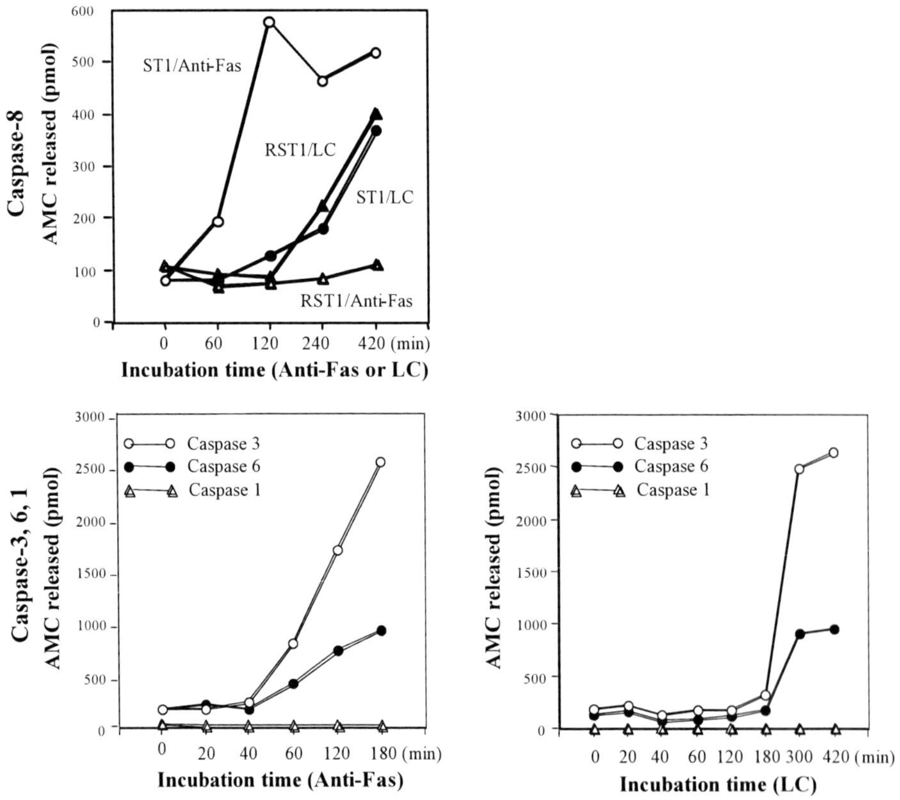

Figure 18. Activation of caspases by lactacystin (LC) Ref. No. [88]. IgM anti-Fas antibody activates caspase-8 in ST1 but not in RST1 (A). LC activates caspase-8 irrespective of Fas sensitivity with a delayed reaction time. LC activates caspase-3 and caspase-6 in an identical manner to Fas-induction (B). Both inducers do not activate caspase-1.

5. Conclusion

ATLL cells are destined to express mFas from the birth because of their cell origin as activated T-cells, and hence they have to establish effective defense mechanisms against natural Fas-L for survival. As a result, the developed ATLL cells have become crafty to escape from apoptosis and possess many devices to inhibit apoptosis cascade. Integration of HTLV-1 in ATLL cells is favorable for this purpose, and its product tax transactivates the genes for apoptosis inhibitors. These anti-apoptotic machineries of ATLL cells are summarized in Figure 19. Since many anticancer drugs kill tumor cells by inducing a common apoptotic program, abnormality of apoptotic signal can also produce multidrug resistance. For instance, it has been reported that Bcl-2 and Bcl-xL overexpression protects cells from the cytotoxic effect of doxorubicin, etoposide, and oxaliplatin in the Jurkat cell model [91], and Bcl-2 and Bcl-xL antisense oligonucleotides not only directly induce apoptosis but also sensitize mesothelioma cells to the cytostatic effect of cisplatin and gemicitabine [92]. In addition, inhibition of survivin expression by using antisense technology and ribozymes not only triggers apoptosis but also enhances chemotherapy-induced and radiotherapy-induced apoptosis in tumor cells but not in normal cells [93,94]. ATLL cells express all these apoptosis inhibitors and the expression correlates with disease progression and prognosis. Strong chemoresistance of ATLL cells and poor prognosis may thus, at least in part, be attributable to this anti-apoptotic machinery. Strategies based on the understanding of this machinery are needed for successful treatment of ATLL, and the combinatory use of the agents that inactivate this machinery with other anticancer drugs might improve the clinical outcome of ATLL.

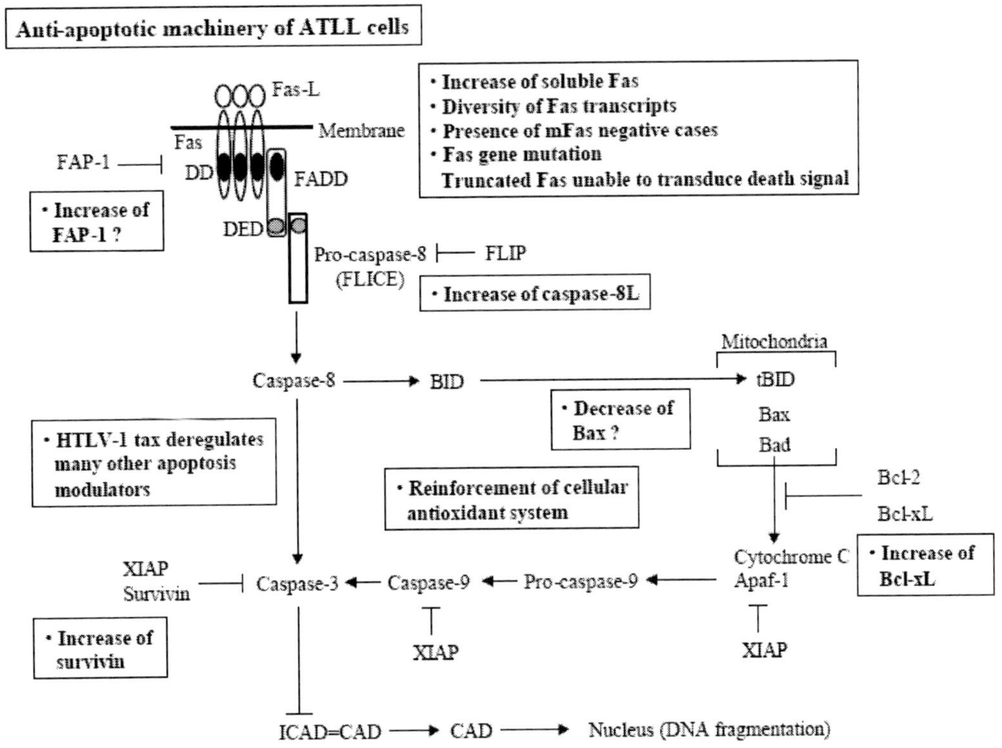

Figure 19. Anti-apoptotic machinery of ATLL cells. All anti-apoptotic devices of ATLL cells described in this paper are schematically summarized in this figure.

REFERENCES

[1] Uchiyama T, Yodoi J, Sagawa K, Takatsuki K, Uchino H: Adult T-cell leukemia: Clinical and hematologic features of 16 cases. *Blood 50*:481-492, 1977.

[2] Yamada Y: Phenotypic and functional analysis of leukemic cells from 16 patients with adult T-cell leukemia/lymphoma. *Blood 61*:192-199, 1983.

[3] Uchiyama T, Hori T, Tsudo M, Wano Y, Umadome H, Tamori S, Yodoi J, Maeda M, Sawami H, Uchino H: Interleukin-2 receptor (Tac antigen) expressed on adult T cell leukemia cells. *J. Clin. Invest. 76*:446-453, 1985.

[4] Poiesz BJ, Ruscetti FW, Gazdor AF, Bunn PA, Minna JD, Gallo RC: Detection and isolation of type C retrovirus particles from fresh and cultured lymphocytes of a patient with cutaneous T-cell lymphoma. *Proc. Natl. Acad. Sci. USA 77*:7415-7419, 1980.

[5] Hinuma Y, Nagata K, Hanaoka M, Nakai M, Matsumoto T, Kinoshita K, Shirakawa S, Miyoshi I: Adult T-cell leukemia: Antigen in an ATL cell line and detection of antibodies to the antigen in human sera. *Proc. Natl. Acad. Sci. USA 78*:6476-6480, 1981.

[6] Yoshida M, Seiki M, Yamaguchi K, Takatsuki K: Monoclonal integration of human T-cell leukemia provirus in all primary tumors of adult T-cell leukemia suggests causative role of human T-cell leukemia virus in the disease. *Proc. Natl. Acad. Sci. USA 81*:2534-2537, 1982.

[7] Hinuma Y, Komoda H, Chosa T, Kondo T, Kohakura M, Takenaka T, Kikuchi M, Ichimaru M, Yunoki K, Sato, Matsuo R, Kakiuchi Y, Uchino H, Hanaoka M: Antibodies to adult T-cell leukemia-virus-associated antigen (ATLA) in sera from patients with ATL and controls in Japan: a nation-wide sero-epidemiologic study. *Int. J. Cancer. 29*:631-635, 1982.

[8] Kinoshita K, Hino S, Amagasaki T, Ikeda S, Yamada Y, Suzuyama J, Momita S, Toriya K, Kamihira S, Ichimaru M: Demonstration of adult T-cell leukemia virus antigen in mild from three sero-positive mothers. *Jpn. J. Cancer Res.* (Gann) *75*:103-105, 1984.

[9] Hino S, Yamaguchi K, Katamine S, Sugiyama H, Amagasaki T, Kinoshita K, Yoshida Y, Doi H, Tsuji Y, Miyamoto T: Mother-to-child transmission of human T-cell leukemia virus type-1. *Jpn. J. Cancer Res. 76*:474-480, 1985.

[10] Gessain A, Barin F, Vernant JC, Gout O, Maurs L Calender A, de The G: Antibodies to human T-lymphotropic virus type-1 in patients with tropical spastic paraparesis. *Lancet 2*(8452):407-410, 1985.

[11] Osame M, Usuku K, Izumo S, Ijichi N, Amitani H, Igata A, Matsumoto M, Tara M: HTLV-1 associated myelopathy, a new clinical entity. *Lancet 1*(8488):1031-1032, 1986.

[12] Yamada Y, Kamihira S, Murata K, Yamamura M, Maeda T, Tsukasaki K, Jubashi T, Atogami S, Sohda H, Taguchi T, Tomonaga M: Frequent hepatic involvement in adult T-cell leukaemia: comparison with non-Hodgkin's lymphoma. *Leuk. Lymphoma 26*:327-335, 1997.

[13] Utsunomiya A, Hanada S, Terada A, Kodama M, Uematsu T, Tsukasa S, Hashimoto S, Tokunaga M: Adult T-cell leukemia with leukemia infiltration into the gastrointestinal tract. *Cancer 61*:824-828, 1988.

[14] Teshima T, Akashi K, Shibuya T, Taniguchi S, Okamura T, Harada M, Sumida I, Hanada M, Niho Y: Central nervous system involvement in adult T-cell leukemia/lymphoma. *Cancer 65*:327-332, 1990.

[15] Shimoyama M and members of The Lymphoma Study Group (1984-1987): Diagnostic criteria and classification of clinical subtypes of adult T-cell leukaemia-lymphoma: a report from The Lymphoma Study Group (1984-1987). *Br. J. Haematol. 79*:428-437, 1991.

[16] Yamada Y, Tomonaga M, Fukuda H, Hanada S, Utsunomiya A, Tara M, Sano M, Ikeda S, Takatsuki K, Kozuru M, Araki K, Kawano F, Niimi M, Tobinai K, Hotta T, Shimoyama M and other members of The Lymphoma Study Group of The Japan Clinical Oncology Group (1994-96). *Br. J. Haematol. 113*:375-382, 2001.

[17] Uchiyama T, Hori T, Tsudo M, Wano Y, Umadome H, Tamori S, Yodoi J, Maeda M, Sawami H, Uchino H: Interleukin-2 receptor (Tac antigen) expressed on adult T cell leukemia cells. *J. Clin. Invest. 76*:446-453, 1985.

[18] Yamada Y, Sugawara K, Hata T, Tsuruta K, Moriuchi R, Maeda T, Atogami S, Murata K, Fujimoto K, Kohno T, Tsukasaki K, Tomonaga M, Hirakata Y, Kamihira S: Interleukin-15 (IL-15) can replace the IL-2 signal in IL-2-dependent adult T-cell leukemia (ATL) cell lines: Expression of IL-15 receptor alpha on ATL cells. *Blood 91*:4265-4272, 1998.

[19] Baba H, Yamada Y, Mori N, Hayashibara T, Harasawa H, Tsuruda K, Sugahara K, Soda H, Takasaki Y, Tawara M, Hirakata Y, Tomonaga M, Kamihira S: Multiple gamma c-receptor expression in adult T-cell leukemia. *Eur. J. Haematol. 68*:362-369, 2002.

[20] Hasegawa H, Nomura T, Kohno M, Tateishi N, Suzuki Y, Maeda N, Fujisawa R, Yoshie O, Fujita S: Increased chemokine receptor CCR7/EBI1 expression enhances the infiltration of lymphoid organs by adult T-cell leukemia cells. *Blood 95*:30-38, 2000.

[21] Yoshie O, Fujisawa R, Nakayama T, Harasawa H, Tago H, Izawa D, Hieshima K, Tatsumi Y, Matsushima K, Hasegawa H, Kanamaru A, Kamihira S, Yamada Y: Frequent expression of CCR4 in adult T-cell leukemia and human T-cell leukemia virus type 1-transformed T cells. *Blood 99*:1505-1511, 2002.

[22] Miyawaki T, Uehara T, Nibu R, Tsuji T, Yachie A, Yonehara S, Taniguchi N: Differential expression of apoptosis-related Fas andtigen on lymphocyte subpopulations in human peripheral blood. *J. Immunol. 149*:3753-3758, 1992.

[23] Kamihira S, Yamada Y, Hirakata Y, Tsuruda K, Sugahara K, Tomonaga M, Maeda T, Tsukasaki K, Atogami S, Kobayashi N: Quantitative characterization and potential function of membrane Fas/APO-1 (CD95) receptors on leukaemic cells from chronic B and T lymphoid leukaemias. *Br. J. Haematol. 99*:858-865, 1997.

[24] Itoh N, Yonehara S, Ishii A, Yonehara M, Mizushima S, Sameshima M, Hase A, Seto Y, Nagata S: The polypeptide encoded by the cDNA for human cell surface antigen Fas can mediate apoptosis. *Cell 66*:233-243, 1991.

[25] Nagata S, Goldstein P: The Fas death factor. *Science 267*:1449-1456, 1995.

[26] Cheng J, Zhou T, Liu C, Shapiro JP, Brauer MJ, Kiefer MC, Barr PJ, Mountz JD: Protection from Fas-mediated apoptosis by a soluble form of the Fas molecule. *Science 263*:1759-1762, 1994.

[27] Liu C, Cheng J, Mountz JD: Differential expression of human Fas mRNA species upon peripheral blood mononuclear cell activation. *Biochem. J. 310*:957-963, 1995.

[28] Papoff G, Cascino I, Eramo A, Starace G, Lynch DH, Ruberti G: An N-terminal domain shared by Fas/Apo-1 (CD95) soluble variants prevents cell death in vitro. *J. Immunol. 156*:4622-4630, 1996.

[29] Casino I, Papoff G, Eramo A, Ruberti G: Soluble Fas/Apo-1 splicing variants and apoptosis. *Frontiers in Bioscience 1*:d12-18, 1996.

[30] Hughes DPM, Crispe IN: A naturally occurring soluble isoforms of murine Fas generated by alternative splicing. *J. Exp. Med. 182*:1395-1401, 1995

[31] Heaney ML, Golde DW: Soluble cytokine receptors. *Blood 87*:847-857, 1996

[32] Van Zee KJ, Kohno T, Fischer E, Rock CS, Moldawer LL, Lowry SF: Tumor necrosis factor soluble receptors circulate during experimental and clinical inflammation and can protect against excessive tumor necrosis factor alpha in vitro and in vivo. *Proc. Natl. Acad. Sci. USA 89*:4845-4849, 1992

[33] Knipping E, Debatin KM, Stricker K, Heilig B, Eder A, Krammer PH: Identification of soluble APO-1 in supernatants of human B- and T-cell lines and increased serum levels in B- and T-cell leukemias. *Blood 85*:1562-1569, 1995

[34] Chinnaiyan AM, O'Rourke K, Tewari M, Dixit VM: FADD, a novel death domain-containing protein, interacts with the death domain of Fas and initiates apoptosis. *Cell 81*:505-512, 1995.

[35] Boldin MP, Goncharov TM, Goltsev YV, Wallach D: Involvement of MACH, a novel MORT1/FADD-interacting protease, in Fas/APO-1- and TNF receptor-induced cell death. *Cell 85*:803-815, 1996.

[36] Mizio M, Chinnaiyan AM, Kischkel FC, O'Rourke K, Shevchenko A, Ni J, Scaffidi C, Bretz JD, Zhang M, Gentz R, Mann M, Krammeer PH, Peter ME, Dixit VM: FLICE, a novel FADD-homologous ICE/CED-3-like protease, is recruited to the CD95 (Fas/APO-1) death-inducing signaling complex. *Cell 85*:817-827, 1996.

[37] Krammer PH: CD95's deadly mission in the immune system. *Nature 407*:789-795, 2000.

[38] Scaffidi C, Fulda S, Srinivasan A, Friesen C, Li F, Tomaselli KJ, Debatin KM, Krammer PH, Peter ME. Two CD95 (APO-1/Fas) signaling pathways. *EMBO J. 17*:1675-1687, 1998.

[39] Li H, Zhu H, Xu CJ, Yuan J: Cleavage of BID by caspase 8 mediates the mitochondrial damage in the Fas pathway of apoptosis. *Cell 94*:491-501, 1998.

[40] Maher S, Toomey D, Condron C, Bouchier-Hayes D: Activation-induced cell death: The controversial role of Fas and Fas ligand in immune privilege and tumor counterattack. *Immunol. Cell. Biol. 80*:131-137, 2002.

[41] Zou H, Henzel WJ, Liu X, Lutschg A, Wang X: Apaf-1, a human protein homologous to C. elegans CED-4, participates in cytochrome c-dependent activationo f caspase-3. *Cell 90*:405-413, 1997.

[42] Enari M, Sakahira H, Yokoyama H, Okawa K, Iwamatsu A, Nagata S: A caspase-activated DNase that degrades DNA during apoptosis, and its inhibitor ICAD. *Nature 391*:43-50, 1998.

[43] Liu X, Zou H, Slaughter C, Wang X: DFF, a heterodimeric protein that functions downstream of caspase-3 to trigger DNA fragmentation during apoptosis. *Cell 89*:175-184, 1997.

[44] Sakahira H, Enari M, Nagata S: Cleavage of CAD inhibitor in CAD activation and DNA degradation during apoptosis. *Nature 391*:96-99, 1998.

[45] Sato T, Irie S, Kitada S, Reed JC: FAP-1: a protein tyrosine phosphatase that associates with Fas. *Science 268*:411-415, 1995.

[46] Irmler M, Thome M, Hahne M, Schneider P, Hofmann K, Steiner V, Bodmer JL, Schroter M, Burns K, Mattmann C, Rimoldi D, French LE, Tschopp J: Inhibition of death receptor signals by cellular FLIP. *Nature 388*:190-195, 1997.

[47] Deveraux QL, Takahashi R, Salvesen GS, Reed JC: X-linked IAP is a direct inhibitor of cell-death proteases. *Nature 388*:300-304, 1997.

[48] Bratton SB, Walker G, Srinivasula SM, Sun XM, Butterworth M, Alnemri ES, Cohen GM: Recruitment, activation and retention of caspases-9 and -3 by Apaf-1 apoptosome and associated XIAP complexes. *EMBO J. 20*:998-1009, 2001.

[49] Tamm I, Wang Y, Sausville E, Scudiero DA, Vigna N, Oltersdorf T, Reed JC: IAP family protein survivin inhibits caspase activity and apoptosis induced by Fas (CD95), Bax, caspases, and anticancer drugs. *Cancer Res. 58*:5315-5320, 1998.

[50] Li F, Ambrosini G, Chu EY, Plescia J, Tognin S, Marchisio PC, Altieri DC: Control of apoptosis and mitotic spindle checkpoint by survivin. *Nature 396*:580-584, 1998.

[51] Ambrosini G, Adida C, Altieri DC: A novel anti-apoptosis gene, survivin, expressed in cancer and lymphoma. *Nat. Med. 3*:917-921, 1997.

[52] Debatin KM, Goldmann CK, Bamford R, Waldmann TA, Krammer PH: Monoclonal-antibody-mediated apoptosis in adult T-cell leukaemia. *Lancet 335*(8688):497-500, 1990.

[53] Debatin KM, Goldmann CK, Waldmann TA, Krammer PH: APO-1-induced apoptosis of leukemia cells from patients with adult T-cell leukemia. *Blood 81*:2972-2977, 1993.

[54] Kamihira S, Yamada Y, Tomonaga M, Sugahara K, Tsuruda K: Discrepant expression of membrane and soluble isoforms of Fas (CD95/APO-1) in adult T-cell leukaemia: soluble Fas isoform is an independent risk factor for prognosis. *Br. J. Haematol. 107*:851-860, 1999.

[55] Shimamoto Y, Kikuchi M, Funai N, Suga K, Matsuzaki M, Yamaguchi M: Spontaneous regression in adult T-cell leukemia/lymphoma. *Cancer 72*:735-740, 1993.

[56] Sugahara K, Yamada Y, Hirakata Y, Matsuo Y, Tsuruda K, Tomonaga M, Maeda T, Atogami S, Tsukasaki K, Kamihira S: Soluble and membrane isoforms of Fas/CD95 in fresh adult T-cell leukemia (ATL) cells and ATL cell lines. *Int. J. Cancer 72*:128-132, 1997.

[57] Niitsu N, Sasaki K, Umeda M: A high serum soluble Fas/APO-1 level is associated with a poor outcome of aggressive non-Hodgkin's lymphoma. *Leukemia 13*:1434-1440, 1999.

[58] Ueno T, Toi M, Tominaga T: Circulating soluble Fas concentration in breast cancer. *Clin. Cancer Res. 5*:3529-3533, 1999.

[59] Tawara M, Maeda T, Yamada Y, Harasawa H, Tsuruda K, Sugahara K, Moriuchi R, Tomonaga M, Kamihira S: Aberrant processing of Fas transcripts in adult T-cell leukemia: a possible role in tumor cell survival. *Cancer Lett. 193*:235-242, 2003.

[60] Nagata S, Suda T: Fas and Fas ligand: lpr and gld mutations. *Immunol. Today. 16*:39-43, 1995.

[61] Fisher GH, Rosenberg FJ, Straus SE, Dale JK, Middleton LA, Lin AY, Strober W, Lenardo MJ, Puck JM: Dominant interfering Fas gene mutations impair apoptosis in a human autoimmune lymphoproliferative syndrome. *Cell 81*:935-946, 1995.

[62] Rieux-Laucat F, Le Deist F, Hivroz C, Roberts IA, Debatin KM, Fisher A, de Villartay JP: Mutations in Fas associated with human lymphoproliferative syndrome and autoimmunity. *Science 268*:1347-1349, 1995.

[63] Maeda T, Yamada Y, Moriuchi R, Sugahara K, Tsuruda K, Joh T, Atogami S, Tsukasaki K, Tomonaga M, Kamihira S: Fas gene mutation in the progression of adult T cell leukemia. *J. Exp. Med. 189*:1063-1071, 1999.

[64] Tamiya S, Etoh K, Suzushima H, Takatsuki K, Matsuoka M: Mutations of CD95 (Fas/Apo-1) gene in adult T-cell leukemia cells. *Blood 91*:3935-3942, 1998.

[65] Bajorath J: Identification of the ligand-binding site in Fas (CD95) and analysis of Fas-ligand interactions. *Proteins 35*:475-482, 1999.

[66] Maeda T, Kamihira S: The role of mutated Fas genes in tumorigenesis. *Adv. Clin. Chem. 36*:109-137, 2001.

[67] Zornig M, Grzeschiczek A, Kowalski MB, Hartmann KU, Moroy T: Loss of Fas/Apo-1 receptor accelerates lymphomagenesis in E mu L-myc transgenic mice but not in animals infected with MoMuLV. *Oncogene 10*:2397-2401, 1995.

[68] Sato T, Irie S, Kitada S, Reed JC: FAP-1: a protein tyrosine phosphatase that associates with Fas. *Science 268*:411-415, 1995.

[69] Arai M, Kannagi M, Matsuoka M, Sato T, Yamamoto N, Fujii M: Expression of FAP-1 (Fas-associated phosphatase) and resistance to Fas-mediated apoptosis in T cell lines derived from human T cell leukemia virus type 1-associated myelopathy/tropical spastic paraparesis patients. *AIDS Res. Hum. Retroviruses 14*:261-267, 1998.

[70] Yamada Y, Sugahara K, Tsuruda K, Nohda K, Hata T, Maeda T, Honda M, Tawara M, Hayashibara T, Joh T, Tomonaga M, Miyazaki Y, Kamihira S: Fas-resistance in ATL cell lines not associated with HTLV-1 or FAP-1 production. *Cancer Lett. 147*:215-219, 1999.

[71] Kamihira S, Yamada Y, Hirakata Y, Tomonaga M, Sugahara K, Hayashi T, Dateki N, Harasawa H, Nakayama K: Aberrant expression of caspase cascade regulatory genes in adult T-cell leukaemia: survivin is an important determinant for prognosis. *Br. J. Haematol. 114*:63-69, 2001.

[72] Horiuchi T, Himeji D, Tsukamoto H, Harashima S, Hashimura C, Hayashi K: Dominant expression of a novel splice variant of caspase-8 in human peripheral blood lymphocytes. *Biochem. Biophys. Res. Commun. 272*:877-881, 2000.

[73] Himeji D, Horiuchi T, Tsukamoto H, Hayashi K, Watanabe T, Harada M: Characterization of caspase-8L: a novel isoform of caspase-8 that behaves as an inhibitor of the caspase cascade. *Blood 99*:4070-4078, 2002.

[74] Sugahara K, Hayashi T, Dateki N, Hirakata Y, Harasawa H, Tomonaga M, Yamada Y, Kamihira S: Possible attenuation of Fas-mediated signaling by dominant expression of caspase-8 aberrant isoform in adult T-cell leukemia cells. *Int. J. Hematol. 76*:50-54, 2002.

[75] Adida C, Haioun C, Gaulard P, Lepage E, Morel P, Briere J, Dombret H, Reyes F, Diebold J, Gisselbrecht C, Salles G, Altieri DC, Molina TJ: Prognostic significance of survivin expression in diffuse large B-cell lymphomas. *Blood 96*:1921-1925, 2000.

[76] Jang M, Cai L, Udeani GO, Slowing KV, Thomas CF, Beecher CW, Fong HH, Farnsworth NR, Kinghorn AD, Mehta RG, Moon RC, Pezzuto JM: Cancer chemopreventive activity of resveratrol, a natural product derived from grapes. *Science 275*:218-220, 1997.

[77] Hayashibara T, Yamada Y, Nakayama S, Harasawa H, Tsuruda K, Sugahara K, Miyanishi T, Kamihira S, Tomonaga M, Maita T. Resveratrol induces downregulation in survivin expression and apoptosis in HTLV-1-infectred cell lines. A prospective agent for adult T cell leukemia chemotherapy. *Nutr. Cancer 44*:192-201, 2002.

[78] Kohno T, Yamada Y, Hata T, Mori H, Yamamura M, Tomonaga M, Urata Y, Goto S, Kondo T: Relation of oxidative stress and glutathione synthesis to CD95(Fas/APO-1)-mediated apoptosis of adult T cell leukemia cells. *J. Immunol. 156*:4722-4728, 1996.

[79] Uchiyama T: Human T cell leukemia virus type 1 (HTLV-1) and human diseases. *Annu. Rev. Immunol. 15*:15-37, 1997.

[80] Brauweiler A, Garrus JE, Reed JC, Nyborg JK: Repression of bax gene expression by the THLV-1 Tax protein: implications for suppression of apoptosis in virally infected cells. *Virology 231*:135-140, 1997.

[81] Mori N, Fujii M, Cheng G, Ikeda S, Yamasaki Y, Yamada Y, Tomonaga M, Yamamoto N: Human T-cell leukemia virus type 1 tax protein induces the expression of anti-apoptotic gene Bcl-xL in human T-cells through nuclear factor-kappaB and c-AMP responsive element binding protein pathways. *Virus Genes 22*:297-287, 2001.

[82] Mori N, Yamada Y, Hata T, Ikeda S, Yamasaki Y, Tomonaga M, Yamamoto N: Expression of survivin in HTLV-1-infected T-cell lines and primary ATL cells. *Biochem. Biophys. Res. Commun 282*:1110-1113, 2001.

[83] Fujimura S, Suzumiya J, Yamada Y, Kuroki M, Ono J: Down regulation of Bcl-xL and activation of caspases during retinoic acid-induced apoptosis in an adult T-cell *Leukemia Cell Line.*

[84] Nakashima K, Kawakami A, Hida A, Yamasaki S, Nakamura H, Kamachi M, Miyashita T, Tanaka F, Izumi Y, Tamai M, Ida H, Furuyama M, Koji T, Nakamura T, Migita K, Origuchi T, Eguchi K: Protection of mitochondrial perturbation by human

T-lymphotropic virus type 1 tax through induction f Bcl-xL expression. *J. Lab. Clin. Med. 142*:341-347, 2003.

[85] Harhaj EW, Good L, Xiao G, Sun SC: Gene expression profiles in HTLV-immortalized T cells: deregulated expression of gene involved in apoptosis regulation. *Oncogene 18*:1341-1349, 1999.

[86] Ruckes T, Saul D, Van Snick J, Hermine O, Grassmann R: Autocrine antiapoptotic stimulation of cultured adult T-cell leukemia cells by overexpression of the chemokine I-309. *Blood 98*:1150-1159, 2001.

[87] Pise-Masison CA, Radonovich M, Mahieux R, Chatterjee P, Whiteford C, Duvall J, Guillerm C, Gessain A, Brqady JN: Transcription profile of cells infected with human T-cell leukemia virus type 1 compared with activated lymphocytes. *Cancer Res. 62*:3562-3571, 2002.

[88] Fenteany G, Standaert RF, Lane WS, Choi S, Corey EJ, Schreiber SL: Inhibition of proteasome activities and subunit-specific amino-terminal threonine modification by lactacystin. *Science 268*:726-731, 1995.

[89] Yamada Y, Sugahara K, Tsuruda K, Nohda K, Mori N, Hata T, Maeda T, Hayashibara T, Joh T, Honda M, Tawara M, Tomonaga M, Miyazai Y, Kamihira S: Lactacystin activates FLICE (caspase 8) protease and induces apoptosis in Fas-resistant adult T-cell leukemia cell lines. *Eur. J. Haematol. 64*:315-322, 2000.

[90] Tan C, Waldmann TA: Proteasome inhibitor PS-341, a potential therapeutic agent for adult T-cell leukemia. *Cancer Res. 62*:1083-1086, 2002.

[91] Ballestrero A, Nencioni A, Boy D, Rocco I, Garuti A, Mela GS, Van Parijs L, Brossart P, Wesselborg S Patrone F: Tumor necrosis factor-related apoptosis-inducing ligand cooperates with anticancer drugs to overcome chemoresistance in antiapoptotic Bcl-2 family members expressing Jurkat cells. *Clin. Cancer Res. 10*:1463-1470, 2004.

[92] Hopkins-Donaldson S, Cathomas R, Simoes-Wust AP, Kurtz S, Belyanskaya L, Stahel RA, Zangemeister-Wittke U: Induction of apoptosis and chemosensitization of mesothelioma cells by Bcl-2 and Bcl-xL antisense treatment. *Int. J. Cancer. 106*:160-166, 2003.

[93] Altieri DC: Validating survivin as a cancer therapeutic target. *Natl. Rev. Cancer 3*:46-54, 2003.

[94] Pennati M, Binda M, Colella G, Folini M, Citti L, Villa R Daidone MG, Zaffaroni N: Radiosensitation of human melanoma cells by ribozyme mediated inhibition of survivin expression. *J. Invest. Dermatol. 120*:648-654, 2003.

In: Cancer Research Perspectives
Editor: Larissa S. Pereira, pp. 219-231
ISBN 978-1-60021-980-1

Chapter VII

Inhibition of RNA Synthesis by 5-Fluorouridine Accounts for its Cytotoxicity on Colorectal Cancer Cells in Vitro

***Pochi R. Subbarayan*[1,*], *Paul Braunschweiger*[2] *and Bach Ardalan*[1]**
Department of Medicine, [1]Division of Hematology and Oncology, [2]Division of Radiation Oncology, University of Miami, Miller School of Medicine, Miami, FL – 33136, USA.

Abstract

Pyrimidine analogue 5-fluorouracil (5-FU) is a standard chemotherapeutic agent in treating colorectal cancer (CRC). Occasionally fluorodeoxyuridine (FUdR) has been used; however, the third analogue fluoro uridine (FUR) has never been used in the clinic. In this study we compared the anti-tumorigenic activity of the above agents *in vitro* and *in vivo*. The cultured cells were protected from the cytotoxic effects of the FUdR by deoxy thymidine and FUR by uridine. Cytotoxicity of these agents as analyzed *in vitro* by cell culture demonstrated FUR to be the most potent anti-tumor agent. *In vivo* we tested the effect of 5-FU and FUR on tumor bearing mice. Intra-peritoneal administration of 5-FU or FUR proved that FUR is fifteen times more effective than 5-FU. Severe inhibitory effect of FUR on TS expression and its RNA mediated cell kill may explain its superiority over the other two fluoropyrimidines tested *in vivo*.

Keywords: colorectal cancer, sluoropyrimidines, thymidylate synthase, 5-FU, FUdR, FUR, animal experiments.

* Correspondence concerning this article should be addressed to: Pochi R Subbarayan, Tel.: +1-305-243-4887 E.mail: spochi@med.miami.edu.

INTRODUCTION

The late Dr. Charles Heidelberger in the early 1950's discovered three fluoropyrimidines namely 5-fluorouracil (5-FU), 5-fluoro-deoxyuridine (FUdR) and 5-fluorouridine (FUR) [10]. Since then, 5-FU remains the most commonly used anti-neoplastic agent in colorectal cancer (CRC). The other two fluoropyrimidines were not used because of synthesis problems and inadequate preclinical and clinical studies.

5-fluororouracil is the main agent used in treatment of CRC. 5-fluorodeoxy uridine is approved for liver directed chemotherapy in patients with liver disease only [1,11,20,25,26]. Currently, 5-FU is used in combination with other anti-neoplastic drugs like CPT-11 or Oxaliplatin to treat patients with colon cancer. 5-FU and FUdR are metabolized to 5-fluoro-2'-deoxyuridine monophosphate (FdUMP). FdUMP competes with dUMP to be the substrate for thymidylate synthase (TS), an important enzyme in the formation of dTMP. Incorporation of fluorinated analogues into DNA causes replication defect resulting in cell death. The lesser-known fluoropyrimidine analogue is 5-fluorouridine (FUR). It is incorporated into RNA thereby affecting translation [20,22,30]. Compared to 5-FU and FUdR, FUR is the most cytotoxic of all the fluoropyrimidine analogues [15].

The mode of anti-tumor activity of 5-FU, FUdR and FUR is not completely understood. *In vitro* studies suggest that concentration and duration of exposure determines the cytotoxicity of 5-FU [3,4,8,9,17,21,24]. Clinical studies demonstrate that administration by 24 hrs infusion of 5-FU and FUdR is superior to bolus administration [1,2,12,16,28,29]. Moreover, 24 hrs high-dose administration of FUdR has better efficacy than 5-FU [1]. Although FUR is the most efficient among the fluoropyrimidine analogues, little information is available regarding its clinical anti-proliferative properties.

Based on the mode of administration, we tried to compare the efficacy of the three fluoropyrimidines *in vitro* and *in vivo*. In this manuscript we present the results of the investigation into the mechanisms of action of 5-FU, FUdR and FUR in *in vitro* cell culture using colorectal cancer cell lines Colo320HSR, CCL221 and HT29. To unravel the mode of action of these drugs we rescued the treated cells with deoxythymidine (dThy) or uridine (Urd). We established time and dose dependent cell kill for fluoropyrimidine analogues on Colo320HSR cells. To determine the effect on transcription, we examined the TS mRNA level in Colo320HSR cells following drug treatment. We also induced tumors in Balb/C mice and challenged with 5-FU or FUR. The anti-tumor activity of 5-FU and FUR was analyzed by clonogenic cell survival assay.

MATERIALS AND METHODS

Cell Lines and Culture Conditions

The human adenocarcinoma cell lines Colo320HSR, CCL221 and HT29 were obtained from American Type Culture Collection, USA. All the cell lines were maintained in RPMI 1640 medium supplemented with 10% FBS (Invitrogen, USA) at 37°C in humidified 5% CO_2 atmosphere.

Table 1. List of primers used for PCR

Primer	Sequence (5' – 3')	Product Length
TS-F	GGG CAG ATC CAA CAC ATC CTC CGC T	970 bp
TS-R	AGG TAA CTG ATA GGT CAC GGA CAG	
β-Actin F	TGA CGG GGT CAC CCA CAC TGT GCC CAT CAT	661 bp
β-Actin R	CTA GAA GCA TTT GCG GTG GAC GAT GGA GGG	

Chemicals, Primers and Enzymes

Cell culture medium and supplements were purchased from Invitrogen, USA. 5-FU, FUdR, FUR, dThymidine and Uridine were obtained from Sigma Chemical Company, USA.

Total RNA was prepared using Tri-Reagent (Sigma, USA). Oligonucleotides for cDNA synthesis and PCR were prepared in the University of Miami Miller School of Medicine DNA core facility. The list of primers used and their respective sequences are given in table 1. M-MLV reverse transcriptase and dNTP mix were purchased from Promega, USA. RNase inhibitor was obtained from Applied Biosystem, USA. All other chemicals were reagent grade.

Cytotoxic and Rescue Assays

1 X 10^5 exponentially growing cells were plated in six well plates. Twenty-four hours later various concentrations of 5-FU, FUdR or FUR were added in 2 ml medium and incubated at standard incubation conditions. Rescue studies were performed by simultaneous addition of 10 μM of deoxythymidine (dThy) or 1 mM of uridine (Urd) to the culture. Seventy-two hours later numbers of surviving cells were determined using Coulter Counter (Coulter Electronics, USA) and IC50 values were calculated. Student T test was used to determine degree of significance in IC50 values following dThy or Urd mediated rescue.

Time and Dose Dependent Chemo Sensitivity Studies

To determine the effects of time and concentration of drugs, 1 X 10^5 exponentially growing Colo320HSR cells were exposed to 1, 5 or 10 μM of 5-FU, FUdR or FUR for 1, 5 or 24 hrs at standard culture conditions. At the end of incubation the drug was washed off and the cells were allowed to recover. The viable number of cells over a period of time was determined using Coulter Counter. All the above experiments were carried out in duplicate and repeated four times.

Reverse Transcriptase PCR for TS and β-Actin mRNAs First Strand cDNA Synthesis

One μg of total RNA was reverse transcribed using M-MLV reverse transcriptase. Each reaction mix contained 0.5 μg of oligo dT_{16} primer per μg of the total RNA used. It was heated to 70°C for 5 min and chilled immediately on ice. The final reaction volume of 25 μl contained 0.5 mM each of dNTP mix, 25 U of RNase inhibitor and 200 U of M-MLV reverse transcriptase. The reaction mixture was incubated at 42°C for 60 minutes and stored on ice.

Second Strand Synthesis and Quantitation of TS mRNA PCR

Second strand synthesis was carried out with Gene Amp PCR kit according to the supplier's instructions. The reaction mixture contained 200 nM each of the gene specific primers (table 1) and 5 μl of the first strand cocktail. β-Actin gene was used as an internal reference. The cycling conditions were 30 sec. denaturation at 94°C, 30 sec. annealing at 60°C and 60 sec. extension at 72°C for 30 cycles. The reaction products were analyzed by electrophoresis through 1.0 % agarose gel and photographed.

In Vivo Effect f 5-FU and FUR

Mouse colorectal cancer cell line CT24.WT [27] was purchased from ATCC, USA. It was maintained in RPMI 1460 medium supplemented with 10% FBS and 1% PS. Five week old Balb/C mice (Harlan Sprague Dawley, USA) were injected with approximately 3 x 10^5 CT26.WT cells in 100-200 μl of PBS. Three weeks later, when tumors were 1.5 cm^2 in size, 2.5 mg FUR or 12.5 mg of 5-FU per kg body weight were injected IP to the tumor bearing mice. Twenty four hours later, the animals were killed in a CO_2 chamber. The tumors were extracted under sterile conditions, rinsed two times in sterile PBS, minced and transferred to sterile ice cold trypsin-EDTA. Following over night incubation in cold trypsin single cell suspension was obtained. Clonogenic assays were performed by plating 50 or 100 cells in duplicate wells of 24 well plates. Two weeks later, formed colonies were counted and recorded. Each experimental set contained at least three animals and were repeated three times. Animal experiments were carried out as per ACUC approved protocol No. 05-070.

RESULTS

FUR and FUDR are 150 Fold More Effective Than 5-FU

Our aim is to compare the antitumorigenic potential of the three uridine analogues. We used cytotoxicity assays to compare their efficacy as chemotherapy agents. The results are presented in Table 2. The data show that nanomolar quantities of FUdR and FUR are sufficient to kill 50% of cells compared to micromolar concentrations of 5-FU. This is in agreement with a previous report [15]. There appears to be cell line dependent variation in the drug dosage. Some cell lines may be intrinsically more resistant to anti-tumor agents. In particular CCL221 is about 1.4 to 2.7 folds more resistant to all the three drugs compared to Colo320HSR and HT29. In contrast the latter two cell lines exhibited almost similar IC50 values (table 2).

Table 2. IC 50 values (μM) of 5-FU, FUdR and FUR for Colo320HSR, CCL221 and HT29 cells

	No rescue	+ 10 μM dThy	*P-Value*	+1 mM Urd	P-Value
5-FU					
Colo320HSR	3.278 + 0.467	5.91 + 0.857	0.041	3.338 + 0.453	0.175
CCL221	8.732 + 1.348	30.710 + 9.861	0.017	18.521+4.221	0.029
HT29	6.062 + 0.536	7.200 + 1.084	0.348	3.548 + 1.549	0.135
FUdR					
Colo320HSR	0.019 + 0.007	194.062 + 63.982	0.0005	0.017 + 0.003	0.781
CCL221	0.029 + 0.007	671.272 + 84.578	0.00000005	0.028 + 0.011	0.0927
HT29	0.014 + 0.004	155.621 + 50.600	0.00039	0.024 + 0.006	0.247
FUR					
Colo320HSR	0.023 + 0.007	0.02 + 0.005	0.738	2.395 + 0.468	0.0001
CCL221	0.052 + 0.009	0.056 + 0.006	0.786	6.861 + 1.419	0.0000073
HT29	0.041 + 0.003	0.059 + 0.010	0.140	2.700 + 0.685	0.008

The IC50 values were determined as described under materials and methods. The values are Mean ± SE from at least four independent experiments done in duplicate. P value indicates the degree of significance between rescue and cytotoxic studies.

Deoxythymidine Protected the Cells from FUDR Whereas Uridine from the Effects Of FUR

10 μM deoxythymidine (dThy) uniformly rescued all three cell lines from the cytotoxic effects of FUdR, but not from FUR. In contrast 1 mM uridine (Urd) was required to protect the cells from the toxic effects of FUR (table 2).

FUR Exhibits Superior Cytotoxicity at Bolus and Infusion Doses

We simulated bolus administration of drugs by short term exposure (1 h) of Colo320HSR cells in culture whereas 5 and 24 hrs replicated infusional regimen. The results of time and dose dependent effect of 5-FU, FUdR and FUR on Colo320HSR are presented in the figure 1 A through I.

5-FU is Most Effective Only at High Dose and Longer Treatment Time

Short time (1 h) exposure of Colo320HSR cells to 5-FU at low (1 μM) to moderate dose (5 mM) did not induce cell death (figure 1A, B). Lower dosage (1 μM) in combination with longer duration (24 h; figure 1C), moderate dosage (5 μM) for intermediate duration (5 h; figure 1B) and high dosage (10 μM) for a short time (1 h; figure 1A) were moderately (2-10%) cytotoxic. A moderate to high dose (5, 10 μM) of 5-FU for a longer time (24 h) inhibited growth by 40-60% (figure 1C).

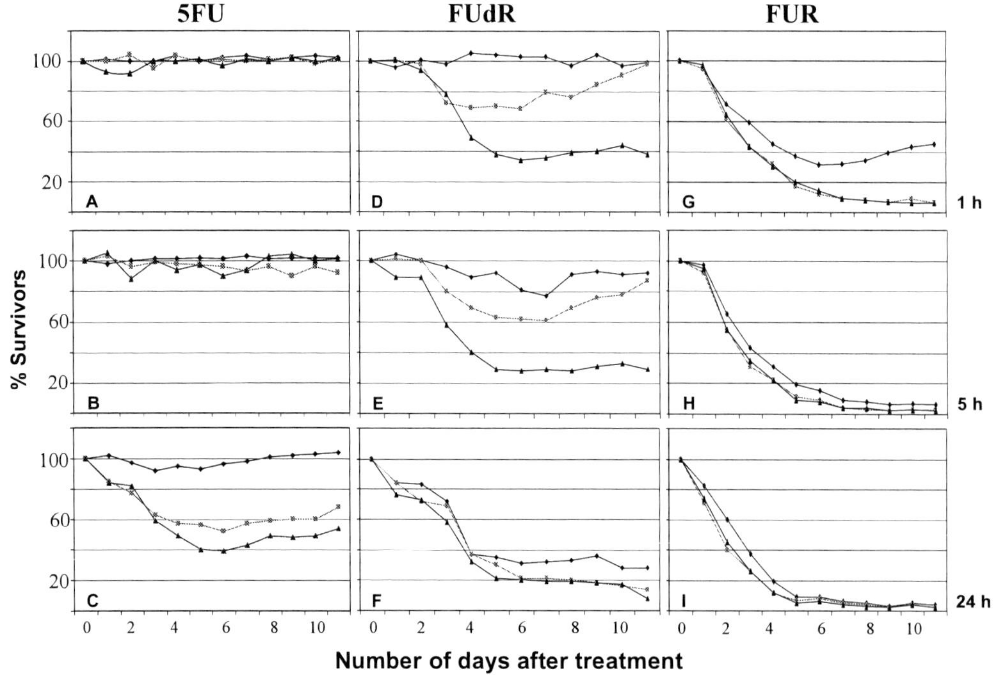

Figure 1. Time and dosage dependent cytotoxic effects of fluoropyrimidines on Colo320HSR cells. FUR at all the conditions tested was found to be cytotoxic. 1 X 10^5 exponentially growing Colo320HSR cells were exposed to 1 μM (closed diamonds), 5 μM (closed squares) or 10 μM (closed triangles) of 5-FU, FUdR or FUR for 1 h (panels A,D,G), 5 h (panels B,E,H), or 24 h (panels C,F,I) at standard incubation conditions. At the end of the incubation period the drug was washed off and the cells were allowed to recover. The viability over a period of time was determined by tryphan blue exclusion assay using Coulter Counter (Coulter Electronics, FL). These experiments were carried out in duplicate and repeated four times.

High Dose of FUDR is Cytotoxic as Bolus and Infusion Regimen

Treatment of Colo320HSR cells for 1 h with 1 μM FUdR was least cytotoxic (figure 1 D), whereas treatment for 5 h killed about 20% of cells (figure 1 E). A moderate dose of 5 μM for 1 or 5 h was effective in inhibiting cell growth by as much as 40% (figure 1D, E). Exposure of cells to a low dose (1 μM) for 24 h (figure 1F), high dose (10 μM) for 1 h (figure 1D) or 5 h (figure. 1E) inhibited growth of 60–70% of cells. Longer treatment period (24 h) at all the concentrations (1, 5, 10 μM) killed most of the cells; i.e. 70-90% growth inhibition (figure. 1 F).

High or Low, Bolus or Infusion of FUR Kills the Most

A combination of low dose (1 μM) of FUR and short exposure time caused 60% growth inhibition (figure 1 G). All other combinations viz, low dose (1 μM) with moderate (5 h; figure 1H) to long (24 h; figure 1I) exposure time, or moderate to higher dose for short (figure 1G), moderate (figure 1H) or long duration (figure 1I) killed most of the cells (80-95% growth inhibition).

FUR Suppressed TS Gene Expression in Cultured Cells Under Short and Long Term Exposure

It is suggested that modified uridine derivative (FUTP) is incorporated into messenger RNA, thus affecting its stability and function. Therefore, we checked the effect of FUR on mRNA synthesis in Colo320HSR cells. 5-FU and FUdR inhibit the activity of the enzyme thymidylate synthase (TS) at protein level. We evaluated the effect of all the three drugs on mRNA synthesis by quantitating TS transcripts using semi-quantitative reverse transcriptase PCR methodology. The house keeping gene β-actin mRNA was used as a control. Results of this experiment are presented in Figures 2 and 3. Two hrs treatment of Colo320HSR cells with 0.1 μM concentration of fluoropyrimidines increased TS expression (figure. 2A lanes 2, 3, 4); whereas, a longer duration of 24 hrs decreased TS transcription in FUdR and FUR treated samples (figure 2 B lanes 3, 4). Exposure of these cells to 1 μM of 5-FU, FUdR or FUR whether for 2 or 24 hrs uniformly inhibited the expression of TS (figure 3 A, B lanes 2, 3, 4).

We also noted that treating cells for 24 hrs with 0.1 μM of FUdR or FUR was more potent in inhibiting TS transcription than 5-FU. One μM of FUR in 2 or 24 h inhibited TS gene expression more than either 5-FU or FUdR (figure 3 A, B lane 4). In the same samples, mRNA quantity of the house-keeping gene β-actin was not affected (figures 2C, D, 3C, D)

FUR is 15 Fold More Effective than 5-FU in its *In Vivo* Anti-Tumor Activity

Having checked the efficacy of these three agents on cultured cells, we tested the effects of 5-FU and FUR on tumor bearing Balb/C mice.figure 4 summarizes the results of this study. Under the same treatment conditions 2.5 mg/kg of FUR killed 78% of cells compared to 26% by 12.5 mg/Kg 5-FU. It is a difference of 3 fold. Accounting for the difference in the dosage between these two anti-tumor agents; FUR is 15 times more potent than 5-FU *in vivo*, which is comparable to the *in vitro* data.

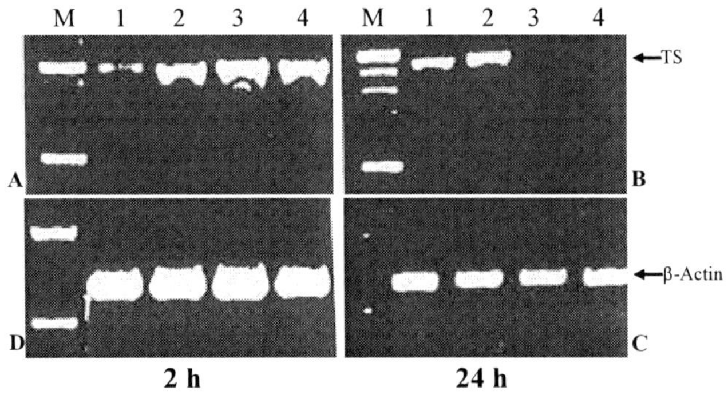

Figure 2. Agarose gel analysis of TS and β-actin RT-PCR products. 0.1 μM of FUdR and FUR suppressed TS gene expression in Colo320HSR cells. Total RNA was isolated from treated cells, cDNA synthesis and PCR for TS and β-actin genes were carried out using gene specific primers (table 1) as described under materials and methods. PCR products were analyzed on 1% agarose gel, stained with ethidium bromide and documented. Lane M. DNA Marker. Lane 1. Untreated control. Lane 2. 5-FU, Lane 3. FUdR, Lane 4. FUR. Panel A and D 2 hrs exposure, Panel B and C 24 hrs exposure.

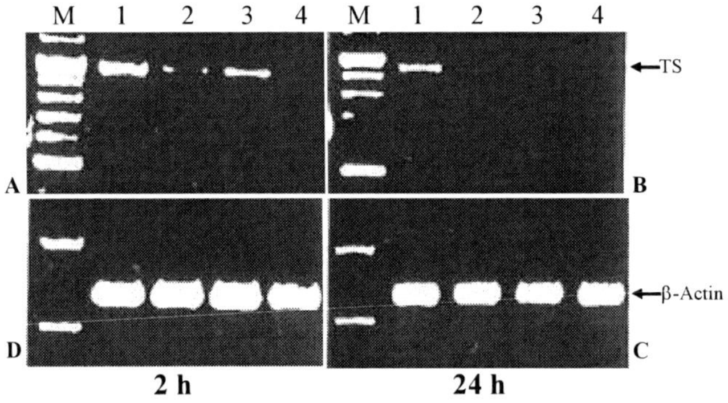

Figure 3. Agarose gel analysis of TS and β-actin RT-PCR products. 1 μM of 5-FU, FUdR and FUR suppressed TS gene expression in Colo320HSR cells. Details of the experiment are as described under Materials and Methods. Lane M. DNA Marker. Lane 1. Untreated control. Lane 2. 5-FU, Lane 3. FUdR, Lane 4. FUR. Panel A and D 2 hrs exposure, Panel B and C 24 hrs exposure.

DISCUSSION

5-FU has been the drug of choice in treating many solid tumors. Its analogue FUdR is only approved for liver directed therapy [1]. Due to its potential toxicity FUR had never been put into clinical trial. In this study we compared the *in vitro* and *in vivo* cytotoxicity of FUR with 5-FU. In the *in vitro* cell culture one hour treatment replicated bolus administration, while 5 and 24 hrs reflected infusion regimen of 5-FU, FUdR and FUR.

As represented in Figure 1 in general, infusion of these drugs is more effective than bolus administration. Previous studies showed an inverse relationship between the duration of exposure and concentration of 5-FU used. High dose (>100 μM) for a short period of time (<6h) or 1 – 10 μM for longer than 72 hrs was found to be effective on a variety of tumor types [3,4,8,9,13,16-18,21,24]. 5-FU is rapidly cleared from the plasma; therefore, infusion ensures a steady supply which leads to effective cytotoxicity. In short 5-FU infusion seems be significantly effective and is in agreement with clinical observations [1,13,16,18,28].

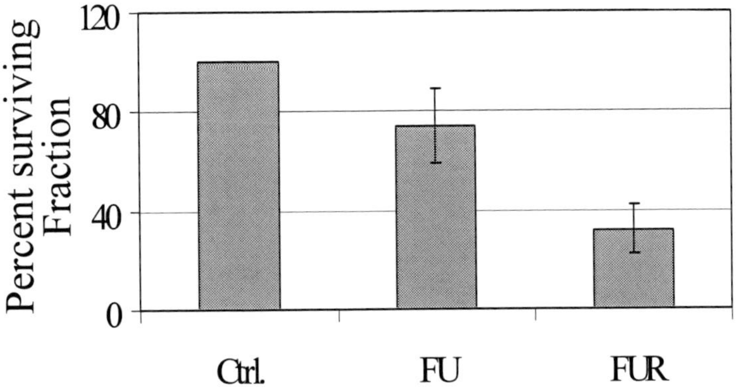

Figure 4. Flurouridine is 15 fold more toxic than 5-FU in its antitumorigenic activity on tumors induced in Balb/C mice. Mouse colorectal cancer cell line CT26.WT was injected S.C. to Balb/C mice. Following tumor formation mice were treated with PBS, 5-FU or FUR. 24 hrs later, tumors were extracted and clonogenic assay performed. At least three animals constituted a group and each experiment was performed three times.

We note that cells were able to recover from the damaging effects of short to moderate exposure to FUdR (figure 1E). However, even low dose (1 μM FUdR) treatment for longer time eliminated this ability (figure 1F). This reinforces the notion that infusion of FUdR is superior to bolus administration. Tumor tissues are reported to be deficient in phosphate donors. Inside the malignant cells FUdR is predominantly converted to 5-FU and eventually to FUMP. 5-FU appears to be more stable in tissue than the extra cellular fluids [12]. Long term exposure to FUdR at all concentrations may lead to the accumulation of more metabolites inside the cultured cells causing maximal damage accounting for the efficacy of FUdR. In contrast, a high dose of FUdR killed 60 – 80% of cells at all the treatment time points. However, 5 and 10 μM of FUdR is not a clinically achievable concentration.

Cytotoxicity and animal data demonstrate 5-fluorouridine (FUR) as a potent anti-tumor agent. Irrespective of the dosage and duration of exposure, FUR killed 60-90% of cells. The cytotoxicity of FUR is rescued by uridine. We also observed that mRNA synthesis is affected by FUR. This data is consistent with the hypothesis that FUR interferes with RNA pathway. Incorporation of fluoro compounds into RNA is attributed to their toxicity. On the other hand tumor bearing mice received significantly low doses of 5-FU and FUdR and exhibited no toxicity (24 hrs exposure). At a relatively low dose, FUR is 15 folds more effective than 5-FU in killing *in vivo* mouse tumor. Taken together the data validate the superiority of FUR as a chemotherapeutic agent.

There is about 500 fold difference in the IC50 values of 5-FU and FUdR and FUR. It may be due to transportation of 5-FU across the plasma membrane. Variation in transport rate in 5-FU across the plasma membrane had been observed in different cell lines. There is a 17 fold difference in the rate of (^{3}H)-uracil uptake in CaCO-2 and LLC-PK1 cells *in vitro* [14].

The same investigators also observed that sodium enhances uracil transport. Once inside the cell a majority of the 5-FU is catabolized to FDHU by the enzyme dihydro pyrimidine dehydrogenase (DPD). The clinical effectiveness of 5-FU had been correlated to balance among DPD, TP/TP and TS. It is reported that more DPD is a cause for treatment failure or requirement of high dose of 5-FU [23]. We speculate that these factors may play a role in the multifold high requirement of 5-FU compared to FUdR or FUR.

In rescue experiments deoxythymidine could partially inhibit the cytotoxicity of 5-FU (Table 2). The reason for failure of dThy to rescue the cells from the cytotoxic effects of 5-FU could lie with its amount used in competition/rescue experiments. Ten μM of dThy is about three folds more than the observed IC50 values for 5-FU. In contrast 10 μM dThy is a few hundred folds more than the IC50 values of FUdR. Therefore, by increasing the concentration of dThy its inhibitory action on 5-FU could have been enhanced.

Uridine could rescue cells from the damaging effects of FUR only. FUR treatment inhibited TS transcription as noted from semi-quantitative RT-PCR analysis. These facts affirm that FUR mainly affects the RNA pathway causing maximum, immediate and irrevocable damage to cells. Therefore, damage to the functional units namely RNA and thereby protein synthesis triggered by FUR might pose lethal and irrecoverable damage to cells.

The inhibitory effect of 5-FU on TS is correlated with its cytotoxicity. The time and dose dependent cytotoxicity of 5-FU may be due to its short half-life or is limited to proliferating cells [19]. Thus, quiescent cells might escape the effect of 5-FU. However, higher concentration and prolonged exposure of 5-FU may result in additional but not yet understood mechanisms that are independent of cell cycle and TS or incorporation into DNA and RNA. Although FUdR is more effective than 5-FU in killing Colo320HSR, from the data it appears that the inhibitory effects of TS gene expression by 5-FU and FUdR are very similar at short exposure time. But, at longer exposure time, FUdR completely inhibited TS transcription. Greater cytotoxicity of FUdR over 5-FU may be due to its partial conversion to stable 5-FU inside the tumor and effective inhibition of dTMP formation. More FdUMP may be formed following FUdR administration than 5-FU. As a result, more TS accumulates shutting down its transcription [5-7]. It is also possible that formed 5-FU metabolize to FUMP which may eventually be incorporated into RNA forming labile transcripts. Therefore, the mechanism of inhibition of TS transcription following fluorodeoxyuridine administration needs further investigation.

Inhibition of TS transcription by FUR is more severe. FUR is not known to bind TS. Therefore, general perturbance in transcription by FUR may be the cause for the loss of TS transcripts. In the present study, FUR inhibited TS transcription but very little difference in β-actin mRNA level was observed. We think that transcriptional interference occurs gradually. In the absence of cellular proliferation β-actin, a house keeping gene might not be transcribed. As a consequence it might take longer to see any change in its quantity. Thus RNA mediated inhibition of tumor growth by FUR makes it an effective alternate to 5-FU and FUdR.

Toxicity data established the LD 50 values for 5-FU, FUdR and FUR to be about 260 mg/Kg, 1400 mg/kg and 160 mg/kg respectively in CBA/J mice [12] and 450 mg/Kg, 2500mg/kg and 175 mg/Kg for CBA mice (Ardalan et. al. unpublished data) administered in

24 hrs. Accordingly FUR is 2.6 times more toxic than 5-FU and FUdR is least toxic. In contrast 2.5 mg/kg of FUR (about 70 fold less than its LD50) is 15 times more potent than 5-FU (12.5 mg/kg = 36 fold less than its LD50). In conclusion, our studies confirm that among the three fluoropyrimidines tested FUR is the most potent anti-tumor agent. Severe inhibitory effect of FUR on gene expression and its RNA mediated cell kill may explain its superiority over 5-FU and FUdR. In contrast FUR was found to be effective in inhibiting cell growth *in vitro* and *in vivo* at all concentrations and modes of administration. The data also show that FUR at a very low dose (i.e. 70 folds less than its LD50 values in mice) is about 15 folds more cytotoxic than 5-FU. Under appropriate dosage, FUR may become less or equi-toxic but an effective alternate to 5-FU.

ACKNOWLEDGEMENT

We wish to thank Dr. Zeming Deng and Philip Lee for their excellent technical help and other lab members for critical reading of the manuscript.

REFERENCES

[1] Ardalan, B. and Lima, M. (2004) A phase II trial of FUdR in patients with advanced pancreatic cancer. *J.Cancer Res.Clin.Oncol. 130*, 561-566.

[2] Ardalan, B., Sridhar, K. S., Benedetto, P., Richman, S., Waldman, S., Morrell, L., Feun, L., Savaraj, N., Fodor, M., and Livingstone, A. (1991) A phase I, II study of high-dose 5-fluorouracil and high-dose leucovorin with low-dose phosphonacetyl-L-aspartic acid in patients with advanced malignancies. *Cancer 68*, 1242-1246.

[3] Aschele, C., Sobrero, A., Faderan, M. A., and Bertino, J. R. (1992) Novel mechanism(s) of resistance to 5-fluorouracil in human colon cancer (HCT-8) sublines following exposure to two different clinically relevant dose schedules. *Cancer Res. 52*, 1855-1864.

[4] Calabro-Jones, P. M., Byfield, J. E., Ward, J. F., and Sharp, T. R. (1982) Time-dose relationships for 5-fluorouracil cytotoxicity against human epithelial cancer cells in vitro. *Cancer Res. 42*, 4413-4420.

[5] Chu, E., Koeller, D. M., Johnston, P. G., Zinn, S., and Allegra, C. J. (1993) Regulation of thymidylate synthase in human colon cancer cells treated with 5-fluorouracil and interferon-gamma. *Mol.Pharmacol. 43*, 527-533.

[6] Chu, E., Voeller, D., Koeller, D. M., Drake, J. C., Takimoto, C. H., Maley, G. F., Maley, F., and Allegra, C. J. (1993) Identification of an RNA binding site for human thymidylate synthase. *Proc.Natl.Acad.Sci.U.S.A 90*, 517-521.

[7] Codacci-Pisanelli, G., van der Wilt, C. L., Pinedo, H. M., Franchi, F., Noordhuis, P., Braakhuis, B. J., van Laar, J. A., and Peters, G. J. (1995) Antitumour activity, toxicity and inhibition of thymidylate synthase of prolonged administration of 5-fluorouracil in mice. *Eur.J.Cancer 31A*, 1517-1525.

[8] Drewinko, B. and Yang, L. Y. (1985) Cellular basis for the inefficacy of 5-FU in human colon carcinoma. *Cancer Treat.Rep. 69*, 1391-1398.

[9] Evans, R. M., Laskin, J. D., and Hakala, M. T. (1980) Assessment of growth-limiting events caused by 5-fluorouracil in mouse cells and in human cells. *Cancer Res. 40*, 4113-4122.

[10] Heidelberger, C. (1965) Fluorinated pyrimidines. Prog.Nucleic Acid *Res.Mol.Biol. 4*, 1-50.

[11] Heidelberger, C., Danenberg, P. V., and Moran, R. G. (1983) Fluorinated pyrimidines and their nucleosides. *Adv.Enzymol.Relat Areas Mol.Biol. 54*, 58-119.

[12] Houghton, J. A., Houghton, P. J., and Wooten, R. S. (1979) Mechanism of induction of gastrointestinal toxicity in the mouse by 5-fluorouracil, 5-fluorouridine, and 5-fluoro-2'-deoxyuridine. *Cancer Res. 39*, 2406-2413.

[13] Kish, J. A., Ensley, J. F., Jacobs, J., Weaver, A., Cummings, G., and Al Sarraf, M. (1985) A randomized trial of cisplatin (CACP) + 5-fluorouracil (5-FU) infusion and CACP + 5-FU bolus for recurrent and advanced squamous cell carcinoma of the head and neck. *Cancer 56*, 2740-2744.

[14] Li, H., Chung, S. J., and Shim, C. K. (2002) Characterization of the transport of uracil across Caco-2 and LLC-PK1 cell monolayers. *Pharm.Res. 19*, 1495-1501.

[15] Link, K. H., Aigner, K. R., Peschau, K., Warthona, M., Schwemmle, K., and Danenberg, P. V. (1988) Concentration and time dependence of the toxicity of fluorinated pyrimidines to HT 29 colorectal carcinoma cells. *Cancer Chemother.Pharmacol. 22*, 58-62.

[16] Lokich, J. J., Ahlgren, J. D., Gullo, J. J., Philips, J. A., and Fryer, J. G. (1989) A prospective randomized comparison of continuous infusion fluorouracil with a conventional bolus schedule in metastatic colorectal carcinoma: a Mid-Atlantic Oncology Program Study. *J.Clin.Oncol. 7*, 425-432.

[17] Moran, R. G. and Scanlon, K. L. (1991) Schedule-dependent enhancement of the cytotoxicity of fluoropyrimidines to human carcinoma cells in the presence of folinic acid. *Cancer Res. 51*, 4618-4623.

[18] O'Connell, M. J., Martenson, J. A., Wieand, H. S., Krook, J. E., Macdonald, J. S., Haller, D. G., Mayer, R. J., Gunderson, L. L., and Rich, T. A. (1994) Improving adjuvant therapy for rectal cancer by combining protracted-infusion fluorouracil with radiation therapy after curative surgery. *N.Engl.J.Med. 331*, 502-507.

[19] Pestalozzi, B. C., McGinn, C. J., Kinsella, T. J., Drake, J. C., Glennon, M. C., Allegra, C. J., and Johnston, P. G. (1995) Increased thymidylate synthase protein levels are principally associated with proliferation but not cell cycle phase in asynchronous human cancer cells. *Br.J.Cancer 71*, 1151-1157.

[20] Pinedo, H. M. and Peters, G. F. (1988) Fluorouracil: biochemistry and pharmacology. *J.Clin.Oncol. 6*, 1653-1664

[21] Ren, Q., van Groeningen, C. J., Hardcastle, A., Aherne, G. W., Geoffroy, F., Allegra, C. J., Johnston, P. G., and Grem, J. L. (1997) Determinants of cytotoxicity with prolonged exposure to fluorouracil in human colon cancer cells. *Oncol.Res. 9*, 77-88.

[22] Rustum, Y. M. (1991) Modulation of fluoropyrimidines by leucovorin: rationale and status. *J.Surg.Oncol.Suppl 2*, 116-123.

[23] Salonga, D., Danenberg, K. D., Johnson, M., Metzger, R., Groshen, S., Tsao-Wei, D. D., Lenz, H. J., Leichman, C. G., Leichman, L., Diasio, R. B., and Danenberg, P. V. (2000) Colorectal tumors responding to 5-fluorouracil have low gene expression levels of dihydropyrimidine dehydrogenase, thymidylate synthase, and thymidine phosphorylase. *Clin.Cancer Res. 6*, 1322-1327.

[24] Santelli, G. and Valeriote, F. (1986) Schedule-dependent cytotoxicity of 5-fluorouracil in mice. *J.Natl.Cancer Inst. 76*, 159-164.

[25] Thomas, D. M. and Zalcberg, J. R. (1998) 5-fluorouracil: a pharmacological paradigm in the use of cytotoxics. *Clin.Exp.Pharmacol.Physiol 25*, 887-895.

[26] van Laar, J. A., Rustum, Y. M., Ackland, S. P., van Groeningen, C. J., and Peters, G. J. (1998) Comparison of 5-fluoro-2'-deoxyuridine with 5-fluorouracil and their role in the treatment of colorectal cancer. *Eur.J.Cancer 34*, 296-306.

[27] Wang, M., Bronte, V., Chen, P. W., Gritz, L., Panicali, D., Rosenberg, S. A., and Restifo, N. P. (1995) Active immunotherapy of cancer with a nonreplicating recombinant fowlpox virus encoding a model tumor-associated antigen. *J.Immunol. 154*, 4685-4692.

[28] Webb, A., Cunningham, D., Scarffe, J. H., Harper, P., Norman, A., Joffe, J. K., Hughes, M., Mansi, J., Findlay, M., Hill, A., Oates, J., Nicolson, M., Hickish, T., O'Brien, M., Iveson, T., Watson, M., Underhill, C., Wardley, A., and Meehan, M. (1997) Randomized trial comparing epirubicin, cisplatin, and fluorouracil versus fluorouracil, doxorubicin, and methotrexate in advanced esophagogastric cancer. *J.Clin.Oncol. 15*, 261-267.

[29] Whitehead, R. P., Benedetti, J. K., Abbruzzese, J. L., Ardalan, B., Williamson, S., Gaynor, E. R., Balcerzak, S. P., and Macdonald, J. S. (2004) A phase II pilot study of high-dose 24-hour continuous infusion of 5-FU and leucovorin and low-dose PALA for patients with colorectal cancer: a Southwest Oncology Group study. *Invest New Drugs 22*, 467-473.

[30] Zhang, Z. G., Harstrick, A., and Rustum, Y. M. (1992) Modulation of fluoropyrimidines: role of dose and schedule of leucovorin administration. *Semin.Oncol. 19*, 10-15.

In: Cancer Research Perspectives
Editor: Larissa S. Pereira, pp. 233-244
ISBN 978-1-60021-980-1

Chapter VIII

DIAGNOSTIC CLASSIFICATION USING GENE EXPRESSION PROFILING IN AML

K. I. Mills[1,2] and A. F. Gilkes[2]

[1]CCRCB, Queen's University Belfast, Lisburn Road, Belfast, BT9 7BL NI, UK
[2]Department of Haematology, School of Medicine, Cardiff University, Cardiff, CF14 4XN, Wales UK.

ABSTRACT

Gene expression profiling initially showed that it could be used to distinguish between the major variants of acute leukaemia. Several studies have now been published that have illustrated the potential of micro array analysis in the diagnosis of haematological malignancy. For acute myeloid leukaemia (AML), in particular, expression profiling has also provided novel insights into disease pathogenesis and shown it could lead to refinements in risk-stratification, prognostic markers, and eventually a more rational and personalised approach to therapy. These gene expression studies will be compared and contrasted in terms of results; with a view to speculating whether arrays can complement current laboratory methodologies for leukaemia diagnosis.

Golub et al. (1999) described the first approach to disease classification based on microarrays. Using an unsupervised, class discovery approach they distinguished between AML and ALL without previous knowledge of the disease of each sample identifying previously unrecognized disease subtypes. The data produced four sub-groups representing AML, T-lineage ALL, and B-lineage ALL (two sub-groups). This demonstrated that a gene expression based cancer classification could discover, and predict, cancer classes without previous biological knowledge and led to the speculation that further sub-classifications could be identified in other haematological or solid tumour diseases.

AML is generally classified by the FAB (French-American-British) classification (Bennett et al. 1976) in which morphology is used to form groupings based on the differentiation status of the immature cells. The WHO (Vardiman, Harris, & Brunning 2002) disease classification of AML takes into account both morphology and the recurrent cytogenetic translocations t(8; 21), t(15; 17) and inv(16), and 11q23 abnormalities to form distinct diagnostic sub-groups. Patients without these chromosomal abnormalities are then grouped on the basis of morphology. Additional genetic mutations are also observed in AML distributed across the cytogenetic or morphology groupings.

Several studies have been done on small numbers of AML patients (less than 60 patients) using the cytogenetically defined groups; these groupings included t(8; 21); t(15; 17), inv(16), 11q23 abnormalities or normal cytogenetics (Debernardi et al. 2003; Gutierrez et al. 2005; Haferlach et al. 2005c; Morikawa et al. 2003; Schoch et al. 2002; Vey et al. 2004; Virtaneva et al. 2001). Schoch et al. (2002) examined 37 samples from three distinct cytogenetic subtypes of AML: t(8; 21), inv(16), and t(15; 17) specifically associated with the four distinct morphological subgroups, AML M2, AML M4Eo, AML M3, and AML M3v. Their analyses, including Significance Analysis of Microarrays (SAM) (Tusher, Tibshirani, & Chu 2001), identified 36 genes whose expression could accurately discriminate between the cytogenetic classes. However, a set of only 13 genes were needed to separate the samples into these distinctive cytogenetic sub-groups.

A similar study (Debernardi et al. 2003) used hierarchical clustering and statistical group comparison to group the major cytogenetic classes and identified 145 genes that could correctly distinguish the chromosomal sub-groups of: t(8; 21), t(15; 17), inv(16), 11q23, and normal karyotype. Members of the class I homeobox A and B gene families were shown to have a distinct up-regulation within the normal karyotype group.

Patients with newly diagnosed AML with high blast counts could be separated into three patient subgroups using un-supervised hierarchical cluster analysis. In general, there was no relationship between the clusters and the FAB classification (Oyan et al. 2006).

AML patients with normal cytogenetics constitute the single largest group in AML although trisomy 8 is the most common numerical aberration observed as either a sole abnormality or part of more complex cytogenetics. Patients with normal karyotype are classified in an intermediate-risk group with a heterogeneous clinical outcome (Grimwade et al. 2001). A comparison of patients with normal cytogenetics versus patients with trisomy 8 as the only cytogenetics abnormality (Virtaneva et al. 2001) showed that the two groups of patients were genetically similar populations. Gene dosage effects were seen however not all of the 29 genes most significantly up-regulated in trisomy 8 samples were mapped to chromosome 8. The most significant differences in expression level between the two groups involved apoptosis genes. A further study (Radmacher et al. 2006) showed that patients with a normal karyotype could be divided into two prognostically relevant subgroups and developed a classification rule to predict outcome for individual patients. A strong association of the outcome classifier with the FLT3 ITD mutation may explain the prognostic significance of the signature. These two studies confirmed that gene expression profiling can be applied to outcome prediction in cytogenetically normal AML.

A microarray study focusing on patients with acute promyelocytic leukaemia (APL, also classified as AML M3) with the t(15; 17) translocation and patients with AML FAB group M1 (AML without maturation characterized by morphologically and phenotypically immature AML blasts and no recurrent chromosomal abnormalities) (Morikawa et al. 2003), and using a multivariate sigma-classifier algorithm, identified 33 genes that could distinguish FAB-M3 with t(15; 17) from the AML M1 sub-group and a further 24 that classify FAB-M1. Unsurprisingly, this showed that two distinct morphologically-defined sub groups (FAB-M1 and FAB-M3) have distinct gene expression signatures. Over-expression of one of these genes, myeloperoxidase, in APL is consistent with the conventional cytochemical staining pattern. Haferlach et al. (2005c) compared patients with variants of APL: AML-M3 or M3v. In contrast to M3, (abnormal pro-myelocytes with heavy granulation and bundles of Auer rods), M3v has a non- or hypogranular cytoplasm and a bi-lobed nucleus. An unsupervised analysis separated these APL samples could be separated from other AMLs with defined cytogenetic abnormalities and those with a normal karyotype. In this well designed study, supervised pair-wise comparison showed discrimination between M3 and M3v, based on gene signatures, with a median classification accuracy of 90%. This discrimination was also identified and expanded in a comparative study of parameters indicative of T-cell lymphoid specification between M3 and M3v (Chapiro et al. 2006). This study suggests a different cellular origin for the two types of disease and subsequent transformation of progenitor populations.

Two studies on larger relatively unselected patient populations were reported in 2004. The first determined expression levels in samples from 116 adults with AML (including 45 with a normal karyotype). They found that 6283 genes had variable expression across most samples and used this gene set to perform an unsupervised two-way, hierarchical cluster analysis (Bullinger et al. 2004). In common with previous studies, they reported that patients with t(15; 17) had a highly specific pattern of expression. Even within this diverse sample population, gene signatures could be obtained for patients with t(8; 21) or inv(16). Those with normal cytogenetics were further sub-divided into two distinct groups, although each group was similar with respect to sex, age and white-cell count, it was noted that FAB M1 or M2 was significantly more common in group I than in group II, whereas FAB subtype M4 or M5 was more common in group II. An unequal distribution of samples with mutations of the FLT3 gene was also observed with statistically more mutations observed in group I. The authors took the opportunity to combine unsupervised and supervised analysis methods by using a training data set to identify a gene list of 133 genes which was then used on a separate test data set to predict clinical outcome. The subgroup of samples predicted to have a poor outcome correlated with significantly shorter survival than those samples predicted to have a good outcome. However, it should be noted that when a similar analysis using prediction analysis of microarrays (PAM) (Tibshirani et al. 2002) was used for samples with normal cytogenetics only, in contrast to the whole population, no difference in outcome could be determined. The authors suggest that this was due to either a relatively small sample or an inherently poorer performance of patients with a normal cytogenetic. Nevertheless, this study showed that potential for gene expression profiling at diagnosis to obtain a risk classification for individual patients.

In a second study on 285 AML patients (Valk et al. 2004), fully characterised for the presence of mutations within the FLT3 ITD or TKD region, NRAS, KRAS or CEBPα and the over-expression of EVI1, data were analysed by SAM (Tusher, Tibshirani, & Chu 2001) and PAM (Tibshirani et al. 2002) in addition to using the Pearson correlation algorithms within the OmniViz software package. The AML samples were subjected to un-supervised ordering and the authors reported that optimal clustering was obtained using 2856 probe sets representing 2008 annotated genes and 146 expressed-sequence tags (ESTs). This analysis produced sixteen distinct groups of patients on the basis of strong similarities in gene-expression profiles. Distinct clusters of t(8; 21), inv(16), and t(15; 17) were readily identified with 1692 probe sets which emphasised the strong effect of these distinctive and recurrent translocations on gene expression. Separate clusters (using 2856 probe sets) were identified containing samples with monosomy 7, mutations of FLT3, or over-expression of EVI1. In addition clusters were defined for 11q23 abnormalities or CEPBα mutations. Patients with t(15; 17) also clustered into one main group although two sub-groups could be identified separating patients with high or low white blood cell count which also correlated with the presence of FLT3 mutations. Several other clusters had distinct gene expression profiles but were not associated with any defined morphological, cytogenetic or mutation status. In addition overall survival data was analysed with the best survival rates being determined for those clusters containing the recurrent translocations (t(8; 21), t(15; 17) and inv(16)). This is perhaps not too surprising as these cytogenetic abnormalities have previously been associated with a favourable prognosis (Grimwade et al. 1998). Interestingly, the molecular signatures associated with FLT3 ITD were not distinctive; and the authors suggested that this type of mutation which occurred across the clusters reflect the heterogeneity of AML.

Serial analysis of gene expression (SAGE) was reported on a small series of 22 AML patients with the most common translocations, (t(8; 21), t(15; 17), t(9; 11), and inv(16)). Around 1100 transcripts were identified which showed that each translocation had a unique expression profile for different functional categories highlighting specific pathways for targeted therapy (Lee et al. 2006).

A more recent study also confirmed that gene expression profiling could identify signatures for novel prognostic and therapeutically relevant groups of AML with a potential impact on therapy (Wilson et al. 2006). Unsupervised clustering algorithms partitioned the AML patients into six distinct and stable groups based on strong similarities in among the 9463 gene expression levels. This study also found significant outcome differences between the clusters for levels of resistant disease and complete remission rates after induction therapy.

In order to expand the molecular characterization of different acute leukaemia's, 90 adult patients with fully characterised acute lymphoblastic leukaemia (ALL) or AML were analysed (Kohlmann et al. 2003) using oligonucleotide microarrays (Affymetrix U95Av2/U133A). Only a small set of differentially expressed genes was needed to accurately discriminate eight clinically relevant acute leukaemia subgroups including those with t(8; 21), t(15; 17), t(11q23)/MLL, or inv(16) as well as precursor B-ALL with t(9; 22), t(8; 14), or t(11q23)/MLL and precursor T-ALL. This approach was expanded in a study (Haferlach et al. 2005b) of 892 patients mainly with AML or ALL but which also included CLL, CML and some non-leukaemia samples. The authors used a combination of un-supervised and supervised statistical methods to identify gene lists that reproduced 12 predefined cytogenetic or morphological leukaemia classification groupings, with 95.1% accuracy, distinct from each other and the non-leukaemia samples. Within AML, specificities of 100% were obtained for t(15; 17), t(8; 21) and inv(16); 97.7% for patients with 11q23 abnormalities and those with complex cytogenetic abnormalities; and 93.7% for the larger and diverse sub-group of "normal cytogenetics and other abnormalities".

The most common genetic abnormality in AML is a mutation within the FLT3 gene. Two types of FLT3 mutations are seen: internal tandem duplications (ITD) in the transmembrane region occur in around 15 – 25% of AML samples; and point mutations in the tyrosine kinase domain (TKD) occur in ~5-10% of cases (Kottaridis et al. 2001; Mills et al. 2005; Moreno et al. 2003; Steudel et al. 2003). FLT3 ITD mutations may have an influence on prognosis (Kottaridis et al. 2001). Other mutations that frequently occur are partial tandem duplications (PTD) within the MLL gene (~5%) (Steudel et al. 2003), point mutations of the CEPBα gene in ~5-10% of patients with normal cytogenetics (Frohling et al. 2004; Snaddon et al. 2003) and the more recently identified point mutations of the NPM gene again in 25-53% of patients with normal cytogenetics (Boissel et al. 2005; Cazzaniga et al. 2005; Schnittger et al. 2005). RAS mutations seen in around 4 – 10% of AML patients are clustered into specific cytogenetic sub-groups and do not influence prognosis (Bowen et al. 2005).

These mutations that occur in AML are usually observed across FAB, cytogenetic or WHO sub-groups. Indeed it is probable the heterogeneity of AML masks the clear identification of a FLT3 specific gene expression profile in the global population studies (Bullinger et al. 2004; Valk et al. 2004). However, if the heterogeneity is removed, such as in the recent study (Gale et al. 2005) which focused only on patients with APL, AML M3 containing the t(15; 17) translocation, then those patients with FLT3 mutations, whether ITD or TKD, clearly clustered differently from patients with wild type FLT3. Interestingly, the TKD mutations formed a separate branch of the mutant cluster, showing an expression profile intermediate between ITD mutants and wild-type FLT3 samples. This study reinforces the scenario, that FLT3 is a secondary, but important mutation, whose genetic effects may be "over-shadowed" when examined in a heterogeneous AML population.

The larger studies showed that patients could be clustered into several groupings mainly based on distinct cytogenetic abnormalities, however gene signatures for patients with FLT3, and in particular MLL and RAS, mutations were more difficult to identify (Bullinger et al. 2004; Schoch et al. 2002; Valk et al. 2004). In a study of patients with normal cytogenetics, a 10-gene signature was identified allowed the correct classification of FLT3-ITD, FLT3-TKD, NRAS-PM, MLL-PTD, and wild-type samples with an accuracy of 83.7%. Their data showed that FLT3-ITD and FLT3-TKD mutations underlie a clinical phenotype distinct from wt specimens (Neben et al. 2005).

The MLL gene is also involved in a wide range of chromosomal translocations involving chromosome 11q23. Often MLL PTD mutations co-occur with FLT3 mutations making the identification of specific gene expression profiles more difficult (Olesen et al. 2005). A study of paediatric AML samples failed to show a distinct expression signature for AML with a MLL-PTD despite clearly identifying the other major cytogenetic types including a sub-group containing patients with rearrangements of the MLL gene (Ross et al. 2004).

About 1/3rd of AMLs have a mutation of the NPM gene within the putative nucleolar localization signal domain. These mutations are frequently associated with normal cytogenetics. Seventy-eight de novo AML samples, characterized for the sub-cellular localization and mutation status of NPM were expression profiled and subjected to unsupervised clustering which clearly distinguished NPM mutants from NPM wild-type AML, with the expression profile dominated by a stem cell molecular signature (Alcalay et al. 2005). NPM mutations dominated in one cluster (78%) and were enhanced in another cluster (61%) in the study by Wilson et al. (2006).

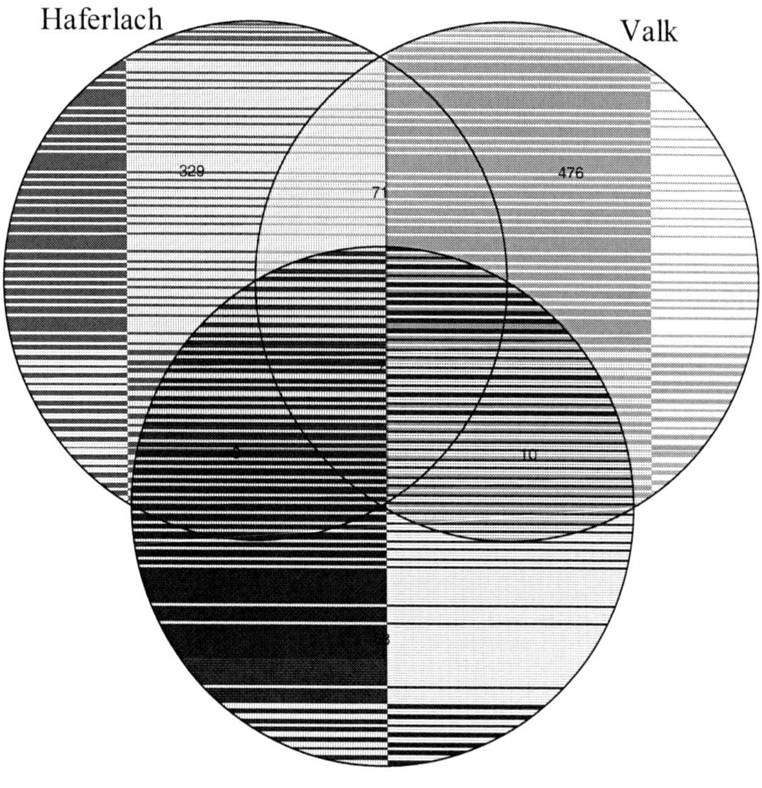

Figure 1. Comparison of genes differentiating between major subgroups in AML between studies. Comparison of the gene lists from three large gene expression studies of AML. (Red: genes identified from the supplementary material for the 6 AML groupings from Haferlach et al. (2005b). Green: genes from the similar supplementary data used for producing 16 clusters from Valk et al. (2004). Blue: 106 genes represented by 149 cDNAs that were used for clustering AML with normal karyotype from Bullinger et al. (2004) and validated by Radmacher et al. (2006).) The genes were translated to only those included on the Affymetrix U133A gene chip. Each study showed that patients could be grouped in several different clusters however the resulting gene lists show very little overlap.

Most of the studies are diverse in terms of sample size, patient characteristics, cytogenetic background or mutational status and each has produced a different molecular classification although certain features are common to each, especially the dominance of the recurrent cytogenetic translocations to form specific subgroups. The potential of gene expression arrays for diagnosis and prognostication was suggested to be supportive of the information obtained by cytogenetic and molecular studies (Dunphy 2006). The larger studies identified gene signatures or lists that could cluster groups into those containing the recurrent translocations but also into several other groupings with a broad, but not exact, relationship to either morphological (i.e. FAB groupings) or mutational status (Bullinger et al. 2004; Valk et al. 2004; Wilson et al. 2006) (Figure 1). However it is often difficult to directly compare gene lists obtained from one study with those from a different study as these studies tend to use different platforms, with samples shipped and stored for differing lengths of time and extracted by different methods. However, recently, the gene expression signatures for clustering AML patients with normal karyotype, obtained using cDNA arrays (Bullinger et al. 2004), into two relevant subgroups was successfully applied to a similar, but independent, group of patient profiles generated with oligonucleotide arrays (Radmacher et al. 2006). This cross-platform analysis using independent patient cohorts confirmed the prognostic significance of the signature.

A small study of 65 diagnostic bone marrow specimens of adult patients with AML, ALL, CML or CLL identified a group of leukaemia-specific genes giving expression profiles distinctly different from normal bone marrow samples. In addition, gene subsets were identified that distinguish between the AML, ALL, CML and CLL patient groups. The results indicated that expression profiling may provide a novel classification of leukaemia patients allowing for more effective treatment (Song et al. 2006). This global approach to leukaemia classification was further developed in a large multi-centre comparison assessing microarray diagnosis with standard diagnostic techniques (Haferlach et al. 2005b). A major step in molecular diagnostic classification was the launch of an international multi-centre clinical research program (MILE: Microarray Innovations in LEukaemia study). The MILE study assesses the application of a microarray test for its potential use in the diagnosis and sub-classification of haematologic malignancies (Haferlach et al. 2005a). The MILE research program was launched in 11 centres: 7 European centres in association with the European Leukaemia Network (ELN) (http://www.leukemia-net.org/index.htm), 3 centres from the USA, and one in Singapore. This study will include 4,400 patients (with all leukaemia types included) and will compare the clinical accuracy of gene expression profiles for 16 acute and chronic leukaemia subclasses with current gold-standard routine diagnostic work-up. The advantage of this study is that each participating centre will use an identical microarray protocol, identical reagents, laboratory equipment, and statistical interpretation. This type of standardisation was recommended by the European Standardisation Working Group for the implementation and analysis of gene expression data (Staal et al. 2006).

Conclusion

The use of microarrays for disease classification has probably been examined more extensively in AML than other types of leukaemia and cancers. The inherent heterogeneity of the disease means that clear clinical benefits have yet to become available, but studies have confirmed that cytogenetic sub-groups have a strong and over-riding influence on gene expression profiles. These studies have also shown that attempts to force current morphological classifications onto a molecular classification may not be successful. The future for gene expression profiling assays, using a defined gene list, is to complement current gold standard diagnostic methods (immunophenotyping, PCR, cytogenetics and FISH). However, if this to be accepted as part of the routine diagnostic workup, co-ordinated, standardised, international and multi-centre protocols need to be developed and tested. Studies, such as the MILE study, suggest that microarray developments are rapidly progressing towards improvements in disease diagnosis and monitoring, and the determination of individualised outcome prediction and personalised treatment regimens.

REFERENCES

Alcalay, M., Tiacci, E., Bergomas, R., Bigerna, B., Venturini, E., Minardi, S. P., Meani, N., Diverio, D., Bernard, L., Tizzoni, L., Volorio, S., Luzi, L., Colombo, E., Lo, C. F., Mecucci, C., Falini, B., & Pelicci, P. G. Acute myeloid leukemia bearing cytoplasmic nucleophosmin (NPMc+AML) shows a distinct gene expression profile characterized by up-regulation of genes involved in stem cell maintenance. Blood 106, 899-902. 14-4-2005.

Bennett, J. M., Catovsky, D., Daniel, M. T., Flandrin, G., Galton, D. A., Gralnick, H. R., & Sultan, C. Proposals for the classification of the acute leukaemias. French-American-British (FAB) co-operative group. *Br.J.Haematol.* *33*[4], 451-458. 1976.

Boissel, N., Renneville, A., Biggio, V., Philippe, N., Thomas, X., Cayuela, J. M., Terre, C., Tigaud, I., Castaigne, S., Raffoux, E., de, B. S., Fenaux, P., Dombret, H., & Preudomme, C. Prevalence, clinical profile and prognosis of NPM mutations in AML with normal karyotype. *Blood.* *26*-7-2005.

Bowen, D. T., Frew, M. E., Hills, R., Gale, R. E., Wheatley, K., Groves, M. J., Langabeer, S. E., Kottaridis, P. D., Moorman, A. V., Burnett, A. K., & Linch, D. C. RAS mutation in acute myeloid leukemia is associated with distinct cytogenetic subgroups but does not influence outcome in patients < 60 yrs. *Blood.* *16*-6-2005.

Bullinger, L., Dohner, K., Bair, E., Frohling, S., Schlenk, R. F., Tibshirani, R., Dohner, H., & Pollack, J. R. Use of gene-expression profiling to identify prognostic subclasses in adult acute myeloid leukemia. *N.Engl.J.Med.* *350*[16], 1605-1616. 15-4-2004.

Cazzaniga, G., Dell'Oro, M. G., Mecucci, C., Giarin, E., Masetti, R., Rossi, V., Locatelli, F., Martelli, M. F., Basso, G., Pession, A., Biondi, A., & Falini, B. Nucleophosmin mutations in childhood acute myelogenous leukemia with normal karyotype. *Blood* *106*[4], 1419-1422. 15-8-2005.

Chapiro, E., Delabesse, E., Asnafi, V., Millien, C., Davi, F., Nugent, E., Beldjord, K., Haferlach, T., Grimwade, D., & Macintyre, E. A. Expression of T-lineage affiliated transcripts and TCR rearrangements in acute promyelocytic leukemia: implications for the cellular target of the t(15; 17). *Blood.* *20*-7-2006.

Debernardi, S., Lillington, D. M., Chaplin, T., Tomlinson, S., Amess, J., Rohatiner, A., Lister, T. A., & Young, B. D. Genome-wide analysis of acute myeloid leukemia with normal karyotype reveals a unique pattern of homeobox gene expression distinct from those with translocation-mediated fusion events. Genes Chromosomes. *Cancer 37*[2], 149-158. 2003.

Dunphy, C. H. Gene expression profiling data in lymphoma and leukemia: review of the literature and extrapolation of pertinent clinical applications. *Arch.Pathol.Lab Med. 130*[4], 483-520. 2006.

Frohling, S., Schlenk, R. F., Stolze, I., Bihlmayr, J., Benner, A., Kreitmeier, S., Tobis, K., Dohner, H., & Dohner, K. CEBPA mutations in younger adults with acute myeloid leukemia and normal cytogenetics: prognostic relevance and analysis of cooperating mutations. *J.Clin.Oncol. 22*[4], 624-633. 15-2-2004.

Gale, R. E., Hills, R., Pizzey, A. R., Kottaridis, P. D., Swirsky, D., Gilkes, A. F., Nugent, E., Mills, K. I., Wheatley, K., Solomon, E., Burnett, A. K., Linch, D. C., & Grimwade, D. The relationship between FLT3 mutation status, biological characteristics and response to targeted therapy in acute promyelocytic leukemia. *Blood Online August 16*. 16-8-2005.

Golub, T. R., Slonim, D. K., Tamayo, P., Huard, C., Gaasenbeek, M., Mesirov, J. P., Coller, H., Loh, M. L., Downing, J. R., Caligiuri, M. A., Bloomfield, C. D., & Lander, E. S. Molecular classification of cancer: class discovery and class prediction by gene expression monitoring. *Science 286*[5439], 531-537. 15-10-1999.

Grimwade, D., Walker, H., Harrison, G., Oliver, F., Chatters, S., Harrison, C. J., Wheatley, K., Burnett, A. K., & Goldstone, A. H. The predictive value of hierarchical cytogenetic classification in older adults with acute myeloid leukemia (AML): analysis of 1065 patients entered into the United Kingdom Medical Research Council AML11 trial. *Blood 98*[5], 1312-1320. 1-9-2001.

Grimwade, D., Walker, H., Oliver, F., Wheatley, K., Harrison, C., Harrison, G., Rees, J., Hann, I., Stevens, R., Burnett, A., & Goldstone, A. The importance of diagnostic cytogenetics on outcome in AML: analysis of 1,612 patients entered into the MRC AML 10 trial. The Medical Research Council Adult and Children's Leukaemia Working Parties. *Blood 92*[7], 2322-2333. 1-10-1998.

Gutierrez, N. C., Lopez-Perez, R., Hernandez, J. M., Isidro, I., Gonzalez, B., Delgado, M., Ferminan, E., Garcia, J. L., Vazquez, L., Gonzalez, M., & San Miguel, J. F. Gene expression profile reveals deregulation of genes with relevant functions in the different subclasses of acute myeloid leukemia. *Leukemia 3*, 402-409. 20-1-2005.

Haferlach, T., Kohlmann, A., Basso, G., Bene, M. C., Downing, J. R., Hernandez, J. M., Hofmann, W. K., Kipps, T. J., te Kronni, T., Liu, W. M., Ro, S., Macintyre, E. A., Mills, K. I., Preudhomme, C., Rassenti, L., de Vos, K., Williams, M., Wieczorek, L., & Foa, R. A Multi-Center and Multi-National Program to Assess the Clinical Accuracy of the Molecular Subclassification of Leukemia by Gene Expression Profiling. *Blood 106*[11], #757. 2005a.

Haferlach, T., Kohlmann, A., Schnittger, S., Dugas, M., Hiddemann, W., Kern, W., & Schoch, C. A global approach to the diagnosis of leukemia using gene expression profiling. *Blood 106*, 1189-1198. 5-5-2005b.

Haferlach, T., Kohlmann, A., Schnittger, S., Dugas, M., Hiddemann, W., Kern, W., & Schoch, C. AML M3 and AML M3 variant each have a distinct gene expression signature but also share patterns different from other genetically defined AML subtypes. Genes Chromosomes. *Cancer 43*[2], 113-127. 2005c.

Kohlmann, A., Schoch, C., Schnittger, S., Dugas, M., Hiddemann, W., Kern, W., & Haferlach, T. Molecular characterization of acute leukemias by use of microarray technology. Genes Chromosomes. *Cancer 37*[4], 396-405. 2003.

Kottaridis, P. D., Gale, R. E., Frew, M. E., Harrison, G., Langabeer, S. E., Belton, A. A., Walker, H., Wheatley, K., Bowen, D. T., Burnett, A. K., Goldstone, A. H., & Linch, D. C. The presence of a FLT3 internal tandem duplication in patients with acute myeloid leukemia (AML) adds important prognostic information to cytogenetic risk group and response to the first cycle of chemotherapy: analysis of 854 patients from the United Kingdom Medical Research Council AML 10 and 12 trials. *Blood 98*[6], 1752-1759. 15-9-2001.

Lee, S., Chen, J., Zhou, G., Shi, R. Z., Bouffard, G. G., Kocherginsky, M., Ge, X., Sun, M., Jayathilaka, N., Kim, Y. C., Emmanuel, N., Bohlander, S. K., Minden, M., Kline, J., Ozer, O., Larson, R. A., LeBeau, M. M., Green, E. D., Trent, J., Karrison, T., Liu, P. P., Wang, S. M., & Rowley, J. D. Gene expression profiles in acute myeloid leukemia with common translocations using SAGE. *Proc.Natl.Acad.Sci.U.S.A 103*[4], 1030-1035. 24-1-2006.

Mills, K. I., Gilkes, A. F., Walsh, V., Sweeney, M., & Gale, R. Rapid and sensitive detection of internal tandem duplication and activating loop mutations of FLT3. *Br.J.Haematol. 130*[2], 203-208. 2005.

Moreno, I., Martin, G., Bolufer, P., Barragan, E., Rueda, E., Roman, J., Fernandez, P., Leon, P., Mena, A., Cervera, J., Torres, A., & Sanz, M. A. Incidence and prognostic value of FLT3 internal tandem duplication and D835 mutations in acute myeloid leukemia. *Haematologica 88*[1], 19-24. 2003.

Morikawa, J., Li, H., Kim, S., Nishi, K., Ueno, S., Suh, E., Dougherty, E., Shmulevich, I., Shiku, H., Zhang, W., & Kobayashi, T. Identification of signature genes by microarray for acute myeloid leukemia without maturation and acute promyelocytic leukemia with t(15; 17)(q22; q12)(PML/RARalpha). *Int.J.Oncol. 23*[3], 617-625. 2003.

Neben, K., Schnittger, S., Brors, B., Tews, B., Kokocinski, F., Haferlach, T., Muller, J., Hahn, M., Hiddemann, W., Eils, R., Lichter, P., & Schoch, C. Distinct gene expression patterns associated with FLT3- and NRAS-activating mutations in acute myeloid leukemia with normal karyotype. *Oncogene 24*[9], 1580-1588. 24-2-2005.

Olesen, L. H., Nyvold, C. G., Aggerholm, A., Norgaard, J. M., Guldberg, P., & Hokland, P. Delineation and molecular characterization of acute myeloid leukemia patients with coduplication of FLT3 and MLL. *Eur.J.Haematol. 75*[3], 185-192. 2005.

Oyan, A. M., Bo, T. H., Jonassen, I., Gjertsen, B. T., Bruserud, O., & Kalland, K. H. cDNA microarray analysis of non-selected cases of acute myeloid leukemia demonstrates distinct clustering independent of cytogenetic aberrations and consistent with morphological signs of differentiation. *Int J Oncol. 28*[5], 1065-1080. 2006.

Radmacher, M. D., Marcucci, G., Ruppert, A. S., Mrozek, K., Whitman, S. P., Vardiman, J. W., Paschka, P., Vukosavljevic, T., Baldus, C. D., Kolitz, J. E., Caligiuri, M. A., Larson, R. A., & Bloomfield, C. D. Independent confirmation of a prognostic gene-expression signature in adult acute myeloid leukemia with a normal karyotype: A cancer and leukemia group B study. *Blood. 2*-5-2006.

Ross, M. E., Mahfouz, R., Onciu, M., Liu, H. C., Zhou, X., Song, G., Shurtleff, S. A., Pounds, S., Cheng, C., Ma, J., Ribeiro, R. C., Rubnitz, J. E., Girtman, K., Williams, W. K., Raimondi, S. C., Liang, D. C., Shih, L. Y., Pui, C. H., & Downing, J. R. Gene expression profiling of pediatric acute myelogenous leukemia. *Blood 104*[12], 3679-3687. 1-12-2004.

Schnittger, S., Schoch, C., Kern, W., Mecucci, C., Tschulik, C., Martelli, M. F., Haferlach, T., Hiddemann, W., & Falini, B. Nucleophosmin gene mutations are predictors of favourable prognosis in acute myelogenous leukemia with a normal kayotype. *Blood. 2*-8-2005.

Schoch, C., Kohlmann, A., Schnittger, S., Brors, B., Dugas, M., Mergenthaler, S., Kern, W., Hiddemann, W., Eils, R., & Haferlach, T. Acute myeloid leukemias with reciprocal rearrangements can be distinguished by specific gene expression profiles. *Proc.Natl.Acad.Sci.U.S.A 99*[15], 10008-10013. 23-7-2002.

Snaddon, J., Smith, M. L., Neat, M., Cambal-Parrales, M., Dixon-McIver, A., Arch, R., Amess, J. A., Rohatiner, A. Z., Lister, T. A., & Fitzgibbon, J. Mutations of CEBPA in acute myeloid leukemia FAB types M1 and M2. Genes Chromosomes. *Cancer 37*[1], 72-78. 2003.

Song, J. H., Kim, H. J., Lee, C. H., Kim, S. J., Hwang, S. Y., & Kim, T. S. Identification of gene expression signatures for molecular classification in human leukemia cells. *Int J Oncol. 29*[1], 57-64. 2006.

Staal, F. J., Cario, G., Cazzaniga, G., Haferlach, T., Heuser, M., Hofmann, W. K., Mills, K., Schrappe, M., Stanulla, M., Wingen, L. U., van Dongen, J. J., & Schlegelberger, B. Consensus guidelines for microarray gene expression analyses in leukemia from three European leukemia networks. *Leukemia. 8*-6-2006.

Steudel, C., Wermke, M., Schaich, M., Schakel, U., Illmer, T., Ehninger, G., & Thiede, C. Comparative analysis of MLL partial tandem duplication and FLT3 internal tandem duplication mutations in 956 adult patients with acute myeloid leukemia. Genes Chromosomes. *Cancer 37*[3], 237-251. 2003.

Tibshirani, R., Hastie, T., Narasimhan, B., & Chu, G. Diagnosis of multiple cancer types by shrunken centroids of gene expression. *Proc.Natl.Acad.Sci.U.S.A 99*[10], 6567-6572. 14-5-2002.

Tusher, V. G., Tibshirani, R., & Chu, G. Significance analysis of microarrays applied to the ionizing radiation response. *Proc.Natl.Acad.Sci.U.S.A 98*[9], 5116-5121. 24-4-2001.

Valk, P. J., Verhaak, R. G., Beijen, M. A., Erpelinck, C. A., Barjesteh van Waalwijk van Doorn-Khosrovani, Boer, J. M., Beverloo, H. B., Moorhouse, M. J., van der Spek, P. J., Lowenberg, B., & Delwel, R. Prognostically useful gene-expression profiles in acute myeloid leukemia. *N.Engl.J.Med. 350*[16], 1617-1628. 15-4-2004.

Vardiman, J. W., Harris, N. L., & Brunning, R. D. The World Health Organization (WHO) classification of the myeloid neoplasms. *Blood 100*[7], 2292-2302. 1-10-2002.

Vey, N., Mozziconacci, M. J., Groulet-Martinec, A., Debono, S., Finetti, P., Carbuccia, N., Beillard, E., Devilard, E., Arnoulet, C., Coso, D., Sainty, D., Xerri, L., Stoppa, A. M., Lafage-Pochitaloff, M., Nguyen, C., Houlgatte, R., Blaise, D., Maraninchi, D., Birg, F., Birnbaum, D., & Bertucci, F. Identification of new classes among acute myelogenous leukaemias with normal karyotype using gene expression profiling. *Oncogene 23*, 9381-9391. 15-11-2004.

Virtaneva, K., Wright, F. A., Tanner, S. M., Yuan, B., Lemon, W. J., Caligiuri, M. A., Bloomfield, C. D., de la, C. A., & Krahe, R. Expression profiling reveals fundamental biological differences in acute myeloid leukemia with isolated trisomy 8 and normal cytogenetics. *Proc.Natl.Acad.Sci.U.S.A 98*[3], 1124-1129. 30-1-2001.

Wilson, C. S., Davidson, G. S., Martin, S. B., Andries, E., Potter, J., Harvey, R., Ar, K., Xu, Y., Kopecky, K. J., Ankerst, D. P., Gundacker, H., Slovak, M. L., Mosquera-Caro, M., Chen, I. M., Stirewalt, D. L., Murphy, M., Schultz, F. A., Kang, H., Wang, X., Radich, J. P., Appelbaum, F. R., Atlas, S. R., Godwin, J., & Willman, C. L. Gene expression profiling of adult acute myeloid leukemia identifies novel biologic clusters for risk classification and outcome prediction. *Blood. 4*-4-2006.

In: Cancer Research Perspectives
Editor: Larissa S. Pereira, pp. 245-257

ISBN 978-1-60021-980-1

Chapter IX

Cystatins in Cancer

***Janko Kos*[1,*] *and Tamara Lah*[2]**
[1]Department of Pharmaceutical Biology, Faculty of Pharmacy, University of Ljubljana, Ljubljana, Slovenia;
[2]Department of GeneticToxicology and Cancer Biology, National Institute of Biology, Ljubljana, Slovenia.

Abstract

Cystatins comprise a large superfamily of related proteins with diverse biological activities. They were initially characterised as inhibitors of lysosomal cysteine proteases, however, in recent years some alternative functions for cystatins have been proposed. In tumours their role was considered as protective since they are capable to impair excessive activity of cysteine proteases, associated with tumour growth, invasion, angiogenesis and metastasis. Knockout or transgenic animal models and clinical investigations of cystatins in body fluids provided the opposite, i.e. cystatins can also promote malignant disease. Their dual relation to progression of cancer, various physiological roles and differences between type I and type II cystatins with regard to possible applications in diagnosis and therapy in cancer are discussed in this review.

Keywords: cystatin; stefin; cathepsin; cancer; prognosis; diagnosis; therapy.

* Correspondence concerning this article should be addressed to: Janko Kos, Department of Pharmaceutical Biology, Faculty of Pharmacy, University of Ljubljana, Aškerčeva 7 SI-1000 Ljubljana, Slovenia. Phone: +386 1 4769 604; Fax: +386 1 4258 031; e-mail: janko.kos@ffa.uni-lj.si.

Introduction

Lysosomal cysteine proteases, the cathepsins, classified as clan C1 [1], were long believed to be responsible for the terminal protein degradation in the lysosomes. This view has changed dramatically when they have been found to be involved in a number of important cellular processes, such as antigen presentation [2], bone resorption [3], apoptosis [4] and protein processing [5], as well as several pathologies such as cancer progression [6], inflammation [7] and neurodegeneration [8].

So far, cathepsin D, an aspartic protease, and cysteine cathespins B, H, L, S and few others [reviewed by Lah and Kos, 9], [10-12] were associated with cancer progression. Their expression varies in different tissues and different developmental stages. Cysteine cathepsins are single-gene products, but the protein products may be polymorphic, due to allelic variants of the gene, alternative RNA splicing and/or post-translational modifications. Similar to other proteases, cathepsins are regulated at every level of their biosynthesis, in addition to the trafficking to lysosomes, which often critically depends of the post-translational modifications. [13,14].

The activity of cysteine cathepsins is controlled by their compartmentalization to lysosomes, activation of pro-enzyme forms and ultimately by their endogenous protein inhibitors [4]. Among them the best characterized are the cystatins, which comprise a superfamily of evolutionary related proteins, each consisting of at least one domain of 100-120 amino acid residues with conserved sequence motifs [4,13,15]. Type I cystatins (the stefins), stefins A and B, are cytosolic proteins, comprised of about one hundred amino acids, lacking disulphide bridges. Type II cystatins are more numerous, comprising at least 14 members [for recent review, see Keppler et al., 14]. They are extracellular proteins, consisting of about one hundred twenty amino acid residues and containing two disulphide bridges. Besides well known cystatins C, D, E/M, F, S, SA, SN this group contains the male reproductive tract cystatins 8 (CRES), 9 (testatin), 11 and 12 (cystatin T), the bone marrow-derived cystatin-like molecule CLM (cystatin 13) and the secreted phosphoprotein SPP-24 (cystatin 14). Type III cystatins, the kininogens, are large multifunctional plasma proteins, containing three type II cystatin-like domains, whereas fetuin and latexin families are constituted by two tandem cystatin domains, however, they are not the subject of the present review.

A broad spectrum of biological roles have been suggested for cystatins, including a role in protein catabolism, regulation of hormone processing and bone resorption, inflammation, antigen presentation and T-cell dependent immune response [16,17] as well as resistance to various bacterial and viral infections. In most cases cystatins function as reversible, tight-binding inhibitors of cysteine proteases, however, they can also act independently of their inhibitory properties [18,19]. Cystatins have been suggested as modulators of the proteolytic system in several diseases, including cancer [9,16,20].

To highlight the function of cystatins in regulation of proteolysis in malignant versus non-malignant cells and tissues and to evaluate their potential for diagnostic and therapeutic interventions represent a significant challenge for basic and translational research in oncology. We review recent finding on the status of type I and type II cystatins (stefins A, B and cystatins C, E/M and F) in cancer with particular emphasis on their suppressive vs. promotional function in the development of malignant diseases.

Cystatins in Tumour Cells and Tissues

Lysosomes normally store about 90-95 % of the lysosomal hydrolases, including cysteine proteases [reviewed by Chapman et al.,3]. It has been observed, that in a variety of tumour cells, these enzymes are translocated from the pericellular lysosomes into plasma membranes [21], destined to secretion and/or are released into the cytosol. Under normal conditions, the lysosomal proteases protect the cell homeostasis, which, however, is altered immediately after cell transformation in carcinogenesis [22].

Cysteine proteases have been implicated in multiple steps of tumour progression, including processes of cell transformation and differentiation, motility, adhesion, invasion, angiogenesis, and metastasis. In most tumour types the levels of expression, protein concentrations and enzymatic activities of cysteine proteases, in particular of cathepsins B and L have been demonstrated to be significantly higher than in their control tissue counterparts [9,23-29].

The increased levels of cathepsins are usually not accompanied by an equal increase of the cystatins what was suggested as the main cause of harmful cysteine cathepsins' dependent proteolytic activity in tumour tissue. However, the balance is selectively altered for type II cystatins which are in most cases downregulated in tumours, whereas type I cystatins, i.e. stefins A and B have been found up-regulated in majority of cases when compared to control tissue counterparts [30]. Higher levels of stefins A and B in tumours have been determined in lung [25,29,31,32], breast [10,33] head and neck [34] prostate cancer [35] as well as in murine lymphosarcomas, hepatomas and Lewis lung carcinomas [36]. These higher levels, up to a certain level, may counter-balance the excessive activity of cysteine cathepsins, associated with the progression of the disease. However, high cytosolic levels of stefins may be relevant for regulation of apoptosis, when initiated via lysosomal cell death pathway [37] inhibiting presumably cathepsin B, which was proposed as a dominant execution protease in the lysosomal apoptotic pathways, induced in a variety of tumour cells by TNF alpha [38].

Type II cystatins are secretory proteins and their lower levels in tissues are expected when compared to stefins. Their role in tumour cells remains protective, however, their lower levels could allow a surplus of harmful tumour associated proteolytic activity. Although several studies reported that the expression of cystatin C is not changed much between malignant and non-malignant tissues [39], some studies provide opposite for cystatin C protein levels. Cystatin C protein concentration was found lower in lung [31] and ovarian [40] tumours and murine HA-1 hepatomas and lymphosarcomas [36]. Chemotherapeutics may increase the level of cystatin C in tumours, as shown for HA-1 hepatoma and lymphosarcoma treated mice [36].

For cystatin E/M a downregulation has been demonstrated in breast tumours [41] although mRNA for cystatin E/M has been reported to be more highly expressed in metastatic oropharingeal squamous cell carcinoma than in the primary tumours [42]. In the study on lung tumours [31] we did not find any difference in cystatin E/M protein levels in primary and secondary lung tumours, and, consistently to the results of Sotiropoulu et al., [41] we found lower protein levels of cystatin E/M in lung tumours when compared to control lung counterparts. The latter is in line with other reports on squamous cell carcinomas of skin, head and neck and lung providing diminished or lost expression of cystatin E/M [43].

Although cystatin F is a type II cystatin, it was found intracellularly in lysosome-like vesicles and due to its inhibitory properties it could effectively impair intracellular endopeptidase activity of cathepsins L, K, V and F [44]. Previously its expression was reported to be restricted to haematopoietic cells, very likely involved in processes of the immune response. The demonstration that cystatin F can be present in primary tumours, together with the reported overexpression of cystatin F mRNA in liver metastatic tumours by Morita et al., [45] suggests a function other that regulation of the immune response. Higher expression of cystatin F was found in human tumour cell lines with high propensity to metastasize in liver [45] and opposite to cystatins E/M and C it higher tumour levels of cystatin F seem to promote the metastatic processes. The latter is supported by the survival analysis of colorectal cancer patients, providing higher risk of death for patients with higher expression of cystatin F. We found cystatin F in tumour cells and histiocytes of lung tumours by immunohistochemical analysis [31], however, using ELISA we were not able to determine its higher concentration in tumours compared to control lung tissue [31].

Both, type I and type II cystatins showed intense immuno-staining in tumour cells and also in the surrounding histiocytes, predominantly macrophages, similarly to that reported for cathepsins B and L, which were found in large amounts in tumour cells and histiocytes in various tumour types [9,27,46]. Functional proteolysis imaging of living carcinoma cells in co-cultures with stromal cells demonstrated that macrophages and fibroblasts could be a major source of harmful tumour-associated proteolytic activity [47] and, therefore, the localization of cystatins in this cell type does not necessarily mean successful inactivation of their targets.

Mueller and Fusenig [48] recently reviewed the current knowledge on the crucial importance of the micro-environment for the progression of the tumour phenotype. They even demonstrated reciprocal up-regulation of proteases between cancer cells and stromal fibroblasts and showed that the stromal cells can enhance or revert the malignant phenotype without affecting tumour cells. This is explained by autocrine and paracrine loops where soluble factors and insoluble ECM components are cleaved by the tumour cell-derived proteases, resulting in an increase in protease production and secretion by the stromal cells, and *vice versa*.

Extracellular Levels of Cystatins

Type II cystatins are secretory proteins and have been detected in significant amounts in various body fluids of cancer patients. In blood, their levels are not drastically changed in comparison to healthy controls and question arises whether these changes may be of any physiological importance. However, at the local level, especially in the extracellular microenvironment the altered levels of these inhibitors could significantly modulate proteolytic activity of secreted or membrane bound cysteine proteases. Minor changes in blood or other fluids may only reflect these local processes. However, cystatin C was found to be increased in sera of patients with B-cell lymphomas, melanoma, colorectal and lung tumours [6,9] and its levels were correlating with the progression of the malignant disease. On the other hand, cystatin C has also been proposed as an accurate marker of glomerular filtration rate (GFR) [49] and its changes may reflect impaired kidney function in cancer patients. Although cancer patients included in cystatin C investigations [50] did not exhibit impaired kidney function, the early, previously undetectable alterations in renal function and their impact on cystatin C level in blood can not be completely excluded [51]. Nevertheless, the reason for the increased levels of cystatin C has to be carefully evaluated before applying this new marker of GFR in clinical use for cancer patients.

Type II cystatins C, E/M and F have also been evaluated in pleural fluids of patients with neoplastic and inflammatory lung disorders [52]. Cystatin C levels did correlate neither with malignant nor with benign diseases. On the other hand, the levels of cystatin E/M were significantly higher in effusions of primary pleural tumours compared to secondary tumours and benign diseases. The levels of cystatin F were increased in parapneumonic effusions and emphysema thoracic effusions. In these groups its levels correlated with the neutrophil count and the inflammatory marker C-reactive protein (CRP) suggesting its association with the inflammatory processes of lung disorders.

Type I cystatins have also been detected in body fluids of cancer patients. Stefin A and stefin B have been detected in ascitic fluid from ovarian carcinoma [53] and in bronhoalveolar fluid of lung cancer patients [54]. Increased serum levels of stefin A in patients with hepatocellular carcinoma and liver cirrhosis correlated with tumour size and with a number of neoplastic lesions [55]. Stefin A, but not stefin B levels were moderately increased also in patients with colorectal or lung cancer [50].

Cystatins in Diagnosis and Prognosis of Cancer

In cancer, the increased levels of cysteine protease activity, not being balanced by a corresponding increase of cysteine protease inhibitors, were suggested to be involved in remodelling and degradation of extracellular matrix proteins, a proteolytic event associated with tumour spread, invasion and metastasis [47]. Enhanced expression of cystatins would be expected to diminish the tumour-associated proteolytic activity and indeed, there is evidence of a suppressive role of tumour-associated cystatins in various cancer types [56-58]. Moreover, higher levels of stefins A, B and cystatin C in tumour tissues have been shown to correlate with a favourable prognosis of cancer patients [9,10,30,34,35,59] – Figure 1.

On the other hand, animal models with excluded expression of particular cystatin did not support a suppressive function for CPI in cancer. In cystatin C [60] and stefin B (Kos et al., unpublished results) knock-out mice, a significantly lower metastatic spread was detected than in wild-type animals. Similarly, higher levels of stefins A, B and cystatin C in body fluids have been associated with a poor prognosis of cancer patients [50] – Figure 2. Alterations in secretion may result in higher extracellular and lower intracellular levels of cystatins and, therefore, a reverse correlation with patient' survival is to be expected. However, cysteine proteases, and consequently their inhibitors, are involved in various physiological processes, including those which may act in a manner opposing tumour progression, such as apoptosis [38], activation of T-cell immune response [3,61], cell migration and seeding [60] and drug resistance processes [62]. Thus, besides their concentration, cell and tissue localisation of cystatins and a number of extrinsic and intrinsic factors could make a critical switch between harmless and harmful.

Different biochemical properties of cystatins provide another reason for their distinct function in cancer processes. In general, all cystatins are tight binding inhibitors of the C1 family of cysteine proteases, including human cathepsins B, H, L, K, S, however, the inhibitory profile of a particular cystatin is rather specific. For example, stefin B is a much weaker inhibitor of cathepsin B than the structurally related stefin A [63]. Also, cystatin F does not inhibit cathepsin B whereas cystatin C, a related type II cystatin, has a high affinity for it [44]. Moreover, in contrast to stefins A and B, the type II cystatins C, E/M and F, possess a second reactive site for inhibiting the C13 family of cysteine proteases (legumain) presumed to be involved in antigen presentation [64]. Besides selective inhibition of cysteine proteases, the secretion of type II but not type I cystatins may specifically regulate the inhibitory potential against intracellular and extracellular targets.

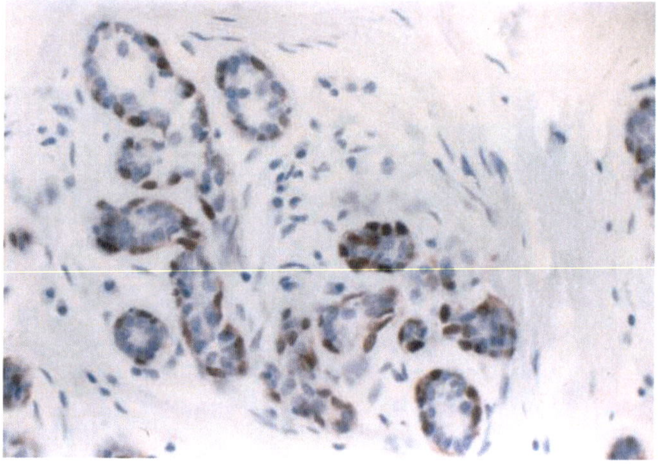

Figure 1. Stefin A immunohistochemical staining in breast carcinoma. Stefin A was immunolabeled, using specific monoclonal antibodies (KRKA, d.d., Slovenia). High expression of stefin A at the invasive edges of malignant tumour islets was observed in the majority, but not all of the tumour samples [30]. Higher levels of stefin A in breast carcinomas were also measured using ELISA (Krka, d.d. Slovenia) and were associated with good prognosis.

Cystatins as Possible Agents in Antitumour Therapy

Proteases, in particular the cysteine cathepsins, the matrix metallo proteases (MMPs) and the uPA/plasmin system, are promising targets for a successful anticancer drug design, because of their involvement in tumour invasion and angiogenesis. There is a substantial amount of the literature showing that the inhibition of one of the above mentioned proteolytic systems leads to the reduced tumour cell invasion as well as tumour regression *in vivo* [12]. Potential candidates for anticancer drugs are endogenous and synthetic protease inhibitors and monoclonal antibodies directed against one or more protease(s). Gene therapy involving antisense oligonucleotides construction and antisense RNA transfection strategies or siRNA silencing could be an additional approach to target protease systems involved in the invasive process.

The role of cysteine proteases in cancer has been very extensively studied during last twenty years, but they have received less attention as possible therapeutic targets compared to the serine or metallo proteases. However, during last years their importance is increasing, partially as a result of failures of metallo protease inhibitors in clinical trials [65]. Recent preclinical studies are promising, it has been shown that cysteine protease inhibitors indeed impaired excessive tumour-associated activity reducing growth, invasion, angiogenesis and metastatic spread [12,57,66-68].

However, there are several factors that greatly limit the general application of cystatins in cancer therapy. Cysteine proteases, causing harmful tumour-associated proteolytic activity, are involved also in several normal physiological processes, like protein turnover, hormone processing and immune response and their total inhibition could result in severe complications. Moreover, cystatins exhibit broad specificity against cysteine proteases, but only some of these proteases are associated with the progression of cancer. The others may possess tumour suppressive functions, such as regulation of anti-tumour immune response or apoptosis and their inhibition would be harmful for cancer patients. Also, in some cases, cystatins do not require the inhibition of cysteine proteases for their activity but bind to cell surface molecules triggering signaling pathways which can also be unfavorable for the patient.

The other problem the application of cystatins in tumour therapy can face is different subcellular localization of the targets, i.e. endosomes/lysosomes, plasma membrane, extracellular fluids, extracellular matrix, cytoplasm or nucleus. Moreover, some tumour-associated proteolytic processes can even take place at different locations. For example, the degradation of extracellular matrix, a crucial step in invasion of tumour cells has been shown to occur extracellularly and intracellularly and cysteine protease inhibitors, capable to inactivate both fractions were the most effective to impair the invasive potential of tumour cells in vitro [47,69].

In our opinion, future approaches in targeting cysteine proteases in anti-tumour therapy should consider two important criteria, first, the selectivity of the inhibitors against the proteases, involved in tumour progressive functions and second, the specific delivery of anti-tumour agents to the spots of harmful proteolytic action. By using advanced methods of molecular and cell biology or chemical synthesis we may expect a number of specific molecules, exploring cystatins' functions and effectively impairing tumour-associated cysteine proteases. On the other hand, the novel delivery systems, including lyposomes and polymeric carriers [70] may be capable to deliver active compounds to the site of action and are believed to achieve the progress in combating cancer.

CONCLUSIONS

There is an accumulating number of studies showing that cystatins are implicated in the progression of various types of cancer. In general, their localisation and regulation of tumour associated proteolytic activity can be recognized by two distinct mechanisms. Type I cystatins, stefins A and B are up-regulated in tumour tissue and, up to a certain level could counter-balance the over-expressed tumour-associated proteolytic activity. Their function as tumour suppressors is supported by survival analysis, which associated their high levels with better outcome of cancer patients. On the other hand, type II cystatins, at least cystatins C and E/M are down-regulated in tumours. Although their role remains protective, their lower levels could allow a surplus of harmful tumour associated proteolytic activity. Outside the cells, higher levels of type II cystatins may impair extracellular activity of cysteine proteases, associated directly or indirectly with the degradation of ECM and resulting in tumour cell invasion and metastasis. However, they can be also involved in processes resulting in tumour regression such as anti-tumour immune response, apoptosis, cell migration and seeding. Higher levels of cystatins in body fluids have been associated with poor prognosis of cancer patients supporting their role in regulation of proteases involved in the regression of tumours. Interestingly, animals with excluded expression of type I or type II cystatins also experience better outcome with regard to tumour growth and metastasis as the wild type ones. Thus, besides their concentration, cell and tissue localisation of cystatins could make a critical switch between harmless and harmful and their application as anti-cancer agents has to be considered with caution and should be directed specifically to cysteine proteases which promote specific stage of tumour progression.

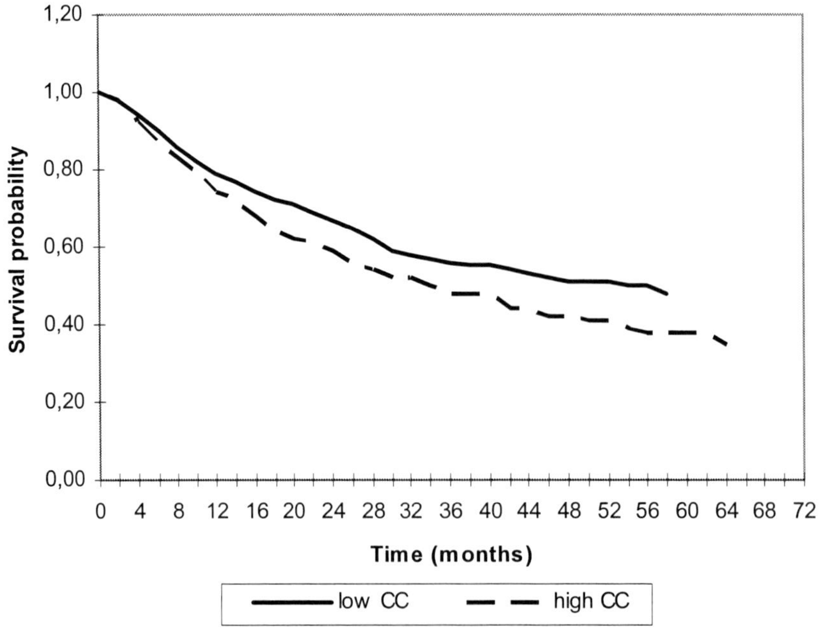

Figure 2. Cystatin C - Prognostic significance in colorectal cancer patients. Cystatin C levels were measured in pre-operative sera from 345 patients [50].

REFERENCES

[1] Barrett, A.J., Rawlings, N.D. and Woessner, J.F. *The Handbook of Proteolytic Enzymes*, 2nd ed. Academic Press, 2004.

[2] Honey, K. and Rudensky, A.Y. (2003) Lysosomal cysteine proteases regulate antigen presentation. *Nat. Rev. Immunol.*, *3*, 472-482.

[3] Chapman, H.A., Riese, R.J., and Shi, G.P. (1997) Emerging roles for cysteine proteases in human biology. *Annu. Rev. Physiol*, *59*, 63-88.

[4] Turk, B., Turk, D., and Salvesen, G.S. (2002) Regulating cysteine protease activity: essential role of protease inhibitors as guardians and regulators. *Curr. Pharm. Des*, *8*, 1623-1637.

[5] Turk, V., Turk, B., and Turk, D. (2001) Lysosomal cysteine proteases: facts and opportunities. *EMBO J.*, *20*, 4629-4633.

[6] Kos, J., Werle, B., Lah, T., and Brunner, N. (2000) Cysteine proteases and their inhibitors in extracellular fluids: markers for diagnosis and prognosis in cancer. *Int. J. Biol. Markers*, *15*, 84-89.

[7] Lang, A., Horler, D., and Baici, A. (2000) The relative importance of cysteine peptidases in osteoarthritis. *J. Rheumatol.*, *27*, 1970-1979.

[8] Felbor, U., Kessler, B., Mothes, W., Goebel, H.H., Ploegh, H.L., Bronson, R.T., and Olsen, B.R. (2002) Neuronal loss and brain atrophy in mice lacking cathepsins B and L. *Proc. Natl. Acad. Sci. U. S. A*, *99,* 7883-7888.

[9] Kos, J. and Lah, T.T. (1998) Cysteine proteases and their endogenous inhibitors: target proteins for prognosis, diagnosis and therapy in cancer (Review). *Oncology Reports* *5*:1349-61.

[10] Levičar, N., Kos, J., Blejec, A., Golouh, R., Vrhovec, I., Frkovič-Grazio, S., Lah, T. (2002). Comparison of potential biological markers cathepsin B, cathepsin L, stefin A and stefin B with urokinase and plasminogen activator inhibitor-1 and clinicopathological data of breast carcinoma patients. *Cancer Det. Prev. 26*: 42-49.

[11] Berdowska I. (2004) Cysteine proteases as disease markers. *Clin. Chim. Acta 342*: 41-69.

[12] Joyce, J.A., Baruch, A., Chehade, K., Meyer-Morse, N., Giraudo, E., Tsai, F.Y., (2004) Cathepsin cysteine proteases are effectors of invasive growth and angiogenesis during multistage tumorigenesis. *Cancer Cell 5*: 443-453.

[13] Rawlings, N.D. and Barrett, A.J. (1990) Evolution of proteins of the cystatin superfamily. *J. Mol. Evol. 30:* 60-71.

[14] Keppler, D. (2005) Towards novel anti-cancer strategies based on cystatin function. *Cancer Letters* 235: 159-176.

[15] Abrahamson, M. (1994) Cystatins. *Methods Enzymol.*, *244*, 685-700.

[16] Henskens, Y.M.C., Veerman, E.C.I., Amerongen, A.V.N. (1996) Cystatins in health and diseases. *Biol. Chem. Hoppe-Seyler 377:* 71-86.

[17] Pierre, P. and Mellman, I.(1998) Developmental regulation of invariant chain proteolysis controls MHC class II trafficking in mouse dendritic cells. *Cell 93:* 1135-1145.

[18] Verdot, L., Lalmanach, G., Vercruysse, V., Hoebeke, J., Gauthier, F., Vray, B. (1999) Chicken cystatin stimulates nitric oxide release from interferon-γ-activated mouse peritoneal macrophages via cytokine synthesis. *Eur. J. Biochem. 266*: 1111-1117.

[19] Giaimo, R., Riccio, M., Santi, S., Galeotti, C., Ambrosetti, D.C. and Melli, M. (2002) New insights into the molecular basis of progressive myoclonus epilepsy. A multiprotein complex with cystatin B. *Human Mol. Genet. 23:* 2941-2950.

[20] Calkins, C.C., Sloane, B.F. (1995). Mammalian cysteine peptidase inhibitors: biochemical properties and possible roles in tumor progression. *Biol. Chem. 376:* 71-80.

[21] Cavallo-Medved, D., Sloane, B.F. (2003) Cell surface cathesin B: understanding its functional signifiance. *Curr. Top. Dev. Biol. 54*; 313-341.

[22] Castino, R., Demoz, M., Isidoro, C. (2003) Destination "lysosome": A target organelle for tumour cell killing? *J. Mol. Recognit. 16:* 337-348.

[23] Trefz, G., Lüthgens, K., Erdel, M., Spiess, E., Ebert, W. (1989) Plasminogen activator and cathepsin B in normal and malignant human lung tissue. *J. Cancer Res. Clin. Oncol. 115*:S50.

[24] Sedo, A., Krepela, E., Kasafirek, E. (1991) Dipeptidylpeptidase IV, prolylendopeptidase and cathepsin B activities in primary human lung tumors and lung parenchyma. *J. Cancer Res. Clin. Oncol. 117*:249-53.

[25] Ebert, W., Knoch, H., Werle, B., Trefz, G., Muley, T., Spiess, E. (1994) Prognostic value of increased lung tumor tissue cathepsin B. *Anticancer Res. 14*:895-0.

[26] Werle, B., Jülke, B., Lah, T., Spiess, E. and Ebert, W. (1997) Cathepsin B fraction active physiological pH of 7.5 is of prognostic significance in squamous cell carcinoma of human lung. *Br. J. Cancer 75:* 1137-1143.

[27] Werle, B., Kraft, C., Lah, T.T., Kos, J., Schanzenbächer, U., Kayser, K., Ebert, W., Spiess, E. (2000) Cathepsin B in infiltrated lymph nodes is of prognostic significance for non-small cell lung cancer patients. *Cancer 89:* 2282-2291.

[28] Krepela, E., Kasafirek, E., Novak, K., Vyklicky, J. (1990) Increased cathepsin B activity in human lung tumors. *Neoplasma 37*: 61-70.

[29] Krepela, E., Prochazkam, J, Karovam, B., Cermakm, J., and Roubkovam, H., (1998) Cysteine proteases and cysteine protease inhibitors in non-small cell lung cancer. *Neoplasma 45:* 318-331.

[30] Lah, TT, Kos,, J, Blejec, A, Frković-Grazio, S, Golouh, R, Vrhovec, I, Turk, V. (1997) The expression of lysosomal proteases and their inhibitors in breast cancer: possible relationship to prognosis of the disease. *Pathology Oncology Research 3/2*: 89-99.

[31] Werle, B., Schanzenbacher, U., Lah, T.T., Ebert, E., Julke, B., Ebert, W., Fiehn, W., Kayser, K., Spiess, E., Abrahamson, M., Kos, J. (2005) Cystatins in non-small cell lung cancer: tissue levels, localisation and relation to prognosis, *Oncology Reports, in press.*

[32] Bianchi, F., Hu, J., Pelosi, G., Cirincione, R., Ferguson, M., Ratcliffe, C. et al., (2004). Lung cancers detected by screening with spiral computed tomography have a malignant phenotype when analyzed by cDNA microarray. *Clin. Cancer. Res. 10*: 6023-28.

[33] Kuopio, T., Kankaanranta, A., Jalava, P. et al. (1998) Cysteine protease inhibitor cystatin A in breast cancer. *Cancer Res. 58*: 432-436.

[34] Strojan, P., Budihna, M., Šmid, L., Svetic, B., Vrhovec, I., Kos, J., Škrk, J. (2000) Prognostic significance of cysteine proteases cathepsins B and L and their endogenous inhibitors stefins A and B in patients with squamous cell carcinoma of the head and neck. *Clin. Cancer Res. 6*: 1052-1062.

[35] Sinha, A.A., Quast, B.J., Wilson, M.J., Fernandes, E.T., Reddy, P.K., Ewing, S.L. et al., (2001) Ratio of cathepsin B to stefin A identifies heterogeneity within Gleason histologic scores for human prostate cancer. *Prostate 48*: 247-284.

[36] Korolenko, T.A., Poteryaeva, O.N., Djanayeva, S.J., Svechnikova, I.G., Kaledin, V.I., Timofeyeva, O.A., Filipenko, M.L., Nowicky, J. (2000) Cystatin C in LS lymphosarcoma and HA-1 hepatoma treated with ukrain and cyclophosphamide and involvement of apoptosis. *Drugs Exptl. Clin. Res. 16*: 285-292.

[37] Jaattela, M. (2004) Multiple cell death pathways as regulators of tumour initiation and progression. *Oncogene 23*: 2746-56.

[38] Foghsgaard, L., Wissing, D., Mauch, D., Lademann, U., Bastholm, L., Boes, M., Elling, F., Leist, M., Jaattela, M. (2001) Cathepsin B acts as a dominant execution protease in tumor cell apoptosis induced by tumor necrosis factor. *J. Cell Biology 153*: 999-1009.

[39] Hirai, K., Yokoyama, M., Asano, G., Tanaka, S. (1999) Expression of cathepsin B and cystatin C in human colorectal cancer. *Hum. Pathol. 30*: 680-686.

[40] Nishikawa, H., Ozaki, Y., Nakanishi, T., Blomgren, K., Tada, T., Arakawa, A., Suzumori, K. (2004) The role of cathepsin B and cystatin C in the mechanisms of invasion by ovarian cancer. *Gynecol. Oncol. 92*: 881-886.

[41] Sotiropoulu, G., Anisowicz, A., Sager, R. (1997) Identification, cloning, and characterisation of cystatin M, a novel cysteine protease inhibitor, down-regulated in breast cancer. *J. Biol. Chem. 272*: 903-910.

[42] Vigneswaran, N., Wu, J., Zacharias, W. Upregulation of cystatin M during the progression of oropharyngeal squamous cell carcinoma from primary tumour to metastasis. *Oral Oncology 39*: 559-568, 2003.

[43] Zeeuwen, P.L., Van Viljmen-Willems, I.M., Egami, H., Schalkwijk, J. (2002) Cystatin M/E expression in inflammatory and neoplastic skin disorders. *Br. J. Dermatol. 147*: 87-94.

[44] Langerholc, T., Zavašnik-Bergant, V., Turk, B., Turk, V., Abrahamson, M., Kos, J. (2005) Inhibitory properties of cystatin F and ist localisation in U937 promonocyte cells. *FEBS Journal 272*: 1535-1545.

[45] Morita, M., Hara, Y., Tamai, Y., Arakawa, H., Nishimura, S. (2000) Genomic construct and mapping of the gene for CMAP (leukocystatin/cystatin F, CST7) and identification of a proximal novel gene BSCv (C20orf3). *Genomics 67*: 87-91.

[46] Lah, T., Kalman, E., Najjar, D., Gorodetsky, E., Brennan, P., Somers, R., Daskal, I.(2000) Cells producing cathepsins D, B and L in human breast carcinoma and teir association with prognosis. *Human Pathol. 31*, 149-160.

[47] Sameni, M., Dosescu, J., Moin, K., Sloane, B.F. (2003) Functional imaging of proteolysis: Stromal and inflammatory cells increase tumor proteolysis. *Molecular Imaging 2*: 159-175.

[48] Mueller, M., Fusenig, N.E. (2004). Friends and foes- bipolar effects of the tumour stroma in cancer. *Nature Reviews Cancer 4*: 839-849.

[49] Finney, H., Newman, D.J., Gruber, W., Merle, P., Price, C.P. (1997) Initial evaluation of cystatin C measurement by particle-enhanced immunonephelometry on the Behring nephelometer systems. *Clin. Chem. 43*: 1016-22.

[50] Kos, J., Krašovec, M., Cimerman, N., Nielsen, H.J., Christensen, I.J., Brunner, N. (2000) Cysteine protease inhibitors stefin A, stefin B, and cystatin C in sera from patients with colorectal cancer : relation to prognosis. *Clin. Cancer Res. 6*: 505-511.

[51] Laterza, O.F., Price, C.P., Scott, M.G. (2002) Cystatin C: An improved estimator of glomerular filtration rate. *Clin. Chem. 48*: 699-707.

[52] Werle, B., Sauckel, K., Nathanson, C.M., Bjarnadottir, M., Spiess, E., Ebert, W., Abrahamson, M. (2003) Cystatins C, E/M and F in human pleural fluids of patients with neoplastic and inflammatory lung disorders. *Biol. Chem. 384*: 281-287.

[53] Lah, T.T., Kokalj Kunovar, M., Kastelic, L., Babnik, J., Stolfa, A., Rainer, S., Turk, V. (1991) Cystatins and stefins in ascites fluid from ovarian carcinoma. *Cancer Lett. 61*: 243-253.

[54] Luetgens, K., Gabrijelčič, D., Turk, V., Ebert, W., Trefz, G., Lah, T. (1993) Cathepsin B and cysteine protease inhibitors in bronchoalveolar lavage fluid of lung cancer patients. *Cancer Det. Prev. 17*: 387-397.

[55] Leto, G., Tuminello, F.M., Pizzolanti, G., Montallo, G., Soresi, M., Gebbia, N. (1996) Lysosomal cathepsins B and L and stefin A blood levels in patients with hepatocellular carcinoma and/or liver cirrosis: potential clinical implications. *Oncology 54*: 79-83.

[56] Lah, T.T., Kokalj-Kunovar, M., Štrukelj, B., Pungercar, J., Barlic-Maganja, D., Drobnič-Kosorok, M., Kastelic, L., Babnik, J., Golouh, R. and Turk, V. (1992) Stefins and lysosomal cathepsin B , L and D in human breast carcinoma. *Int. J. Cancer 50:* 36-44.

[57] Cox, J.L., Sexton, P.S., Green, T.J., Darmani, N.A.(1999) Inhibition of B16 melanoma metastasis by overexpression of the cysteine protease inhibitor cystatin C. *Melanoma Res. 9*: 369-374.

[58] Ervin, H., and Cox, J.L. (2005) Late stage inhibition of hematogenous melanoma metastasis by cystatin C over-expression. *Cancer Cell International 5*: 1-8.

[59] Strojan, P., Oblak, I., Svetic, B., Šmid, L., Kos, J. (2004) Cysteine protease inhibitor cystatin C in squamous cell carcinoma of the head and neck: relation to prognosis. *Brit. J. Cancer 90*: 1961-1968.

[60] Huh, C.G., Häkansson, K., Nathanson, C.M., Thorgeirsson, U.P., Grubb, A., Abrahamson, M. and Karlsson, S. (1999) Decreased metastatic spread in mice homozygous for a null allele of the cystatin C protease inhibitor gene. *J. Clin. Pathol. Mol. Pathol. 52*: 332-340.

[61] Kos, J., Sekirnik, A., Kopitar, G., Cimerman, N., Kayser, K., Stremmer, A., Fiehn, W. and Werle, B. (2001) Human cathepsin S in patients with lung cancer: relation to prognosis. *Brit. J. Cancer. 85:* 1193-1200.

[62] Zheng, X., Chou, P.M., Mirkin, B.L., Rebbaa, A. (2004) Senescence-initiated reversal of drug resistance: specific role of cathepsin L. *Cancer Res. 64*: 1773-1780.

[63] Tate, S., Ushioda, T., Utsonomiya-Tate, N., Shibuya, K., Ohyama, Y., Nakano, Y., Kaji, H., Inagaki, F., Samejima, T., Kainosho, M. (1995) Solution structure of human cystatin A variant, cystatin A2-98 M65L, by NMR spectroscopy. A possible role of the interactions between the N- and C-termini to maintain the inhibitory active form of cystatin A. *Biochemistry 34*: 14637-14648.

[64] Alvarez-Fernandez, M., Barrett, A.J., Gerhartz, B., Dandi, P.M. Ni, J., Abrahamson, M. (1999) Inhibition of mammalian legumain by some cystatins is due to a novel second reactive site. *J. Biol. Chem. 274*: 19195-19203.

[65] Coussens, L.M., Fingleton, B., Matrisian, L.M. (2002) Matrix metalloprotease inhibitors and cancer: trials and tribulations. *Science 295*: 2387-2392.

[66] Konduri, S.D., Yanamandra, N., Siddique, K., Joseph, A., Dinh, D.H., Olivero, W.C. et al. (2002) Modulation of cystatin C expression impairs the invasive and tumorigenic potential of human glioblastoma cells. *Oncogene 21*: 8705-8712.

[67] Gondi, C.S., Lakka, D.H., Dinh, D.H., Olivero, W.C., Gujrati, M., Rao, J.S. (2004) RNAi-mediated inhibition of cathepsin B and uPAR leads to decreased cell invasion, angiogenesis and tumor growth in gliomas. *Oncogene 23*: 8486-8496.

[68] Ulbrich, C., Heechen, C., Aicher, A., Sasaki, T., Bruhl, M.R., Farhadi, M.R. et al. (2005). Cathepsin L is required for endothelial progenitor cell-induced neovascularisation. *Nat. Med. 11*: 206-213.

[69] Premzl, A., Zavašnik Bergant, V., Turk, V., Kos, J. (2003) Intracellular and extracellular cathepsin B facilitate invasion of MCF-10A neoT cells through reconstituted extracellular matrix in vitro. *Exp. Cell Res. 283*: 206-214.

[70] Cegnar, M., Kristl, J., Kos, J. (2005) Nanoscale polymer carriers to deliver chemotherapeutics to tumours. *Expert Opinion on Biol. Therapy 5*: 1557-1569.

INDEX

B

C

D

E

F

G

H

I

J

K

L

M

N

O

P

S

U

V

W

X

Y